W9-BZJ-019

Spirituality
in Nursing

STANDING ON HOLY GROUND

Spirituality
in Nursing

STANDING ON HOLY GROUND

Third Edition

Mary Elizabeth O'Brien
SFCC, PhD, MTS, RN, FAAN

School of Nursing
The Catholic University of America
Washington, DC

JONES AND BARTLETT PUBLISHERS
Sudbury, Massachusetts
BOSTON   TORONTO   LONDON   SINGAPORE

World Headquarters

Jones and Bartlett Publishers	Jones and Bartlett Publishers	Jones and Bartlett Publishers
40 Tall Pine Drive	Canada	International
Sudbury, MA 01776	6339 Ormindale Way	Barb House, Barb Mews
978-443-5000	Mississauga, Ontario L5V 1J2	London W6 7PA
info@jbpub.com	Canada	United Kingdom
www.jbpub.com		

Jones and Bartlett's books and products are available through most bookstores and online booksellers. To contact Jones and Bartlett Publishers directly, call 800-832-0034, fax 978-443-8000, or visit our website www.jbpub.com.

Substantial discounts on bulk quantities of Jones and Bartlett's publications are available to corporations, professional associations, and other qualified organizations. For details and specific discount information, contact the special sales department at Jones and Bartlett via the above contact information or send an email to specialsales@jbpub.com.

Copyright © 2008 by Jones and Bartlett Publishers, Inc.

All rights reserved. No part of the material protected by this copyright may be reproduced or utilized in any form, electronic or mechanical, including photocopying, recording, or by any information storage and retrieval system, without written permission from the copyright owner.

The authors, editor, and publisher have made every effort to provide accurate information. However, they are not responsible for errors, omissions, or for any outcomes related to the use of the contents of this book and take no responsibility for the use of the products and procedures described. Treatments and side effects described in this book may not be applicable to all people; likewise, some people may require a dose or experience a side effect that is not described herein. Drugs and medical devices are discussed that may have limited availability controlled by the Food and Drug Administration (FDA) for use only in a research study or clinical trial. Research, clinical practice, and government regulations often change the accepted standard in this field. When consideration is being given to use of any drug in the clinical setting, the health care provider or reader is responsible for determining FDA status of the drug, reading the package insert, and reviewing prescribing information for the most up-to-date recommendations on dose, precautions, and contraindications, and determining the appropriate usage for the product. This is especially important in the case of drugs that are new or seldom used.

Production Credits
Executive Editor: Kevin Sullivan
Acquisitions Editor: Emily Ekle
Associate Editor: Amy Sibley
Editorial Assistant: Patricia Donnelly
Production Director: Amy Rose
Production Editor: Carolyn F. Rogers
Senior Marketing Manager: Katrina Gosek
Associate Marketing Manager: Rebecca Wasley
Manufacturing and Inventory Coordinator: Amy Bacus
Composition: Auburn Associates, Inc.
Cover Design: Kristin E. Ohlin
Cover Image: © Tomasz Slowinski/ShutterStock, Inc.
Printing and Binding: Malloy, Inc.
Cover Printing: Malloy, Inc.

Library of Congress Cataloging-in-Publication Data
O'Brien, Mary Elizabeth.
  Spirituality in nursing : standing on holy ground / Mary Elizabeth O'Brien. — 3rd ed.
    p. ; cm.
  Includes bibliographical references and index.
  ISBN-13: 978-0-7637-4648-3 (pbk. : alk. paper)
  ISBN-10: 0-7637-4648-7 (pbk. : alk. paper)
  1. Nursing—Religious aspects—Christianity. 2. Nursing ethics. 3. Nurse and patient. 4. Spirituality. I. Title.
  [DNLM: 1. Nurse-Patient Relations. 2. Spirituality. 3. Christianity. 4. Nursing Care—ethics. 5. Philosophy, Nursing. 6. Religion and Medicine.   WY 87 O135s 2007]
  RT85.2.O37 2007
  610.73'01—dc22
                                                                                   2007005323

6048

Printed in the United States of America
11 10 09   10 9 8 7 6 5 4 3

Dedication

This book is dedicated to the many patients, family members, and caregivers, including nurses, physicians, chaplains, firefighters, and police officers, who so generously shared their beliefs and experiences in the hope of clarifying the importance of spirituality in nursing. Some have crossed over to a new life; others continue to live courageously, finding meaning and hope in the experience of illness or in ministering to those who are ill. Their words, quoted extensively in the following pages, are their legacy. I am privileged to be the storyteller.

God called to Moses out of the bush: . . .
"Remove the sandals from your feet, for the place on
which you are standing is holy ground."

Exodus 3:4–5

*The nurse's smile warmly embraces the cancer patient arriving for a
chemotherapy treatment.*
> *This is holy ground.*

*The nurse watches solicitously over the pre-op child who tearfully
whispers, "I'm scared."*
> *This is holy ground.*

*The nurse gently diffuses the anxieties of the ventilator-dependent
patient in the ICU.*
> *This is holy ground.*

*The nurse lovingly sings hymns to the anencephalic infant dying in
the nurse's arms.*
> *This is holy ground.*

*The nurse slips a comforting arm around the trembling shoulders of the
newly bereaved widow.*
> *This is holy ground.*

*The nurse tenderly takes the hand of the frail elder struggling to accept
life in the nursing home.*
> *This is holy ground.*

*The nurse
reverently touches and is touched by
the patient's heart,
the dwelling place of the living God.*

*This is spirituality in nursing,
this is the ground of the practice of nursing,
this is holy ground!*

▦ Preface

As the third millennium begins, our society is looking more and more to its spiritual traditions and philosophies for understanding, guidance, and comfort. This is witnessed by the fact that the concept of spirituality, encompassing numerous definitions, is being widely explored in such media as books, newsmagazines, and television documentaries. The nursing community, also, has experienced a resurgence of interest in spirituality, especially in relation to the spiritual needs of those who are ill.

The purpose of this book is to explore the relationship between spirituality and the practice of nursing from a number of perspectives, including nursing assessment of patients' spiritual needs, the nurse's role in the provision of spiritual care, the spiritual nature of the nurse–patient relationship, the spiritual history of the nursing profession, and the contemporary interest in spirituality within the nursing profession. The work is undergirded by the author's research in spirituality and nursing over the past two decades. The book's subtitle and theme, "Standing on Holy Ground," which describes the nurse's posture in providing spiritual care, was derived from nursing studies of the spiritual needs of chronically and acutely ill adults and children experiencing the sequelae of such conditions as cancer (including leukemia and lymphoma), cardiovascular disease, diabetes, depression, arthritis, Alzheimer's disease, chronic renal failure, and HIV infection and AIDS. The research included both formal and informal interviewing and observing of patients at home as well as in the hospital setting. The spiritual needs of fragile patient populations—the poor, the elderly, and ventilator-dependent patients in the intensive care unit—were also explored. Data on the spiritual needs and concerns of patients' family members were obtained through interaction with significant others.

In order to expand the database of patient spiritual needs appropriate to nursing intervention, qualitative interviews were conducted with a cadre of contemporary nurses from a variety of clinical backgrounds, including medical–surgical nursing, perioperative nursing, critical care nursing, emergency nursing, community health nursing, psychiatric–mental health nursing, pediatric nursing, gerontological nursing, and parish nursing; the group included nurse clinicians, nurse educators, nurse administrators, and nurse researchers. In addition to providing data on patient spiritual needs, numerous reports of spiritual care provided by practicing nurses were documented. The data derived from patient, family, and nurse interviews are supplemented by materials excerpted from the author's journal maintained both during the research and while serving as a chaplain intern in a research-oriented medical center. Pseudonyms are used in all instances where naming of study respondents is warranted.

The book presents study findings and implications for care in chapters on nurse–patient interaction, the nurse's role in spiritual care, the spiritual needs of acute and chronically ill persons, the spiritual needs of ill children and the families of those who are ill, the spiritual needs of the frail older adult, spiritual needs in mass casualty disasters, the spirituality of parish nursing, and spiritual needs in death and bereavement.

In this third edition of *Spirituality in Nursing: Standing on Holy Ground,* two new chapters have been added, one exploring spiritual well-being and quality of life at the end of life and the other describing an author-developed middle-range theory of spiritual well-being in illness. The former chapter contains empirical data from three studies examining the spiritual and religious concerns of persons at or near the end of life. The latter chapter describes the development of a middle-range theory of spiritual well-being in illness that nurses may use to guide both practice and research with individuals suffering from a variety of acute or chronic illnesses.

Chapter 3, "Nursing Assessment of Spiritual Needs," contains a number of tools to assess patients' spiritual beliefs, behaviors, and concerns. The author has included a Spiritual Assessment Scale with established validity and reliability, which can be used by nurses in both practice and research, in addition to qualitative tools constructed for specialized research efforts. Finally, a chapter chronicling a spiritual history of nursing describes the spiritual care activities of selected nursing figures from the pre-Christian and early Christian eras to the present. This chapter is grounded in the nursing and theological literature documenting the historical role of the nurse in the provision of spiritual care.

It is understood that the text of a book dealing with spiritual issues must, to a large degree, be influenced by the personal spiritual and religious élan of the writer. Thus, it is important to acknowledge that the author's Christian philosophy of life inspired, guided, and supported the writing of *Spirituality in Nursing.* Although an effort has been made to include examples of patient needs, supported by both data and literature, relative to other religious affiliations, the overall orientation of the work is derived primarily from the Judeo-Christian tradition. It is believed, nonetheless, that nurse readers whose spirituality is guided by another religious ethic will find meaning and inspiration in the poignant nursing examples of spiritual care and compassion as well as in the case examples of patients' spiritual needs.

■ Contents

■ Text Credits

The Scripture quotations are from the New Revised Standard Version Bible: Catholic Edition, Copyright © 1993 and 1989 by the Division of Christian Education of the National Council of the Churches of Christ in the U.S.A. Used by permission. All rights reserved.

Chapter 2, page 50, quote by John Cardinal O'Connor from the unpublished document *The Way of Life*, as cited in the Sisters of Life brochure. Used with the permission of John Cardinal O'Connor.

Chapter 3, pages 70–71; Chapter 6, page 139; and Chapter 7, page 164, quotes from M. E. O'Brien (1982), "The Need for Spiritual Integrity" in H. Yura and M. Walsh (Eds.), *Human Needs and the Nursing Process*, Vol. 2. Norwalk, CT: Appleton Century Crofts. Used with permission of the editors.

One section of Chapter 3, Nursing Assessment of Spiritual Needs, describing the patient spiritual assessment and care mandated by the Joint Commission for Accreditation of Healthcare Organization (JCAHO), has been reprinted from *A Nurse's Handbook of Spiritual Care: Standing on Holy Ground*, p. 15, Jones and Bartlett Publishers, 2004, used with permission of the publisher.

Major sections of Chapter 4, A Middle-Range Theory of Spiritual Well-Being in Illness, have been taken from Chapter 5, Conceptual Models of Parish Nursing Practice: A Middle-Range Theory of Spiritual Well-Being in Illness, in *Parish Nursing: Healthcare Ministry within the Church*, Jones and Bartlett Publishers, 2003, used with permission of the publisher.

Other Jones and Bartlett Titles by Mary Elizabeth O'Brien

*Prayer in Nursing: The Spirituality
of Compassionate Caregiving*

Parish Nursing: Healthcare Ministry within the Church

*A Nurse's Handbook of Spiritual Care:
Standing on Holy Ground*

1 ✦ Spirituality in Nursing: Standing on Holy Ground

*God called to Moses out of the bush: "Moses, Moses!" And he said, "Here I
am." "Come no closer," God said. "Remove the sandals from your feet, for
the place on which you are standing is holy ground."*

EXODUS 3:4–5

Perhaps no scriptural theme so well models the spiritual posture of
nursing practice as the Old Testament depiction of Moses and the
burning bush. In the biblical narrative, God reminded Moses that,
when he stood before his Lord, the ground beneath his feet was holy. When
the nurse clinician, nurse educator, nurse administrator, or nurse researcher
stands before a patient, a student, a staff member, or a study participant,
God is also present, and the ground on which the nurse is standing is holy. For
it is here, in the act of serving a brother or sister in need, that the nurse truly
encounters God. God is present in the nurse's practice of caring just as surely
as He was present in the blessed meeting with Moses so many centuries ago.
In an editorial in the *Journal of Christian Nursing*, Judy Shelly reminded us
that "the holy ground we as nurses are called to enter may be . . . difficult . . .
we face pain, suffering, fear, communication barriers, cultural and ethnic
prejudice, injustice, impossible working conditions and constant obstacles"
(2003, p. 3). However, Shelly adds, although we may at times "feel inadequate
and defeated . . . God is with us. He offers us his peace" (p. 3). This, I believe,
is the gift and the grace of our nursing vocation of "standing on holy ground."
This is the blessing; the precious knowledge that, however great or small our
nursing task may be, God is with us and will give us His peace.

This introductory chapter addresses the nurse's spiritual posture,
"standing on holy ground," while also offering a historical perspective on the
spiritual ministry of nursing. The overall relationship between spirituality
and nursing practice is explored; the concepts of spirituality—as distinguished from religiosity or religious practice—and nursing are defined with
a view to understanding their meaning for the contemporary nurse. Nursing
practice is examined in relation to the nurse's spiritual stance in caring for

1

patients, the nurse's participation in the provision of holistic care, and the nurse's role as healer. Finally, a practice model, labeled a "Nursing Theology of Caring," is described.

The empirical data on the spiritual concerns and needs of the ill in the present chapter, as well as those in the following chapters, are derived from nursing research with persons suffering from a multiplicity of illness conditions in a variety of settings. The author conducted both formal and informal interviewing and observation with these patients, their family members, and their nurse caregivers. The interview and observational data are supplemented by materials excerpted from journals maintained during the conduct of the research and also during a hospital chaplaincy experience.

THE SPIRITUAL MINISTRY OF NURSING: A HISTORICAL PERSPECTIVE

In a small but classic volume, *The Nurse: Handmaid of the Divine Physician*, written in the early 1940s, Franciscan Sister Mary Berenice Beck articulated what a great number of nurses of her era, especially those of the Judeo-Christian tradition, understood as the spirituality of their practice. Historically, nursing was viewed in large part as a vocation of service, incorporating a clearly accepted element of ministry to those for whom the nurse cared. A nurse's mission was considered to be driven by altruism and empathy for the sick, especially the sick poor. The practicing nurse of the early and middle 20th century did not expect much in terms of worldly rewards for her efforts. She envisioned her caregiving as commissioned and supported by God; to Him alone were the thanks and the glory to be given. This vision of nursing as a spiritual ministry is reflected in Sr. Mary Berenice's nurse's prayer:

> I am Thine Own, great Healer, help Thou me to serve Thy sick in
>   humble charity;
> I ask not thanks nor praise, but only light to care for them in every
>   way aright.
> My charges, sick and well, they all are Thine.
>
> (1945, p. xvii)

Other nursing authors of the time also supported the concept of nursing as a calling, with a decidedly spiritual element undergirding its practice. As nurse historian Minnie Goodnow (1916) asserted, "Nursing is not merely an occupation, temporary and superficial in scope; it is a great vocation" (p. 17). She added, "It [nursing] is so well known to be difficult that it is seldom undertaken by a woman who has not, in the depths of her conscious-ness, an earnest purpose to serve humanity" (p. 17). And, in the introduction to a basic fundamentals of nursing textbook, *The Art, Science and Spirit of Nursing* (1954), author Alice Price observed, "Nursing is possessed of a spir-itual quality, in that its primary aim is to serve humanity, not only by giving curative care to the bodies of the sick and injured, but by serving the needs of the mind and spirit as well" (p. 3). For the Christian nurse, the frequently quoted scriptural text supporting practice was that of Matthew 25:35–40, "For I was . . . sick and you took care of me. . . . I tell you, just as you did it to one of the least of these . . . you did for me."

A condition that kept the original spiritual ministry of nursing alive in this country was the fact that many early to mid-20th century nurses received their education in nursing schools affiliated with one of the predominant religious denominations. Prior to the development of con-temporary undergraduate and graduate programs in nursing, the three-year diploma schools that were the norm were generally not associated with academic institutions. Rather they were sponsored by individual hospitals, many of which were religiously affiliated. These schools tended to be small and insular in character, taking on the spiritual élan of the hospital with which they were connected. This was evident in the rituals of passage such as "capping" and graduation that were often conducted in places of worship with the blessing of a cleric included as part of the ceremony.

In the latter half of the 20th century, however, although some U.S. nurs-ing schools did retain a strong spiritual milieu as a characteristic feature, many of the newer university- and college-affiliated programs began to focus on the professional character of nursing. Nursing publications and confer-ences described the characteristics of a profession, and much debate cen-tered around how nursing incorporated specified professional criteria, particularly the criterion of autonomy of practice. These discussions were ap-propriate, as advanced health care technology and burgeoning knowledge generated by the behavioral sciences resulted in the practicing nurse re-quiring and receiving ever more sophisticated education related to patient care. For a time, at least, the proverbial pendulum appeared to swing toward the *science*, rather than the *art*, of nursing. This represented a concerted ef-fort to bring nursing practice up to standard alongside medical practice and that of other caregiving professions.

During the 1970s and 1980s, however, despite the fact that curricula in baccalaureate and newly emerging master's and doctoral programs in nurs-ing were becoming increasingly more complex in terms of the biological and behavioral sciences, many were beginning to acknowledge the need for holistic health care. With the advent of the concept of holism, came a reawakening of the importance of the ill person's spiritual nature and a heightened concern for spiritual needs. In identifying a model for holistic nursing, nurse clinician and researcher Cathie Guzzetta (1988) described holistic concepts as incorporating "a sensitive balance between art and science, analytic and intuitive skills, and the ability and knowledge to choose from a wide variety of treatment modalities to promote balance and interconnectedness of body, mind and spirit" (p. 117). Thus, in the holistic nursing model, patients' spiritual nature and needs are brought into equal focus with their cognitive and physiological needs.

Recently, an abundance of literature, both professional and lay, has begun to address the spiritual component of the human person. Books and articles abound relating to such topics as prayer, spiritual counseling, "near-death" experiences, interactions with angels, and volunteer activities undertaken for spiritual motives. Many individuals in our society are seeking to find transcendent meaning in their lives. It is not surprising, then, that nurses, now more solidly entrenched in their professional identities, should follow suit. As theorist Barbara Barnum (1994) pointed out, whereas nursing's focus during the past two decades has been on the "biopsychosocial" model of care, more recently nurse scholars have demonstrated a renewed interest in the spiritual dimension of caregiving (p. 114). Barnum's assertion is reflected in an increase in the nursing literature in conceptual and research-based articles related to the association between spirituality and health/illness. One example is the work of Jean Watson (1995) who observed, "At its most basic level nursing is a human-caring, relational profession. It exists by virtue of an ethical-moral ideal, and commitment to provide care for others" (p. 67). Watson's comment reflects a contemporary understanding of the spiritual ministry of nursing practice.

SPIRITUALITY AND NURSING PRACTICE

In order to provide some basis for beginning a discussion of spirituality and contemporary nursing practice, there must be a common understanding of the concepts of spirituality and nursing. Spirituality, as a personal concept, is generally understood in terms of an individual's attitudes and beliefs related to transcendence (God) or to the nonmaterial forces of life and of nature. Religious practice or religiosity, however, relates to a person's beliefs and behaviors associated with a specific religious tradition or denomination. Nurses need to have a clear understanding of this distinction or they may neglect spiritual needs in focusing only on a patient's religious practice (Emblen, 1992, p. 41).

Spirituality

Spirituality, as related to holistic nursing, is described by Dossey (1989) as "a broad concept that encompasses values, meaning, and purpose; one turns inward to the human traits of honesty, love, caring, wisdom, imagination, and compassion; existence of a quality of a higher authority, guiding spirit or transcendence that is mystical; a flowing, dynamic balance that allows and creates healing of body-mind-spirit; and may or may not involve organized religion" (p. 24). Pamela Reed (1992) presented a paradigm with which to explore spirituality in nursing by defining spirituality as "an expression of the developmental capacity for self-transcendence" (p. 350). Nurse anthropologist Madeleine Leininger (1997, p. 104) identified spirituality as a relationship with a supreme being that directs one's beliefs and practices.

Spirituality viewed as a human need has been described as "that dimension of a person that is concerned with ultimate ends and values. . . . Spirituality is that which inspires in one the desire to transcend the realm of the material" (O'Brien, 1982, p. 88). For many individuals, especially those adhering to the Western religious traditions of Judaism, Christianity, and Islam, the concept of transcendence incorporates belief in God. This is reflected explicitly in the conceptualization of spirituality articulated by nurse Ruth Stoll (1989) who asserted, "Through my spirituality I give and receive love; I respond to and appreciate God, other people, a sunset, a symphony and spring" (p. 6). Prayers as a meaning in life have been identified as indications of spirituality (Meraviglia, 1999); spirituality may thrive, however, outside the sphere of organized religion (Kendrick and Robinson, 2000).

Three characteristics of spirituality posited by Margaret Burkhardt (1989) include "unfolding mystery," related to one's attempt to understand the meaning and purpose of life; "harmonious interconnectedness," or an individual's relationship to other persons and/or to God; and "inner strength," which relates to one's personal spiritual resources and "sense of the sacred" (p. 72). Spirituality is proposed as a "cornerstone" of holistic nursing by Nagai-Jacobson and Burkhardt (1989) who suggested that questions appropriate to exploring a patient's spirituality might include how the individual understands God and what things give meaning and joy to life (p. 23). Each nurse needs to understand his or her own spirituality, keeping in mind that this personal belief system may differ significantly from that of a patient and family.

The nursing literature offers no one clear definition of spirituality. As pointed out by Verna Benner Carson in the *Journal of Christian Nursing* (1993), "Definitions of spirituality represent a variety of worldviews and the opinions of people from divergent walks of life" (p. 25). Common to most descriptions of spirituality, as reflected in the nursing literature, are the elements of love; compassion; caring; transcendence; relationship with God; and the connection of body, mind, and spirit.

Nursing

Writing in the early 1950s, Alice Price, RN (1954), offered a definition of nursing that incorporated not only the concept of the patient's spiritual nature, but the altruistic vocation of the nurse as well. She described nursing as neither pure science nor true art, but as a combination of both. "Nursing, as a profession, will embrace more than an art and a science; it will be a blending of three factors: of art and science, and the spirit of unselfish devotion to a cause primarily concerned with helping those who are physically, mentally or spiritually ill" (p. 2). Price ultimately defined nursing as "a service to the individual which helps him to regain, or to keep, a normal state of body and mind; when it cannot accomplish this, it helps him gain relief from physical pain, mental anxiety or spiritual discomfort" (p. 3). Although Nurse Price was writing some 25 to 30 years prior to the widespread acceptance of the term *holistic nursing,* her vision of the professional nurse's role clearly included attention to the needs of a patient's spirit, as well as to the needs of the body and the mind.

In their book *Introduction to Nursing,* written 40 years after publication of Price's 1954 text, coauthors Lindberg, Hunter, and Kruszewski (1994) argued that, presently, because of the continual growth and development of the profession, no single definition of nursing can be accepted (p. 7). The authors presented excerpts of nursing definitions articulated by a cadre of theorists from Florence Nightingale in 1859 to Martha Rogers in 1970 but, ultimately, suggested that each practicing nurse develop a definition of his or her own. Lindberg and colleagues did, however, express the hope that, whatever one's definition, it will contain an emphasis on caring or nurturing as a motivating factor for choosing nursing (p. 7).

Following the suggestions of Price in 1954 and Lindberg, Hunter, and Kruszewski in 1994, a current working definition of nursing follows:

> Nursing is a sacred ministry of health care or health promotion provided to persons both sick and well, who require caregiving, support, or education to assist them in achieving, regaining, or maintaining a state of wholeness, including wellness of body, mind, and spirit. The nurse also serves those in need of comfort and care to strengthen them in coping with the trajectory of a chronic or terminal illness, or with experiencing the dying process.

The spiritual dimensions of the definition relate to two concepts: first, the sacred ministry of caring on the part of the nurse; and second, the ultimate goal of the patient's achievement of a state of wholeness, including the wellness of body, mind, and spirit. These concepts are next explored in terms of the nurse's spiritual posture, the patient's spiritual wholeness, and the nurse–patient spiritual interaction.

THE NURSE'S SPIRITUAL POSTURE: STANDING ON HOLY GROUND

Sister Macrina Wiederkehr (1991) advised, "If you should ever hear God speaking to you from a burning bush, and it happens more often than most of us realize, take off your shoes for the ground on which you stand is holy" (p. 2). How appropriate, it seems, to envision practicing nurses, who must come together with their patients in caring and compassion, as standing on holy ground. God frequently speaks to us from a "burning bush," in the fretful whimper of a feverish child, in the anxious questions of a preoperative surgical patient, and in the frail moans of a fragile elder. If we "take off our shoes," we will be able to realize that the place where we stand is holy ground; we will respond to our patients as we would wish to respond to God in the burning bush.

But what does it really mean to "take off one's shoes"? Sister Macrina asserted that it means stripping away "whatever prevents us from experiencing the holy" (1991, p. 3). She added that God speaks to us in many "burning bushes of today" and that "the message is still one of holy ground"; it is a message that is often missed "because of [our] unnecessary shoes" (p. 3). In the contemporary conduct of nursing practice, nursing education, nursing administration, and nursing research, some of us may admit to having a number of unnecessary pairs of shoes littering our professional closets. First, there are running shoes, which many of us wear as we rush pell-mell from task to task in order to manage the day. As we fly about, feet barely touching the ground, it is easy to forget, in the busyness, that where we are standing is a holy place. Another often-relied-on pair of shoes are sturdy walking brogues, which provide protection against unwanted intrusions. Unfortunately, their insulated soles, which keep us safe and secure, may also prevent our feet from feeling the holy ground on which we walk. And then there are old, favorite loafers, well worn and cozy. When we are wearing these shoes, we can so rest in their comfort that we need not be troubled by any disturbing bumps in the holy ground. We nurses probably have, I am sure, many more unnecessary pairs of shoes that prevent our feet from experiencing holy ground. But recollections of times past when, literally or figuratively, we have been able to take off our shoes, even if only briefly, well validate the Old Testament message.

A personal experience recorded in the author's journal describes the powerful spiritual impact of physically removing a pair of shoes during the course of a worship service.

> I had been invited to attend an early morning church service at "Gift of Peace," a home for persons with terminal illness operated by Mother Teresa's Missionaries of Charity. On arrival, I settled quietly into a back corner of the small chapel. There were no pews; the sisters sit or kneel on the floor. As I began to observe the sariclad Missionaries of Charity entering the chapel, I noticed, with some astonishment, that none were wearing shoes; they were all barefoot. I knew that the sisters wore sandals when they cared for patients but these had apparently been put aside as they came to kneel before their Lord. Not wanting to violate the spiritual élan of the service, I proceeded, as inconspicuously as possible, to slip out of my own sandals. Somehow, becoming shoeless in church, a condition I had not experienced before, provided a powerful symbol for me. I felt that I was truly in the presence of God, of the Holy Mystery, before whose overwhelming compassion and care it seemed only right that I should present myself barefoot, in awe and reverence. Near the end of the service, as I went forward and stood before the altar in bare feet to receive the sacrament of the Eucharist, I sensed in the deepest recesses of my soul that I was indeed "standing on holy ground." That memory will, I pray, serve as a poignant reminder that whenever I stand before a suffering patient, I am, there also, just as surely in the presence of God, and I must take care to remove whatever unnecessary "shoes" I happen to be wearing at the time. I need to allow the "bare feet" of my spirit to touch the "holy ground" of my caregiving, so that I shall never fail to hear God's voice in the "burning bush" of a patient's pain.

HOLISTIC NURSING: THE BODY, MIND, AND SPIRIT CONNECTION

At times one hears an individual described as being truly healthy. The assumption underlying such a remark may relate not so much to the physical health or well-being of the person as to the fact that he or she is perceived as solidly grounded spiritually. One can be possessed of a healthy attitude toward life, even if suffering from a terminal illness. In order to achieve such a spiritual grounding in the face of physical or psychological deficit, the individual must be closely attuned to the body, mind, and spirit connection; one must understand and accept the value of the spiritual dimension in the overall paradigm of holistic health.

As our society advanced scientifically during the past half-century, it became increasingly more difficult for some in the health care community to give credence to the importance of the spiritual nature of the human person, especially in relation to health/illness issues. More recently, however, caregivers are recognizing that sensitivity to a patient's spiritual needs is critical if they are to provide truly "holistic" health care. Nurse and minister Ann Robinson (1995) believes that nurses must "embrace the spirituality of the human community" in order to support their patients' holistic health behaviors (p. 3).

Authors Dossey and Keegan (1989) defined the concept of holism, which undergirds holistic health and holistic nursing care, including the body, mind, and spirit connection, as "the view that an integrated whole has a reality independent of and greater than the sum of its parts" (p. 4). They described holism as consisting of a philosophy of positive, interactionally based attitudes and behaviors that can exist not only in one who is well but also in one who is seriously or terminally ill (p. 5). Nurses practicing care supportive of such holism need to envision the spiritual needs of a patient as deserving of attention equal to that provided in response to physical and psychosocial concerns.

Overall, holistic nursing is supported by and alternately supports the intimate connection of body, mind, and spirit. Nursing of the whole person requires attention to the individuality and uniqueness of each dimension, as well as to the interrelatedness of the three. In *The Wholeness Handbook*, Emeth and Greenhut (1991) described the body, mind, and spirit elements: The body is the physical substance of a person that can be perceived in empirical reality; the mind is that dimension of an individual that conceptualizes; and the spirit is the life principle that is shared with all humanity and with God. "It is the dimension of personhood that drives us to create, love, question, contemplate and transcend" (pp. 27–28).

For the nurse seeking to provide holistic health care, then, the spiritual dimension and needs of the person must be carefully assessed and considered in all therapeutic planning. Spiritual care cannot be separated from physical, social, and psychological care (Lo and Brown, 1999; O'Connor, 2001). Often it is uniquely the nurse, standing either literally or figuratively at the bedside, who has the opportunity and the entreé to interact with patients on that spiritual level where they strive to create, love, question, contemplate, and transcend. Here, truly, the nurse is standing on holy ground.

THE NURSE AS HEALER

The nurse, standing as he or she does on the holy ground of caring for the sick, is well situated to be the instrument of God's healing. In the sacred interaction between nurse and patient, the spiritual healing dimension of holistic health care is exemplified and refined. The nurse stands as God's surrogate and as a vehicle for His words and His touch of compassionate care.

Healing has been described variously as facilitating openness to the "communication of the Holy Spirit, whose message is always wholeness" (Johnson, 1992, p. 21); "the process or act of curing or restoring to health or wholeness, the body, the mind and the spirit" (Haggard, 1983, p. 235); and "to make whole" (Burke, 1993, p. 37). The concept of the nurse as healer incorporates the characteristics of all three definitions; that is, the nurse healer must listen to the voice of God; desire to restore health either of body or of spirit; and attempt to assist the patient in achieving wholeness and integrity of body, mind, and spirit. For the nurse of the Judeo-Christian tradition, spiritually oriented scriptural models of healing abound in both the Old and the New Testaments.

Yahweh's healing power is reflected in Old Testament Scripture in such narratives as Elijah's healing of the widow's son (1 Kings 17:17–23) and Elisha's cleansing of Naaman's leprosy (2 Kings 5:1–14). In the New Testament account of the ministry of Jesus, 41 healings are identified (Kelsey, 1988, p. 43). Jesus healed by word and by touch, sometimes even using physical materials such as mud and saliva. Always, Jesus' healings were accompanied by love and compassion for the ill persons or their families, as in the case of Jairus' young daughter, who her parents thought to be dead. Jesus comforted Jairus with the words, "The child is not dead but sleeping" (Mark 5:39). And then, "He took her by the hand and said to her, 'Talitha cum,' which means 'Little girl, get up!' And immediately the girl got up and began to walk about" (Mark 5:41).

In her doctoral dissertation entitled "Biblical Roots of Healing in Nursing," Maria Homberg (1980) posited that an established biblical tradition reflecting the healing power of such concepts as respect for human dignity and positive interpersonal relationships has parallels in contemporary nursing (p. 2). Homberg suggested that the biblical history of healing can be used by nurse educators to support the importance of these concepts. Dossey (1988) identified the characteristics of a nurse healer as having an awareness that "being present" to the patient is as essential as technical skills, respecting and loving all clients regardless of background or personal characteristics, listening actively, being nonjudgmental, and viewing time with clients as times of sharing and serving (p. 42). These characteristics reflect the spiritual nature of healing described in the Old and the New

Testament Scriptures. Finally, nurse educator Brenda Lohri-Posey says that to become a "compassionate healer" a nurse must "recognize the ability to be a healer" and understand that "healing occasions are unique for each patient" and that "the healing occasion" may change a nurse's "beliefs about pain and suffering" (2005, p. 37).

The Nurse As Wounded Healer

When a nurse is described as a healer, one tends to focus on his or her ability to relieve suffering. The label "healer" evokes the concept of a strong and gifted individual whose ministry is directed by care and compassion; this is an appropriate image. What may be forgotten in such a description is the fact that sometimes the gift of healing has emerged from, and indeed has been honed by, the healer's own experiences of suffering and pain. In chapter 5, which explores the nurse's healing role as an "anonymous minister," a gerontological nurse practitioner, Sharon, describes using her own pain in counseling patients: "I may not talk about my pain . . . [but] I understand where they're coming from if they're hurting." Sharon, who imagined this experience as being "united in suffering" with those she cared for, reflected Henri Nouwen's (1979) classic conceptualization of the wounded healer. Nouwen described the wounded healer as one who must look after personal wounds while at the same time having the ability to heal others. The wounded healer concept is derived from a Talmudic identification of the awaited Messiah:

> He is sitting among the poor covered with wounds. The others unbind all their wounds at the same time and bind them up again, But he unbinds one at a time and binds it up again, saying to himself: "Perhaps I shall be needed; if so, I must always be ready so as not to delay for a moment."
>
> TRACTATE SANHEDREN
> (as cited in Nouwen, 1979, p. 82)

The nurse, as any person who undertakes ministry, brings into the interaction personal and unique wounds. Rather than hindering the therapeutic process, the caregiver's wounds, when not unbound all at once, can become a source of strength, understanding, and empathy when addressing the suffering of others. The nurse as a wounded healer caring for a wounded patient can relate his or her own painful experiences to those of the ill person, thus providing a common ground of experience on which to base the initiation of spiritual care.

A NURSING THEOLOGY OF CARING

In the previous pages the nurse is described as having the opportunity to heal and to facilitate wholeness, and in the process, to be in the posture of standing on holy ground. But what is it that initiates and supports such nursing practice? What theological or spiritual understanding and beliefs guide the nursing activities of contemporary practitioners? Perhaps these questions can best be answered in the exploration of a nursing theology of caring. The theology of caring encompasses the concepts of being, listening, and touching and was derived from the author's clinical practice with a variety of acutely and chronically ill patients. The nursing theology of caring is supported by the Christian parable of the Good Samaritan:

> A man was going down from Jerusalem to Jerico, and fell into the hands of robbers who stripped him, beat him and went away leaving him half dead. . . . But a Samaritan, while traveling . . . saw him and was moved to pity. He went to him and bandaged his wounds, having poured oil and wine on them. Then he put him on his own animal, brought him to an Inn, and took care of him.
>
> (Luke 10:30, 33–34)

The Gospel relates Jesus' parable of the Good Samaritan, told in response to a question posed by a scholar of the law who asked, "Teacher, " he said, "what must I do to inherit eternal life?" (Luke 10:25). Jesus said to him, "What is written in the Law?" In response to Jesus' question, the scholar replied, "You shall love the Lord your God with all your heart . . . and your neighbor as yourself" (Luke 10:27). To justify himself, however, the scholar added, "And who is my neighbor?" (Luke 10:29). Jesus related the parable of the Good Samaritan in reply. At the conclusion of the parable, Jesus asked the scholar, of all those who had seen the beaten man, which one was truly a neighbor. The scholar replied, "The one who showed him mercy." Jesus said to him, "Go and do likewise" (Luke 10:36–37).

In a commentary on the parable of the Good Samaritan, Kodell (1989) noted that Jesus' story was intended to challenge a prevailing but discriminating attitude in the society of the time—the fact that a Samaritan, a member of an ethnic group despised by some, could behave so lovingly. The parable, Kodell pointed out, exemplified the love commandment: while the lawyer suggests that not all persons are his neighbors, Jesus' reply indicates that one must consider everyone a neighbor regardless of nationality or religious heritage and affiliation (p. 62). This Gospel narrative provides nurses with a model of unequivocal concern and nondiscrimination in providing care to those in need; it reflects the conceptual framework to support a nursing theology of caring.

Prior to discussing a theology of caring, on which nursing practice may be based, the key concepts of theology and caring will be explored briefly.

Theology

The term *theology* comes originally from the Greek words *theos* meaning "God," and *logos* or "science." The contemporary meaning of theology is "an intellectual discipline, i.e., an ordered body of knowledge about God" (Hill, 1990, p. 1011). The study of theology is often described according to Anselm of Canterbury's conceptualization as "faith seeking understanding." In this context, faith is viewed as "a stance of the whole person towards God, characterized by radical trust, hope, love and commitment" (Fehr, 1990, p. 1027). Each nurse's personal understanding of theology will be informed by myriad factors: religious or denominational heritage, formal and informal religious education, religious and spiritual experience, and current faith practices.

Caring

James Nelson (1976), in his exploration *Rediscovering the Person in Medical Care*, reported that "Underneath . . . important assumptions about the unity of the person and the individual's and community's participation in the healing process lies a fundamental truth: the importance of caring" (p. 62). Nelson added that in health care facilities (clinics, hospitals, nursing homes) staff have a primary interest in "curing" certain disease and illness conditions. Ministers and nurses must, however, remember the importance of their vocational call to care (p. 62). Nelson defined caring as "an active attitude which genuinely conveys to the other person that he or she does really matter. . . . It is grounded in the sense of uniqueness and worth which, by the grace of God, the other has" (p. 63).

One of the earliest nursing theorists of caring is Madeleine Leininger, who defined the concept as referring to "direct (or indirect) nurturant and skillful activities, processes and decisions related to assisting people in such a manner that reflects behavior attributes which are empathetic, supportive, compassionate, protective, succorant, educational and otherwise dependent upon the needs, problems, values and goals of the individual or group being assisted" (1978, p. 489). In her later writings, Leininger described caring as the central focus or dimension of nursing practice (Leininger, 1980, 1988, 1991). Nurse authors Eriksson (1992); Montgomery (1992); and Benner,

Tanner, and Chesla (1996) also identified caring as a central concept of nursing, as did Simone Roach (1992), who postulated five attributes of the concept: "compassion, competence, confidence, conscience, and commitment" (p. 1). In their practice, nurses have always embraced the concept of caring as integral to the essence of the profession (Picard, 1995; Pinch, 1996). And ultimately, through the manifestation of caring nursing practice, nurses engender the kind of trust and confidence in their patients that leads to the promotion of good health (Bishop & Scudder, 1996, p. 41).

The following section, "Dimensions of Caring," encompasses the characteristics of caring as identified in the theological and health care literature and the goal of a healing outcome as understood in the clinical practice of nursing. Patient examples are drawn from the author's journal chronicling a chaplaincy experience at a research medical center.

DIMENSIONS OF CARING

For the nurse practicing spiritual caring, three key activities may serve as vehicles for the carrying out of the theological mandate to serve the sick: being with patients in their experiences of pain, suffering, or other problems or needs; listening to patients verbally express anxieties or emotions, such as fear, anger, loneliness, depression, or sorrow, which may be hindering the achievement of wellness; and touching patients either physically, emotionally, or spiritually to assure them of their connectedness with others in the family of God.

In and of themselves the acts of being with, listening to, or touching a patient may not constitute spiritual care. These behaviors, however, grounded in a nurse's spiritual philosophy of life such as that articulated in the parable of the Good Samaritan, take on the element of ministry; they constitute the nurse's theology of caring.

Being

> *Being with a sick person without judgement creates space for meaning to emerge and for the holy to be revealed.*
>
> E. EMETH and J. GREENHUT (1991, p. 65)

A description from the author's journal of an experience with a young cancer patient reflects the importance of being with a patient in need.

This morning a young man, Michael, who was facing mutilating surgery in hope of slowing the progress of advanced rhabdomyosarcoma, asked to talk to me; he said, "I need you to help me understand why this is happening. I need you to help me deal with it." I sought consultation both in prayer and from my own spiritual mentor before the meeting. I entered Michael's room, however, with much trepidation; how could I possibly help him "understand why" God seemed to be allowing his illness. As it turned out, Michael was the one who helped me. As soon as I sat down, he said, "There are some things I've been thinking about that I need to tell you," and the conversation continued with Michael sharing much about his own faith and his attempt to understand God's will in his life. As I prepared to leave, Michael got up, hugged me, and said, "Our talk has helped a lot"; we prayed together for the coming surgery. Simply being with Michael as he struggled with the diagnosis of cancer in light of his own spirituality constituted the caring. I did not have, nor did I need, any right words; I only needed to be a caring presence in Michael's life.

Emeth and Greenhut (1991), in their discussion of understanding illness, described the importance of being with patients and families, especially when, as with Michael, they need to ask questions for which there are no answers. "We cannot answer the question, 'Where is God in this experience?' for anyone else; rather, we must be willing to be with others in their experience as they live with the questions and wait for their personal answers to emerge. This 'being with' is at the heart of health care" (p. 65).

Listening

Many people are looking for an ear that will listen. . . . He who no longer listens to his brother will soon no longer be listening to God either. . . . One who cannot listen long and patiently will presently be talking beside the point and never really speaking to others, albeit he be not conscious of it.

DIETRICH BONHOEFFER (1959, p. 11)

The concept of listening is an integral part of being with a person, as was learned from interaction with Michael. However, as his illness progressed, there were also times when being with Michael in silence was a significant dimension of caring. In some situations, however, active listening, with responsive and sensitive feedback to the person speaking, is important in providing spiritual care. Ministering to Philip, a young man diagnosed with anaplastic astrocytoma, revealed the importance of such listening. Philip, because of his neurological condition, had difficulty explaining his thoughts, especially in regard to spiritual matters, yet he very much wanted to talk. Philip described himself as a born-again Christian, a fact of which he was very proud.

> On my first visit Philip showed me a well-worn Bible in which he had written comments on favorite Scripture passages. As our meetings continued, I began to realize that if I opened the Bible and focused on a particular passage, Philip's speech was helped by looking at the words. I tried to listen carefully, to follow and comprehend Philip's thoughts on the Scripture and its meaning in his life. Our sharing was validated one day when Philip reached out and took my hand and said, "I'm glad you're here; I really like our talking about God together."

In a discussion of spirituality and the nursing process, Verna Carson (1989) recognized the importance of such listening. "The ability to listen is both an art and a learned skill. It requires that the nurse completely attend to the client with open ears, eyes and mind" (p. 165). And, in a poignant case study entitled *A Lesson Learned by Listening,* palliative care nurse Katie Jantzi affirmed the importance of listening to a dying patient, reminding us that patients are our "best teachers" (2005, p. 41).

Touching

And there was a leper who came to Him, and knelt before Him saying: "Lord, if you choose you can make me clean." He stretched out His hand and touched him saying: "I choose. Be made clean." Immediately his leprosy was cleansed.

MATTHEW 8:2–3

The Christian Gospel message teaches us compellingly that touch was important to Jesus; it was frequently used in healing and caring interactions with His followers. Loving, empathetic, compassionate touch is perhaps the most vital dimension of a nursing theology of caring. At times the touch may be physical: the laying on of hands, taking of one's hand, holding, or gently stroking a forehead. At other times a nurse's touch may be verbal: a kind and caring greeting or a word of comfort and support. Physical touch has been described in the nursing literature as encompassing five dimensions of caring: physical comfort, emotional comfort, mind–body comfort, social interaction, and spiritual sharing (Chang, 2001).

Perhaps one of the most rewarding experiences with the use of caring touch occurred during an interaction with Erin, a 9-year-old newly diagnosed with acute lymphocytic leukemia.

> Erin was about to begin chemotherapy and was terrified at the thought of having IVs started; the staff asked if I would try to help calm her during the initiation of treatment. One of the pediatric oncology nurses pulled up a stool for me next to Erin so that I could hold and comfort her during the needle insertion. After the procedure was finished and I was preparing to leave, Erin trudged across the room dragging her IV pole, wrapped her arms around me, and said, "Thank you for helping me to get through that!"

It is not surprising that Carson (1989) identified touch, associated with being with a patient, as critical to the provision of spiritual caring. She suggested that the nurse's "presence and ability to touch another both physically and spiritually" is perhaps his or her most important gift (p. 164). And, in describing the power of "compassionate touch," Minister Victor Parachin asserts, "Whenever we reach out with love and compassion to touch another life, our contact makes the burden a little lighter and the pain more bearable. . . . By reaching out and touching someone through deed or word, we provide the extra push that person needs to carry on, rather than give up" (2003, p. 9). "The human touch," Parachin concludes, "can make the difference between life and death" (p. 9).

Ultimately the activities of being, listening, and touching, as exemplified in Jesus' parable of the Good Samaritan and in a nursing theology of caring, will be employed in a variety of ways as needed in the clinical setting. This is what constitutes the creativity of nursing practice; this is what constitutes the art of the profession of nursing.

Nursing, as a profession, has developed significantly during the past half-century. The vocation or spiritual calling to care for the sick, somewhat diminished during nursing's heightened concern with professionalism, is experiencing a reawakening among contemporary nurses. This may be related to the interest in spiritual and religious issues manifested in the larger society. Nursing, as an occupation, encompasses a unique commitment to provide both care and compassion for those one serves. The subject of spirituality in nursing practice includes concern not only with the personal spiritual and religious needs of the patient and nurse, but with the spiritual dimension of the nurse–patient interaction as well.

REFERENCES

Barnum, B. S. (1994). *Nursing theory: Analysis, application, evaluation.* Philadelphia: J. B. Lippincott.

Beck, M. B. (1945). *The nurse: Handmaid of the divine physician.* Philadelphia: J. B. Lippincott.

Benner, P., Tanner, C. A., & Chesla, C. A. (1996). *Expertise in nursing practice: Caring, clinical judgment and ethics.* New York: Springer.

Bishop, A. H., & Scudder, J. R. (1996). *Nursing ethics: Therapeutic caring presence.* Sudbury, MA: Jones and Bartlett.

Bonhoeffer, D. (1959). *Life together.* New York: Harper & Brothers.

Burke, B. H. (1993, September). Wellness in the healing ministry. *Health Progress,* 33–39.

Burkhardt, M. A. (1989). Spirituality: An analysis of the concept. *Holistic Nursing Practice, 3*(3), 69–77.

Carson, V. B. (1989). Spirituality and the nursing process. In V. B. Carson (Ed.), *Spiritual dimensions of nursing practice* (pp. 150–179). Philadelphia: W. B. Saunders.

Carson, V. B. (1993, Winter). Spirituality: Generic or Christian. *Journal of Christian Nursing,* 24–27.

Chang, S. O. (2001). The conceptual structure of physical touch in caring. *Journal of Advanced Nursing, 33*(6), 820–827.

Dossey, B. M. (1988). Nurse as healer: Toward an inward journey. In B. M. Dossey, L. Keegan, C. E. Guzzetta, & L. G. Kolkmeier (Eds.), *Holistic nursing: A handbook for practice* (pp. 39–54). Rockville, MD: Aspen.

Dossey, B. M. (1989). The transpersonal self and states of consciousness. In B. M. Dossey, L. Keegan, L. G. Kolkmeier, & C. E. Guzzetta (Eds.), *Holistic health promotion: A guide for practice* (pp. 23–35). Rockville, MD: Aspen.

Dossey, B. M., & Keegan, L. (1989). Holism and the circle of human potential. In B. M. Dossey, L. Keegan, L. G. Kolkmeier, & C. E. Guzzetta (Eds.), *Holistic health promotion: A guide for practice* (pp. 3–21). Rockville, MD: Aspen.

Emblen, J. D. (1992). Religion and spirituality defined according to current use in nursing literature. *Journal of Professional Nursing, 8*(1), 41–47.

Emeth, E. V., & Greenhut, J. H. (1991). *The wholeness handbook: Care of body, mind and spirit for optimal health.* New York: Continuum.

Eriksson, K. (1992). Nursing: The caring practice, "Being There." In D. A. Gaut (Ed.), *The presence of caring in nursing* (pp. 201–210). New York: National League for Nursing Press (Pub. No. 15-2465).

Fehr, W. L. (1990). The history of theology. In J. A. Komonchak, M. Collins, & D. A. Lane (Eds.), *The new dictionary of theology* (pp. 1027–1035). Collegeville, MN: The Liturgical Press.

Goodnow, M. (1916). *Outlines of nursing history*. Philadelphia: W. B. Saunders.

Guzzetta, C. E. (1988). Nursing process and standards of care. In B. M. Dossey, L. Keegan, C. E. Guzzetta, & L. G. Kolkmeier (Eds.), *Holistic nursing: A handbook for practice* (pp. 101–126). Rockville, MD: Aspen.

Haggard, P. (1983, Fall). Healing and health care of the whole person. *Journal of Religion and Health, 22*(3), 234–240.

Hill, W. J. (1990). Theology. In J. A. Komonchak, M. Collins, & D. A. Lane (Eds.), *The new dictionary of theology* (pp. 1011–1027). Collegeville, MN: The Liturgical Press.

Homberg, M. (1980). *Biblical roots of healing in nursing*. Unpublished doctoral dissertation, Teacher's College, Columbia University. Ann Arbor, MI: University Microfilms International.

Jantzi, K. (2005). A lesson learned by listening. *Journal of Christian Nursing, 22*(1), 41.

Johnson, R. P. (1992). *Body, mind, spirit: Tapping the healing power within you*. Liguori, MO: Liguori.

Kelsey, M. T. (1988). *Psychology, medicine and Christian healing*. San Francisco: Harper & Row.

Kendrick, K. D., & Robinson, S. (2000). Spirituality: Its relevance and purpose for clinical nursing in a new millennium. *Journal of Clinical Nursing, 9*(5), 701–705.

Kodell, J. (1989). *The gospel according to Luke*. Collegeville, MN: The Liturgical Press.

Leininger, M. M. (1978). *Trans-cultural nursing: Concepts, theories and practice*. New York: John Wiley & Sons.

Leininger, M. M. (1980). Caring: A central focus of nursing and health care services. *Nursing and Health Care, 1*(3), 135–143.

Leininger, M. M. (1988). *Care: The essence of nursing and health*. Detroit: Wayne State University Press.

Leininger, M. M. (1991). Foreword in D. A. Gaut & M. M. Leininger (Eds.), *Caring: The compassionate healer*. New York: National League for Nursing Press (Pub. No 15-2401).

Leininger, M. M. (1997). Transcultural spirituality: A comparative care and health focus. In M. S. Roach (Ed.), *Caring from the heart: The convergence of caring and spirituality* (pp. 99–118). New York: Paulist Press.

Lindberg, J. B., Hunter, M. L., & Kruszewski, A. Z. (1994). *Introduction to nursing: Concepts, issues, and opportunities*. Philadelphia: J. B. Lippincott.

Lo, R., & Brown, R. (1999). Holistic care and spirituality: Potential for increasing spiritual dimensions of nursing. *Australian Journal of Holistic Nursing, 6*(2), 4–9.

Lohri-Posey, B. (2005). Becoming a compassionate healer. *Journal of Christian Nursing, 22*(4), 34–37.

Meraviglia, M. G. (1999). Critical analysis of spirituality and its empirical indicators: Prayers and meaning in life. *Journal of Holistic Nursing, 17*(1), 18–33.

Montgomery, C. L. (1992). The spiritual connection: Nurses' perceptions of the experience of caring. In D. A. Gaut (Ed.), *The presence of caring in nursing* (pp. 39–52). New York: National League for Nursing Press (Pub. No. 15-2465).

Nagai-Jacobson, M. G., & Burkhardt, M. A. (1989). Spirituality: Cornerstone of holistic nursing practice. *Holistic Nursing Practice, 3*(3), 18–26.

Nelson, J. B. (1976). *Rediscovering the person in medical care*. Minneapolis: Augsburg.

Nouwen, H. J. (1979). *The wounded healer*. Garden City, NY: Image Books.

O'Brien, M. E. (1982). The need for spiritual integrity. In H. Yura & M. Walsh (Eds.), *Human needs and the nursing process* (Vol. 2, pp. 82–115). Norwalk, CT: Appleton Century Crofts.

O'Connor, C. I. (2001). Characteristics of spirituality, assessment and prayer in holistic nursing. *Nursing Clinics of North America, 36*(1), 33–46.

Parachin, V. M. (2003). The power of compassionate touch. *Journal of Christian Nursing, 20*(2), 8–9.

Picard, C. (1995). Images of caring in nursing and dance. *Journal of Holistic Nursing, 13*(4), 323–331.

Pinch, W. J. (1996). Is caring a moral trap? *Nursing Outlook, 44*(2), 84–88.

Price, A. L. (1954). *The art, science and spirit of nursing*. Philadelphia: W. B. Saunders.

Reed, P. G. (1992). An emerging paradigm for the investigation of spirituality in nursing. *Research in Nursing and Health, 15*, 349–357.

Roach, S. (1992). *The human act of caring*. Ottowa: Canadian Hospital Association.

Robinson, A. (1995). Spirituality and risk: Toward an understanding. *Holistic Nursing Practice, 8*(2), 1–7.

Shelly, J. A. (2003). Walking on holy ground. *Journal of Christian Nursing, 20*(3), 3.

Stoll, R. I. (1989). The essence of spirituality. In V. B. Carson (Ed.), *Spiritual dimensions of nursing practice* (pp. 4–23). Philadelphia: W. B. Saunders.

Watson, J. (1995, July). Nursing's caring-healing paradigm as exemplar for alternative medicine. *Alternative Therapies, 1*(30), 64–69.

Wiederkehr, Sr. M. (1991). *Seasons of your heart*. New York: HarperCollins.

2 ✸ A Spiritual History of Nursing

Nursing is an art, and if it is to be made an art, it requires as exclusive a devotion, as hard a preparation, as any painter's or sculptor's work. For what is having to do with dead canvas or cold marble compared with having to do with the living body, the temple of God's spirit.

FLORENCE NIGHTINGALE, 1867
(cited in Baly, 1991, p. 68)

Recently there has been a resurgence of nursing publications directed toward the spiritual concerns of those who are ill. To better understand practicing nurses' contemporary interest in spirituality and the spiritual vocation of nursing, it is important to walk briefly in the world of our ancient and medieval past, as well as to examine the post-Reformation period, to explore the powerful and compelling spiritual history of nursing up to the modern era.

It is said that we stand on the shoulders of those who have gone before us; in the stories of the pre-Christian and early Christian caregivers are found many strong shoulders on which to stand. They are exemplary models whose ministries of love and care for the sick speak eloquently to us as nurses today. The spirit and spirituality of these pioneer nurses provide a foundation and a vision that informs, strengthens, and supports contemporary caregiving as nursing moves into the 21st century.

In this chapter, selected caregivers to the sick, whose activities prefigure the role and posture of the modern nurse, are described. The spiritual attitudes and behaviors of these individuals and communities are presented chronologically, beginning with the pre-Christian era, and continuing through the early and later Christian period, up to the present day. The common thread unifying the persons and communities discussed is their concern with the spiritual as well as the physical and psychosocial needs of those who are ill or infirm; these caregivers viewed nursing the sick as a religious vocation supported by the individual's personal spiritual belief system. This chapter is based on the extant nursing and theological literature that documents the historical role of the nurse in providing spiritual care.

NURSING IN THE PRE-CHRISTIAN ERA

Whatsoever they receive for their wages . . . they do not keep as their own,
but bring into the common treasury for the use of all, nor do they neglect
the sick who are unable to contribute their share.

PHILO, writing of the "Essenes"
(cited in Robinson, 1946, p. 6)

Prior to discussing the Christian influence on care of the sick, health care in the pre-Christian era should be examined briefly. Medicine and nursing in ancient civilizations provided the foundations on which many of the health care practices of Christian nurses rested. These ancient cultures also influenced the concept of Christian charity in relation to caring for those who are ill (Bullough & Bullough, 1987). Archeological study of the pre-Christian cultures has revealed two related yet distinct types of nurses. One group consisted of skilled women who "nursed for hire"; more commonly identified, however, were "nurses" whose positions were those of slaves in wealthy households (Dolan, Fitzpatrick, & Herrmann, 1983, p. 81). These nurses practiced their art according to the established medical models of their respective societies.

Nursing might be explored in a number of early cultures. In Babylonia, the "Code of Hammurabi" suggested that nursing care was provided for patients between physician visits (Walsh, 1929, p. x). Early Buddhist discoveries in China of the curative value of many plants led to nursing therapeutics employing herbology (Sellew & Nuesse, 1946, p. 6). Hindu medical practice in India included a role for the male nurse (Grippando, 1986, p. 3). In Ireland, ancient druidic priests and priestesses advised on care and healing in illness (Dolan, Fitzpatrick, & Herrmann, 1983, p. 40). The four key societies, however, whose spiritual and cultural contributions are most frequently cited as supporting the art and the science of modern medicine and nursing are those of Egypt, Greece, Rome, and Israel.

Egypt

Egyptian medicine contained a strong element of religious magic in its origins; however, the practice of embalming taught the Egyptians human anatomy, from which they were able to derive surgical procedures (Deloughery, 1977, p. 7). Egyptian history boasts the first physician, Imhotep, as well as the first medical textbook, *Ebers Papyrus* (Frank, 1959, p. 9).

The Egyptians were concerned about public health problems such as famine and malnutrition. While offering prayers and sacrifices to religious deities, they also took preventive measures such as storing grain against future need. Researchers have determined that a school for the education of Egyptian physicians existed as early as 1100 B.C., and as a result a number of practical therapeutic remedies for care of the sick were developed. Nurse historians Dietz and Lehozky (1967) concluded, thus, that "undoubtedly some form of instinctive nursing care must have existed at this time" (p. 10).

Greece

History documents the fact that "nursing in the Greco-Roman era was largely the responsibility of members of the patient's own family or that of slaves employed to provide specific skills. The spiritual rationale for providing nursing care was duty to and love for a relative" (Swaffield, 1988, pp. 28–30). The consummate ancient Greek physician, of course, was Hippocrates (460–370 B.C.), who instructed caregivers to "use their eyes and ears, and to reason from facts rather than from gratuitous assumptions" (Deloughery, 1977, p. 8). Hippocrates cautioned those who tended the sick to be solicitous to their patients' spiritual well-being and "to do no harm" (Frank, 1959, p. 17).

Although Hippocrates did not identify nursing as a profession, many of his prescribed therapies fall within the realm of nursing practice. Some examples include the teachings that "fluid diet only should be given in fevers"; "cold sponging [should be used] for high temperatures"; and "hot gargles [should be taken] for acute tonsillitis" (Dietz & Lehozky, 1967, p. 16).

Researchers have explored the characteristics and role of the "nurse" in Greek life by studying the literature, art, and culture of Grecian society. From a study of the early Greek world, Gorman (1917) determined that the nurse "though usually a slave, was sometimes manumitted; that a preference was frequently shown at Athens for the foreign-bred nurse; and, that, on occasion, free women resorted to nursing as a means of gaining a livelihood" (p. 15). The nurse's role was considered a noble one among the Greeks of the era, and, Gorman pointed out, "instances of love and devotedness of nurses are not wanting in the [Greek] literature" (p. 30).

It is also noted that Greek religious mythology introduced the concept of women's involvement in the healing arts, in the tale of Aesculapius, the god of healing: "One of his five children, Hygeia, became the Goddess of Health and another, Panacea (from whom comes our word for 'cure all'), the Restorer of Health" (Deloughery, 1977, p. 9).

Rome

Rome did not offer great advances in medical and nursing practice prior to Christianity but depended greatly on the knowledge of the Greek physicians. Prior to the advent of Greek medicine, care of the sick in Roman households was guided primarily by the use of natural or folk remedies. For example, in the writings of the early Roman scholar, Cato the Elder, is found "advice for the treatment and care of gout, colic, indigestion, constipation, and pain in the side" (Bullough & Bullough, 1969, p. 24). Religion was influential in nursing the sick; Roman gods were offered libations in petition for favors related to health and illness needs. Following the conquest of Corinth many Roman youth began to study in Athens and personally achieved the skills of Greek healing (Pavey, 1952, p. 78). Together with this professional education, however, appreciation and respect for the favor of the gods continued as an important adjunct to therapeutic procedures. Prayer to a god, or to several gods, was considered a critical adjuvant therapy in nursing a sick Roman.

Israel

The Hebrew people of Israel identified in their Mosaic Law much concern for the provision of nursing care for the ill and infirm. There were religious proscriptions concerning general health and hygiene: "Rules of diet and cleanliness, and hours of work and rest" (Sellew & Nuesse, 1946, p. 35). Sellew and Nuesse observed that "Since these rules were enforced by the group and not left to the will of the individual, they were, in effect, rules of public health" (p. 34). Robinson (1946) asserted that the people of Israel actually "laid the foundations of public health nursing on enduring principles, [as they] naturally regarded visiting the sick ('*bikkur holim*') as a religious duty incumbent upon all" (p. 4). The Israelites articulated specific rules regarding the nursing of those with contagious diseases, and were particularly noted for their care of children and of the elderly. Another religious tradition of the Hebrew people related to nursing of the sick encompassed the concepts of "hospitality" and "charity" for anyone in need. This resulted in a system of "houses for strangers," supported by each citizen tithing a tenth of his or her possessions toward charitable work (Pavey, 1952, p. 29).

Finally, the Old Testament Scriptures contain references to the "nurse"; one who "appears at times as a combination servant, companion and helpmate" (Bullough & Bullough, 1969, p. 14). An example from Genesis 24, verse 59, describes Rebekah's going forth to meet Isaac, her future husband, accompanied by her nurse, Deborah: ". . . they allowed Rebekah and her nurse to leave, along with Abraham's servant and his men." Grippando (1986) asserted that "Deborah was the first nurse to be recorded in history" (p. 3).

CHRISTIANITY AND CARE OF THE SICK
Early Christian Nurses

> *Then Jesus went about all the cities and villages, teaching in their synagogues, and proclaiming the good news of the Kingdom, and curing every disease and sickness.*
>
> MATTHEW 9:35

In the early Christian Church, nursing of the sick or injured was accorded a place of honor and respect, associated as it was with one of the primary messages of Jesus: to love one's neighbor. Scripture describes many instances of Christ's healing the sick; His teaching regarding the need for each individual's care for brothers and sisters is reflected especially in the parable of the Good Samaritan (Luke 10:30–36).

Nurse historian Josephine Dolan (1973) pointed out that the way in which Jesus interacted with the sick provides our example. "Instead of 'saying the word' and healing the sick, Christ gave individual attention to the needs of all by touching, anointing, and taking the hand" (p. 47). She concluded, "The least gesture of human kindness" was important to Jesus, and even "a cup of cold water given in His name did not pass unrewarded" (p. 47). Thus, Christ, in His own ministry of healing and teaching, prepared the way for his early followers to serve, with care and tenderness, the needs of their ill brothers and sisters. Central among the early Christians involved in nursing the sick were those persons identified as having a diaconal role in the young church.

Deacons and Deaconesses

> *I give you a new commandment, that you love one another . . . by this everyone will know that you are my disciples.*
>
> JOHN 13:34–35

Among the first "titled" followers of Jesus for whom care of the sick and infirm was an identified task were the deacons and deaconesses, the term *deacon* being derived from the Greek verb *diakonen* meaning "to serve." These men and women were obliged, by their positions, to visit and nurse the sick (Frank, 1959).

And whoever gives even a cup of cold water to one of these little ones in the name of a disciple, truly, I tell you, none of these will lose their reward.

(Matthew 10:42)

Following the exhortation of Jesus to give "a cup of cold water" in His name, these early disciples of Christianity opened their homes, as well as their hearts, to those in need of physical and emotional care. "The Deacons and Deaconesses were especially zealous in seeking out cases of need, and not only nursed the sick by a system of visiting, but brought them into their own homes to be cared for" (Nutting & Dock, 1935, Vol. 1, p. 118). These settings, precursors to the modern hospital, were called diakonias, associating, again, the diaconate with the work of nursing. The diakonias were, in the very early days of the Church, called "Christrooms," suggesting a direct association with Jesus' teaching, "I was a stranger and you took me in" (Dolan, 1973, p. 56). A well-known deacon, Lawrence, was asked to bring the treasures of the Church before a Roman prefect, prior to his trial for being a Christian. He brought to the prefect a group of the "halt, the blind, and the very ill who were unable to care for themselves, and presented them . . . as the treasures of the Church" (Walsh, 1929, p. 2). For his trouble, Lawrence was roasted on a gridiron in martyrdom.

An early Christian woman, Phoebe, described as a friend of St. Paul, is identified as a deaconess in the New Testament. "I commend to you our sister Phoebe, a deacon of the Church . . . for she has been a benefactor of many" (Romans 16:1–2). Phoebe, who lived around 55 A.D., was known as a woman of great dignity and social status; she is said to have spent many hours nursing the poor in their homes (Grippando, 1986, p. 4).

These deacons and deaconesses and their later counterparts, the Roman matrons, were the earliest forerunners of professional nursing in the Christian Church.

Roman Matrons

A number of Roman matrons who had converted to Christianity served the early Church around the third and fourth centuries. These women were able to use their power and wealth to support the charitable work of nursing the sick. The matrons founded hospitals and convents, living ascetic lives dedicated to the care of the ill and infirm. Three of the most famous Roman matrons were Saints Helena, Paula, and Marcella.

St. Helena, or Flavia Helena, was empress of Rome and mother of Constantine the Great. After embracing Christianity, she devoted her life to care of the sick poor. She is identified as having started the first "gerokomion" or home for the aged infirm in the Roman Empire (Dolan, 1973).

St. Paula, a learned woman of her time, founded the first hospice for pilgrims in Bethlehem (Frank, 1959). Paula also built hospices for the sick along the roads to the city; she both managed the institutions and personally nursed the tired and the sick for almost 20 years. St. Jerome wrote of her, "She was oft by them that were sick, and she laid their pillows aright; and . . . she rubbed their feet and boiled water to wash them. And it seemed to her that the less she did to the sick in service, so much the less service she did to God" (Jameson, 1855, as cited in Nutting & Dock, 1935, Vol. 1, p. 141).

St. Marcella, who has been described as the leader of the Roman matrons (Pavey, 1952, p. 102), was known as a scholar and a deeply spiritual woman. She founded a community of religious women whose primary concern was care of the sick poor. Marcella instructed her followers in the care of the sick, while also devoting herself personally to charitable works and prayer.

Although individual deacons, deaconesses, and Roman matrons cared for many of the sick, especially the sick poor, during the early Christian era, it was with the advent and rise of monasticism that the work of nursing began to become institutionalized.

Early Monastic Nurses

The care of the sick is to be placed above and before every other duty, as if indeed Christ were being directly served by waiting on them.

Rule of ST. BENEDICT, 529 A.D.

The monasticism of the fourth, fifth, and sixth centuries was born out of a desire of many Christian men and women to lead lives of sanctity, withdrawing from the world to be guided by the vows of poverty, chastity, and obedience. At first the monks' daily work consisted primarily of prayer and manual labor. This began to change with the advent of such communities as that of St. Benedict of Nursia, whose rule was written in 529 A.D. Although early monasteries, such as those of Benedict, were centers of learning, eventually "nursing of the sick became a chief function and duty of community life" (Donahue, 1985, p. 127). In this era, twin communities of men and women also developed. Three of the most famous abbesses who ruled these groups were St. Radegunde at Poitiers (559 A.D.); St. Hilda of Whitby (664 A.D.); and St. Brigid (487 A.D.), who was the first woman to rule an abbey in Ireland (Donahue, 1985, pp. 129–130).

St. Radegunde, daughter of a Thuringin king, initially took poor patients into her own palace to nurse them. She later founded Holy Cross Monastery, with a community of more than 200 nuns (Goodnow, 1916). Radegunde also established a hospice where she herself cared for the patients; she is reputed to have cared lovingly and tenderly especially for those afflicted with leprosy. Radegunde's work is said to have encouraged many other women to make a life commitment to caring for the sick.

St. Hilda, a cultured and scholarly woman, directed her monastic community in the care of the sick; she nursed the sick poor, including lepers, herself. Hilda also supported a group of associate members of the monastery, called oblates, who assisted in the nursing of those who came under her care (Seymer, 1949).

St. Brigid, who became one of the most famous abbesses in Ireland, was the daughter of an Ulster chieftain and also a disciple of St. Patrick. Brigid founded the great monastery of Kildare, where the ill were received with charity and compassion. Dolan (1973) related that "In Fifth Century Ireland, when leprosy was an incurable scourge . . . they [lepers] came in droves to Kildare to be bathed and treated by Brigid" (p. 60). Brigid became known as the "Patroness of Healing."

Although the monastic communities initiated a more formalized nursing care program for the physically ill and infirm, a greatly neglected and significantly stigmatized population in need of support were those suffering from mental illness or other cognitive impairments.

Mental Illness in the Middle Ages
Dymphna of Belgium

> *The people of Gheel have learned from childhood to live with the patients; their reception and care have been passed on from generation to generation.*
>
> "Foster Family Care in Gheel," 1991, p. 15

Dymphna, the seventh century Irish saint, identified to this day as the patroness of the mentally ill, devoted her life to care of the sick poor in the manner of the early monastic nurses ("Foster Family Care," 1991; Matheussen, Morren, & Seyers, 1975). According to legend, Dymphna traveled to Gheel, Belgium, to assist the Irish missionaries. Once there, she focused her compassion and care especially on persons with impaired mental health. Dymphna was martyred at a young age, but after her death the Belgian women of Gheel believed that she could still intercede for the needs of the ill. Thus, a church and small clinic were erected in Dymphna's honor in the town. Many pilgrims traveled there hoping for a cure and, as the clinic could not house all of these visitors, local Gheel families began offering hospitality to mentally challenged pilgrims (Dolan, Fitzpatrick, & Herrmann, 1983, pp. 59–60). The practice has continued for centuries, and today the Flemish community of Gheel, with its own psychiatric hospital under the supervision of the Belgian government, is considered a model for home health care of the mentally ill ("Foster Family Care," 1991).

At this point in Christian nursing history, the concept of free-standing institutions or hospitals to care for both the mentally and physically ill was beginning to emerge. These early facilities were staffed primarily by men and women inspired by religious motives to care for their less fortunate brothers and sisters.

Medieval Hospital Nursing

Augustinian nuns began their attendance at the Hotel Dieu; for twelve hundred years immured within these walls; alive yet not of this world; aloof from the human race, with the breath of God upon their faces. To and fro they walked the wards, back and forth throughout the days and years and centuries.

ROBINSON (1946, p. 50)

Two of the most famous medieval Christian hospitals built outside monastic walls were the Hotel-Dieu of Lyon (542 A.D.) and the Hotel-Dieu of Paris (650 A.D.). The title *Hotel-Dieu,* or "House of God," was often chosen as the name for a French hospital of the era (Grippando, 1986, p. 10). In the beginning, these "hospitals" served as almshouses and orphanages, as well as facilities for care of the sick. Goodnow (1916) reported that the early nurses in these facilities were "religious women who devoted their lives to charity" (p. 29).

The Hotel-Dieu of Lyon eventually added to its cadre of women nurses a group of men called "brothers" who also assisted with the care of the sick. The hospital was designed to care for pilgrims, orphans, the poor, and the sick. It was one of the first hospitals to separate those with contagious illnesses from those with more ordinary ills (Nutting & Dock, Vol. 1, 1935).

The Hotel-Dieu of Paris began as a hostel providing care for a small number of the sick poor. After a brief period, the group of women who had ultimately been constituted as a religious community known as the Augustinian Sisters took over the hospital (Dietz & Lehozky, 1967, p. 25). The

Sisters lived under a very strict rule; following profession of religious vows their entire world became the hospital where they both lived and worked with no thought of ever returning home even to visit. The Sisters gave excellent care to the patients; for each the work was her life. As Nutting and Dock (1935) observed, "Their home is the 'Hotel-Dieu.' From the day of their profession they live and die there" (Vol. 1, p. 296).

Although these early hospitals served the civilian populations until about the 10th century, it was recognized with the undertaking of the Crusades that casualties generated by the wars would overwhelm existing nursing facilities. It was anticipated that following the conflicts large numbers of wounded crusaders would return home weakened and battle scarred, many in need of extensive nursing care. Thus an entirely new cadre of nurses was created whose mission was centered on the care of wounded crusaders; these nursing communities were called the military nursing orders.

Military Nursing Orders

> *To the Knights Hospitallers of St. John of Jerusalem:*
> *With regard to the hospital which thou hast founded in the city of*
> *Jerusalem . . . that House of God . . . shall be placed under the protection*
> *of the Apostolic See.*
>
> Bull of POPE PASCAL II
> 15 February 1113

Out of the 11th-, 12th-, and 13th-century Crusades to the Holy Land came the military nursing orders, orders of men who were committed by their religious ministry to the care of those wounded in battle. The three major groups were the Knights Hospitallers of St. John of Jerusalem, the Teutonic Knights, and the Knights of St. Lazarus. The three general classes of members in the orders were knights, priests, and serving brothers (Kalisch & Kalisch, 1995). The knights participated in the Crusades and helped to care for the injured, the priests served the religious needs in camps and hospitals, and the serving brothers were responsible for general care of the sick (Pavey, 1952, pp. 163–164). All members of the orders, however, professed religious commitment of their lives as exemplified in the Rule of the Order of St. John of Jerusalem, as written by its first grand master, Raymond du Puy:

> Firstly, I ordain that all the brethren engaging in the service of the sick
> shall keep with God's help the three promises that they have made
> to God, . . . poverty, chastity, obedience . . . and to live without any

property of their own, because God will require of them at the last judgement the fulfillment of these three promises.

(Austin, 1957, p. 73)

The largest of the orders, the Knights Hospitallers of St. John of Jerusalem, is thought to have been created around 1050 A.D. to staff the two Jerusalem hospitals organized to care for those wounded in the Crusades: one for men, dedicated to St. John; the other for women, dedicated to St. Mary Magdalene (Seymer, 1949). Historians assert that the order was originated under the guidance of Peter Gerard, a deeply religious man. An associated order for women was also created to nurse the sick, under Agnes of Rome (Jensen, Spaulding, & Cady, 1959). The knights of St. John were characterized by a specific dress: a black robe with white linen cross.

A second community, the German order of Knights Hospitallers or Teutonic Knights, was founded in 1191 A.D. at the time of the Third Crusade. These knights, who followed the rule of the Knights of St. John, taking the usual vows of poverty, chastity, and obedience, also took a vow of care of the sick (Donahue, 1985, p. 155). The Teutonic Knights were in charge of many German hospitals and later became a separate organization under the Rule of St. Augustine (Jensen, Spaulding, & Cady, 1959).

The Knights of St. Lazarus were organized primarily to care for the lepers in Jerusalem; they also admitted lepers to their order. There were two categories of knights: warriors and hospitallers. The latter group had a special commitment to care for those with leprosy. The community's first grand master was himself a leper (Seymer, 1949). It might be suggested here that the military nursing orders of the 11th, 12th, and 13th centuries— which were founded specifically to care for the Crusaders, the soldiers of the day, fallen or injured in battle—were indeed the forebears of contemporary military nurses in this country and throughout the world. Members of the early military nursing orders, as military nurses today, took an oath of obedience and promised a willingness to risk their lives in order to care for those wounded in war (see O'Brien, 2003, "Navy Nurse: A Call to Lay Down My Life").

During the period of the Crusades and afterward, while the military nursing orders cared for those wounded in war, medieval monastics continued to provide nursing care for civilians. Some of these monastic nurses were highly respected and honored for their care and compassion, as well as for their healing powers. One of the most respected healers of medieval monasticism, who currently has a following among some contemporary nurses, is Hildegard of Bingen.

Medieval Monastic Nursing

Hildegard of Bingen

> *I raise my hands to God, that I might be held aloft by God, just like a*
> *feather which has no weight from its own strength and lets itself be*
> *carried by the wind.*

Letter from HILDEGARD to Guibert of Gembloux
(cited in Fox, 1987, p. 348)

Sometimes described as the "Sybil of the Rhine" (Livingstone, 1990, p. 241), Hildegard of Bingen (1098–1179), German abbess, visionary, musician, writer, and nurse, was one of the most outstanding of the medieval monastic women. At the age of 8, she was given over to the care of the Anchoress Jutta who lived in a hermitage within the walls of the great Benedictine Monastery at Disibodenberg. While yet in her teens, Hildegard took the Benedictine veil and some 20 years later was herself named abbess of the small group of women who had joined her at the monastery. Hildegard ultimately broke away from the abbey at Disibodenberg and founded two new monasteries for women: Rupertsberg and its daughter house at Ebingen.

Hildegard was told by God to relate what she "saw and heard" in her many visions; her first book of visions was entitled *Scivias* or "Know the Ways [of the Lord]" (Lachman, 1993). Hildegard's writings were numerous and included works on medicine and nursing, as well as theology; she had learned a great deal about illness and healing during an internship of nursing in the Disibodenberg infirmary. Two of her medical books written around 1159 were entitled *Physica* and *Liber Composite Medicinae*. The former described anatomy and physiology; the latter explained the symptoms and cure of illness and disease.

In her books, Hildegard described diseases of "various organs of the body, pallor and redness of the face, bad breath, and indigestion" (Sellew & Nuesse, 1946, p. 125). She was continually sought out by those with various ailments and frequently provided cures; she was even thought to perform miracles (Jensen, Spaulding, & Cady, 1959, p. 77). For Hildegard, diseases and cures were all associated with "the four qualities of heat, dryness, moistness and cold . . . fire, air, water and earth, and, the humors and personality types to which these elements give rise" (Bowie & Davies, 1992, p. 48). For example, she wrote in her "Third Vision: On Human Nature", "I noticed how the humors in the human organism are distributed or altered by various qualities of the wind and air. . . ." (Fox, 1987, p. 56).

For centuries, Hildegard of Bingen's work, in its original Latin, lay forgotten. Then in the early 1960s, her Benedictine Sisters began to translate the writings into German. During the last decade, especially, Hildegard's extensive contributions to medicine, nursing, and theology have been recognized in this country as well. Barbara Lachman (1993), who has spent 20 years studying the life and writings of Hildegard, identified the mystic's early awareness of the body–mind connection. "Hildegard reminds us . . . that the body can be afflicted with sickness and torments only the spirit can heal" (p. 10). This concept is most timely in light of our present-day emphasis on holistic health care, uniting rather than isolating the needs and problems of body, mind, and spirit.

Among other outstanding monastic nurses of the Middle Ages, and their tertiaries, who contributed notably to the healing arts were Francis and Clare of Assisi, Elizabeth of Hungary, and Catherine of Siena.

Francis and Clare of Assisi

> Great was his [Francis'] compassion for the sick, and great his care for their needs. He entered into the feelings of all the sick, and gave them words of sympathy when he could not give words of help.
>
> > *Life of St. Francis*
> > BROTHER THOMAS OF CELANO, 1228 A.D.
> > (cited in Austin, 1957, p. 86)

While distinguished as the primary founder of mendicant monasticism, Francis of Assisi (1184–1224) is also considered by many nursing caregivers as a patron of those who tend the sick. Francis is best known for his care and compassion for those suffering from leprosy, the most fearful and stigmatizing illness of his time. Francis not only requested that his Friars Minor visit and care for lepers, but also spent much time personally caring for those with the disease. Virtually every biography of Francis recounts his conversion experience, describing how one day, as a young man, Francis Bernardone was moved to dismount from his horse and embrace a leper approaching him in the road (Dennis, Nangle, Moe-Lobeda, & Taylor, 1993; Green, 1987). Following this epiphany, Francis began to visit "leper houses." "There the lepers were always waiting for him . . . knowing that he brought love" (Maynard, 1948, p. 43). Sabatier (1894) recounted the story of one particularly difficult victim of leprosy who was always dissatisfied with his care and blaspheming God. When the Brothers described this behavior to Francis, their leader went to the leper and said, "I will care for you myself"; "St. Francis made haste to heat some water with many sweet smelling herbs; next he took off the leper's clothes and began to bathe him" (p. 142).

In the *Life of St. Francis*, written by Brother Thomas of Celano in 1228, Francis' great compassion for the sick is noted. "He entered into the feelings of all the sick, and gave them words of sympathy when he could not give words of hope" (cited in Austin, 1957, p. 86). In 1262, St. Bonaventure, then the eighth superior general of the Friars Minor, graphically described Francis' commitment to the sick. "Thence that lover of utterest humility betook himself unto the lepers, and abode among them, with all diligence serving them all for the love of God. He would bathe their feet, and bind up their sores . . . yea, in his marvelous devotion, he would even kiss their ulcerated wounds, he that was soon to be a Gospel physician" (*Legenda Maior S. Francisci*, St. Bonaventure, as cited in Austin, 1957, p. 86).

Clare of Assisi (1194–1253), daughter of a wealthy Italian family who gave up all to follow Jesus in the way of her beloved Francis, is also considered a model for those who commit their lives to the care of the sick. St. Clare's "Rule" for her original group of "Poor Ladies" mentions only care of the ill within the community. "All are obliged to serve and provide for their Sisters who are ill just as they would wish to be served themselves" (*Rule of St. Clare*, 1252, cited in Armstrong & Brady, 1982, p. 220). The literature, however, recounts numerous instances of Clare and her Sisters caring for the sick poor of the area, especially lepers. Robinson (1946) reported that "Francis sent the diseased and deformed to Clare and her nuns, who nursed them in little huts of mud and branches, grouped around the convent" (p. 41). The veracity of this account is reinforced by Nutting and Dock (1935, Vol. 1) who also described "little mud huts" where the "Poor Clarisses" "received and nursed the sick which Francis sent to them, so that finally San Damiano became a sort of hospital, and nursing one of the chief interests of the community" (p. 215). Clare is said to have cared personally for many of the sick sent by Francis.

Elizabeth of Hungary

> *It was not alone by presents or with money that the young [Elizabeth] testified her love for the poor of Christ, it was still more by personal devotion, by those tender and patient cares, which are assuredly, in the sight of God and of the sufferers, the most holy and most precious alms.*
>
> Life of St. Elizabeth of Hungary
> COUNT DE MONTALEMBERT
> (cited in Austin, 1957, p. 91)

One of the most distinguished Franciscan tertiaries, noted for her compassion for the sick, especially for lepers, was Elizabeth of Hungary (1207–1231). Elizabeth was a princess of Thuringia who, after her husband's death in the Crusades, entered the Third Order of St. Francis and committed her life to the care of the sick poor. She is especially remembered as a "builder of hospitals" (Robinson, 1946, p. 42), having established no less than five institutions during her short life.

While she lived in a castle, it is reported that Elizabeth daily walked to the local village ". . . distributing alms to the poor, feeding the hungry, nursing the sick . . . [and placing] her compassionate hands on the bodies of the lepers" (Robinson, 1946, p. 42). A number of folk tales relate Elizabeth's ministry to the sick poor. One story (described by both Robinson, 1946, and Nutting and Dock, 1935, Vol. 1) asserts that on a cold winter day early in her ministry, when Elizabeth was walking toward the village with a large bundle of food under her cloak, she was accosted by her husband, angry that she was spending so much time and money on her work with the ill. When he ordered Elizabeth to open her cloak, she was found to be carrying an armload of magnificently blossoming red and white roses, thus validating the saintly nature of her mission. Nutting and Dock (1935, Vol. 1) reported that after her husband's death Elizabeth's entire life was dedicated to nursing. "Twice a day she went to the hospitals to care for the most wretched patients, bathing them, dressing their wounds and taking them nourishment" (p. 221). Elizabeth's life's work is perhaps best summarized in the comments of Theodoric of Thüringen, written in 1725:

> She busied herself with works of charity and mercy; and, those whom poverty, sickness or infirmity had oppressed more than others . . . she placed in her hospital and most humbly ministered to their wants with her own hands. She arranged their baths, put them to bed, and covered them, saying to her servants: "How well it is for us that thus we bathe and cover our Lord."
>
> (Austin, 1957, p. 90)

Elizabeth of Hungary died at the young age of 24 and was buried in the chapel of one of her hospitals, which she had dedicated to St. Francis.

Catherine of Siena

> Then in her sacred saving hands
> She took the sorrows of the lands,
> With maiden palms she lifted up
> The sick times blood-embittered cup,
> And in her virgin garment furled
> The faint limbs of a wounded world,
> Clothed with calm love and clear desire
> She went forth in her souls attire,
> A missive fire.

ALGERNON SWINBURNE
(1911, p. 162)

Historian of nursing James Walsh (1929) poignantly described Catherine of Siena's commitment to the sick poor:

> According to . . . legend, her devotion to the ailing poor was so pleasing to the Master, who had gone about healing the ailing, that she had a number of visits from celestial personages. Above all the Christ Child was so much interested in this young woman, who, when scarcely more than a child, had insisted on devoting herself to His ailing poor, that He put a ring on her finger as an indication of the fact that she was to be His heavenly spouse.

(Walsh, 1929, pp. 121–122)

Catherine of Siena (1347–1380), known to contemporary health care providers as the "Patroness of Nursing," entered the Tertiaries of St. Dominic while still in her teens. Catherine, like Elizabeth, also died young, at the age of 34, yet during her life she became renowned as a teacher, nurse, and mystic (Sellew & Nuesse, 1946, pp. 129–130). Catherine worked extensively with the ill, especially lepers, and when Siena was overwhelmed with the Black Plague epidemic in 1372, she is said to have "walked night and day in the wards, only resting for a few hours now and then in an adjacent house" (Nutting & Dock, 1935, Vol. I, p. 230).

An anecdote is told about an indigent woman of Siena suffering from leprosy who was so diseased that no caregiver, even in the hospital, had the courage to assist her. "When Catherine heard of this . . . she hastened to the hospital, visited the leper, kissed her, and offered not only to supply all her necessities, but also to become her servant during the remainder of her life"

(Raymond of Capua, 1853, pp. 93–94). In summarizing St. Catherine's extraordinary commitment to the sick, Blessed Raymond of Capua (1853) wrote, "Catherine was wonderfully compassionate to the wants of the poor, but her heart was even more sensitive to the sufferings of the sick (cited in Austin, 1957, p. 94).

POST-REFORMATION NURSING: THE CATHOLIC AND PROTESTANT NURSING ORDERS

Nurse historian Patricia Donahue (1985) reported that in the 16th century alone "more than 100 female [religious] orders were founded specifically to do nursing" (p. 216). The growth of nursing communities continued, though more slowly, during the 17th, 18th, and 19th centuries, with a few new groups being founded in the early to mid-20th century. Some orders have survived and attained a notable history and tradition in the care of the ill and infirm; others were short-lived with little historical information available about them. For the present exploration, a select group of two Catholic and two Protestant communities with significant historical involvement with nursing and health care activities, and which still continue this ministry today, are discussed. These groups are the Daughters of Charity of St. Vincent de Paul and the related American communities of Sisters of Charity, who also adhere to the spirit and spirituality of Vincent de Paul; the Sisters of Mercy; the Kaiserswerth Deaconesses; and the Nightingale nursing community. Although not formally constituted as a religious order, Florence Nightingale and her nursing community, who served in the Crimean War, undertook their work out of spiritual motivation. Florence Nightingale was a staunch Christian who viewed the work of nursing the sick as a vocation. This conviction sustained her work in the hospital in Scutari and informed her leadership of the group of nurses who accompanied her to the battlefield hospital.

Briefly described also are five smaller women's religious communities that continue to maintain a significant commitment to nursing as a contemporary ministry. These include the Sisters of Bon Secours, the Servants for Relief of Incurable Cancer, the Medical Mission Sisters, the Missionaries of Charity, and the Sisters of Life.

Daughters of Charity of St. Vincent de Paul

One of the largest and best known of the early religious communities of women are the Daughters of Charity founded in Paris, France, in 1633 by St. Vincent de Paul, in conjunction with St. Louise de Marillac. Some years after ordination to the priesthood, Vincent became concerned about the lack of care for the poor and needy, especially the sick poor, in 17th-century France. His personal spirituality was centered on seeing Christ in the person of the poor; he was much attracted to the Lukan Gospel of Jesus, especially such passages as Luke 4:18. "The Spirit of the Lord . . . has sent me to bring glad tidings to the poor, to proclaim liberty to captives, recovery of sight to the blind. . . ." (Maloney, 1992, p. 14).

In 1617, Vincent began gathering together a band of laity to visit and care for the sick and the poor, naming them the Confraternity of Charity. As some of the women, later named the Ladies of Charity, encountered the overwhelming needs of the sick, both in hospitals where they observed the exhaustion of the overworked Augustinian nuns and in the homes of the poor, they recognized a great need for more nursing Sisters. One of the women, Louise de Marillac, a wealthy widow, was directed by Vincent to become the first leader of the small community. "She would give the Dames de Charité instructions. She accompanied them on their rounds helping them, advising them, assisting them in their duties and making suggestions about other ways of giving care to patients" (Dolan, 1973, p. 100).

The Daughters of Charity were formally established as a religious community dedicated to serving the "poorest of the poor" in 1633. The first Sisters "nursed the sick poor in their homes" as well as caring for patients in the famous Hotel-Dieu in Paris (Daughters of Charity National Health Services, 1994, p. 1). Many of the early Daughters were young Frenchwomen raised in rural areas. "They wore the French peasant costume, a heavy coarse dress of blue woolen cloth with a full skirt and tight fitting waist, a blue apron of washable material, and a large white linen headdress . . . [T]hey were not nuns but 'pious women of the world' prepared to nurse on the battlefields in time of war or to be sent to care for the sick in any disaster" (Sellew & Nuesse, 1946, pp. 198–199).

Dock and Stewart (1920) noted that St. Vincent de Paul would not let the Daughters pronounce permanent vows; they took vows for one year only, as they do today. The vows can, however, be renewed indefinitely on an annual basis. Vincent's advice to his Sisters "if they were to be useful as nurses, was uncompromising in the extreme: 'My daughters,' he said, 'You are not religious in the technical sense, and if there should be found some marplot among you to say, it is better to be a nun, Ah! then, my daughters, your company will be ready for extreme unction. Fear this, my daughters, and while you live permit no such change; never consent to it. Nuns must needs have a cloister, but the Daughters of Charity must needs go everywhere" (p. 102). Vincent directed also that the Daughters were to have neither convent nor cell; his emphasis in this regard has been preserved in a well-known quote from the community's rule:

> Your convent will be the house of the sick; your cell, a hired room; your chapel, the parish church; your cloister, the streets of the city, or the wards of the hospital.
>
> (Daughters of Charity, 1993)

Stepsis and Liptak (1989) observed that, given the Church's history, in the era of mandating cloistered community life for all women religious "the successful efforts of Saint Vincent de Paul and Saint Louise de Marillac to create and maintain a noncloistered congregation of women in France, during the seventeenth century and beyond . . . were monumental" (p. 18). They added, "Vincent's attempt at bridging the gap between cloistered and active religious community became the American model" (p. 19). A historical overview of Vincent's vision for health care identifies the "essential attributes" as including such characteristics as "spiritually rooted," "holistic," "integrated," "flexible," and "creative" (Sullivan, 1997, p. 49).

Today the Daughters of Charity comprise one of the largest international Catholic religious communities of women in existence, with approximately 28,000 Daughters worldwide. Some 1,400 Daughters are involved in a variety of ministries in the United States, with health care, education, and social ministry being the major categories of service.

In the United States, the Daughters of Charity National Health Services (DCNHS) is one of the most extensive health care systems in the world, with Sisters serving primarily in the arenas of administration, nursing, and pastoral care. In addition to ministering in hospitals and nursing homes, the Daughters serve the sick poor in settings such as "free clinics in poor neighborhoods in the cities, in rural areas, with migrant workers in the deep south, and in drug treatment centers" (Daughters of Charity, 1995, p. 1).

A related but separate group of U.S. communities of followers of Vincent de Paul are the Sisters of Charity. Communities of Sisters of Charity are located in a multiplicity of geographical locations in the United States; the sisters carry out various ministries, nursing being a central ministry of a number of the groups.

Sisters of Charity

The American Sisters of Charity, also followers of the vision of Vincent de Paul, were founded in 1809 by Elizabeth Bayley Seton (1774–1821), whose father had been a prominent physician. After Elizabeth's husband died as a young man, the widow determined to commit her life to the service of others by teaching children and caring for the sick. Elizabeth, then an Episcopalian, served the poor first with the Protestant Sisters of Charity. After converting to Catholicism, she opened a small school near Emmitsburg, Maryland, gradually expanding the services as other committed women came to join her.

Mother Elizabeth Seton and her young community adopted the rule of Vincent de Paul for the French Daughters of Charity, with some modifications for the American milieu of the era; their habit, a black dress, was modeled after Mother Seton's widow's costume (Dolan, Fitzpatrick, & Herrmann, 1983, p. 138). Mother Seton was interested in her American Sisters of Charity being formally united with the international community of Daughters of Charity, founded by St. Vincent in France. After Mother Seton's death in 1821, the Emmitsburg community of Sisters of Charity sought unification with the French Daughters. In 1850, the Emmitsburg Sisters became formally affiliated with the Daughters of Charity in France; they "passed under the authority of the Superior General of that Order, assuming the garb of the French sisterhood; the headdress was the celebrated white linen coronet as given by Saint Vincent de Paul" (Stepsis & Liptak, 1989, p. 292).

Prior to the unification of the Emmitsburg Sisters with the Daughters of Charity in Paris, however, some of the women who had come to join Mother Seton but wanted to maintain their American rule of life and dress branched out from the motherhouse to establish other communities of Sisters of Charity. Two of the largest of the new groups with direct Emmitsburg roots were the New York Sisters of Charity and the Sisters of Charity of Cincinnati. These Sisters were responsible for the founding and administration of many hospitals, as well as the carrying out of other nursing and social ministries. Nurse historian Minnie Goodnow (1916) pointed out that while indeed nursing was only one branch of the American Sisters of Charity's ministry, it was an important one:

> In 1832, during a great cholera epidemic, they [Sisters of Charity] nursed under the city authorities in New York, Philadelphia and Baltimore. They have always had many hospitals and asylums of their own. (p. 144)

Currently many different groups belonging to the Elizabeth Seton Federation, the offspring of Mother Elizabeth Seton's original Emmitsburg community, are involved in U.S. health care activities (see Stepsis & Liptak, 1989).

Sisters of Mercy

Another nursing community with a long history and tradition in the administration of U.S. hospitals and schools of nursing is the Sisters of Mercy. The Sisters of Mercy was founded in 1831 in Dublin, Ireland, by Mother Catherine McAuley (Grippando, 1986, p. 17). Catherine, wealthy from an inheritance she received at age 40, had a great concern for the poor, especially the sick poor, living in the slums of Dublin. With her fortune, she erected a building with classrooms, dormitories, a clinic, and a chapel, labeling it the "House of Mercy." Her original plan was to create a "corps" of Catholic social service workers. She began initially to work with a group of laywomen who would visit the sick in their homes, but ultimately, at the suggestion of the Bishop of Dublin, she began to organize the women into a religious community. Catherine faced opposition from family and friends. Nevertheless she persisted, and "in January 1832 seven women who had worked with Catherine McAuley were clothed in the habit of the Institute" (Walsh, 1929, p. 189).

Walsh (1929) reported that, although the Sisters began by visiting the sick in their homes, "after a time [Mother Catherine] obtained permission to visit the wards of several Dublin hospitals with her nuns to bring consolation to the patients. This was an innovation . . . very greatly appreciated by the poor sufferers. Patients became ever so much more tractable. Above all, the morale of the sick improved, and with it their resistive vitality" (p. 189). The Sisters of Mercy were sent to the Crimea by the English government and labored with Florence Nightingale (Frank, 1959, p. 94). The difficulty of the conditions at the hospital in Scutari was described by Goodnow (1916), who also lauded the work of the Sisters of Mercy in the setting. Citing a war office report, Goodnow wrote:

> The superiority of an ordered system is beautifully illustrated in the Sisters of Mercy. One mind appears to move all, and their intelligence, delicacy and conscientiousness invest them with a halo of extreme confidence. The medical officer can safely consign his most critical cases to their hands. (p. 89)

Sisters of Mercy came to the United States from Ireland around 1854 and began establishing schools and hospitals. By 1928, there were 140 convents in America, and by 1965, the Mercy congregations in the United States had merged into one "federation," which ultimately evolved into the present Institute of the Sisters of Mercy of the Americas. This institute includes Mercy communities in North, South, and Central America, as well as Guam, the Caribbean, and the Philippines (Sisters of Mercy of the Americas, "Sisters of Mercy Founded," 1995, pp. 4–5).

Presently the Sisters of Mercy of the Americas "sponsor or co-sponsor approximately 140 hospitals or health-related facilities throughout the United States," as well as hospitals and health clinics in Belize, Guam, Guyana, Peru, and the Philippines (Sisters of Mercy of the Americas, "Mercy Health Care," 1995, p. 1).

Kaiserswerth Deaconesses

The Kaiserswerth Deaconesses, an important Protestant community of women with a primary ministry of nursing the sick, was founded by a young Lutheran minister, Theodor Fliedner, around 1836 in Kaiserswerth, Germany (Kalisch & Kalisch, 1995). Pastor Fliedner, who was concerned about the overall social and health care needs of his poor parishioners, enlisted his wife, Frederika Munster, to gather a group of women who would visit and nurse the sick poor in their homes. The Fliedners attempted to attract a group of young women of good character; in this era, prior to Florence Nightingale, nurses were generally considered to be prostitutes, alcoholics, and generally unseemly women.

Frank (1959) described the education of the Kaiserswerth Deaconesses. "Their course of training lasted three years, their uniform was simple, and they were taught domestic duties associated with caring for the sick" (p. 95). Nutting and Dock (1935, Vol. 2) quoted Pastor Fliedner's own description of the essentials of the Deaconess vocation. "In organization the work is a free religious association, not dependent on state or church authorities. It takes its stand on the mother nature of the church founded by Christ" (p. 33). The four key branches of the Deaconesses' work were described as "Nursing; relief of the poor; care of children; and work among unfortunate women" (Nutting & Dock, 1935, Vol. 2, pp. 33–34).

In commenting on the Deaconesses' religious commitment, Woolsey (1950) observed, "The Deaconess Vows are taken for five years . . . however, women are expected to declare that they intend to adopt the office of Deaconess for life. Those trained as nurses are more apt . . . to regard [the] vows and retain their connection with the order . . . and the settled resolution, no doubt, is one of the elements that contributes to make them good nurses" (pp. 30–31).

The Kaiserswerth Deaconesses began their work in the United States in 1849 when four deaconesses were sent to Pennsylvania. "They were to assume responsibility for the Pittsburgh Infirmary [Passavant Hospital]. This was the first Protestant Church hospital in the United States" (Dolan, 1973,

p. 123). The Pittsburgh infirmary was founded by Lutheran minister William Passavant, a founder of the Lutheran deaconess movement in this country. The American Lutheran Deaconess Foundation continued to grow in the years following Passavant's initiation, spreading to such places as Philadelphia, New York, and Baltimore (Olson, 1992, see "Lutheran Deaconesses in America," pp. 243–339).

The role of the contemporary Lutheran deaconess is to "serve God's people through spiritual care and works of mercy" ("Just What Is a Deaconess?", 1994). Central to diaconal ministry are the concepts of "agape love and love of neighbor" as well as a sense of "mercifulness and community" (Zetterlund, 1997, p. 11). Deaconess roles are encompassed in such professions as nursing, social work, parish ministry, chaplaincy, counseling, and missionary work. A deaconess may serve within a Lutheran Church congregation, she may be employed by a caregiving institution such as a hospital or nursing home, or she may accept a domestic or foreign missionary assignment.

Three Lutheran deaconess communities that provide diaconal education in the United States are the Evangelical Lutheran Deaconess Association community motherhouse at Gladwyne, Pennsylvania; the Center for Diaconal Ministry of the Lutheran Deaconess Association at Valpariso University, Valpariso, Indiana; and the Deaconess Program at Concordia University, River Forest, Illinois. Deaconess education programs may vary but generally include the study of theology and ministry as well as liberal arts and courses to prepare the future deaconess for a professional role. A year-long deacon internship is usually included in the program of study. Following diaconal education, a woman may be consecrated in the role of deaconess within the Lutheran Church.

Nightingale Nurses: Mission to the Crimea

The Nightingale Pledge

I solemnly pledge myself before God and in the presence of this assembly:
To pass my life in purity and to practice my profession faithfully.
I will abstain from whatever is deleterious and mischievous, and will not take or knowingly administer any harmful drug.
I will do all in my power to elevate the standard of my profession, and will hold in confidence all personal matters committed to my keeping, and all family affairs coming to my knowledge in the practice of my profession.
With loyalty will I endeavor to aid the physician in his work, and devote myself to the welfare of those committed to my care.

(cited in Kalisch & Kalisch, 1995, p. 117)

Although, as noted earlier, Florence Nightingale's community (1820–1910) is not considered a religious "order," it was, however, the first Christian community of nurses sent by the English government in 1854 to care for the wounded soldiers during the Crimean War. Nightingale trained under Pastor Fliedner at his Deaconess School in Kaiserswerth, as well as under the Daughters of Charity of St. Vincent de Paul in France. In exploring the historical roots of spirituality in nursing, Patricia Maher observed that prior to the 19th century "there was little beside spiritual care with which to heal. Within an overtly religious society, spiritual care was seen as a formidable and credible endeavor and people were suspicious of medical care for good reason" (2006, p. 419). Florence Nightingale, Maher asserts, "was one of the first to bring spirituality and science together to improve the care of the sick" (p. 419).

Nurse historian Deloughery (1977) offered a glimpse of Nightingale's personal spirituality in reporting that in 1847, "after a busy 'social summer,' . . . she went into retreat for ten days in the convent of the Trinita dei Monti, where she absorbed much of the spirit of the Church and where her religious belief greatly matured" (p. 52). Deloughery added that Nightingale, a member of the Church of England, "remained deeply religious throughout her life" (p. 52). Central to Florence Nightingale's spirituality was her belief in the greatness of God, as the "Spirit of Truth" (Widerquist, 1992, p. 49). Nightingale felt spiritually called to model the greatness and generosity of God in service to the sick; her first experience of this vocational call occurred immediately before her 17th birthday (Selanders, 1993, p. 8). At the age of 24, Florence wrote to her friend and mentor, Dr. Samuel Howe, to ask "if there would be anything unsuitable or unbecoming to a young Englishwoman, if she should devote herself to works of charity in hospitals and elsewhere as the Catholic Sisters do?" Howe replied, "Go forward if you have a 'vocation' for that way of life . . . and God be with you" (Dolan, 1973, p. 167). Florence Nightingale sought to instill her sense of "spiritual vocation" into the team of "Nightingale Nurses" who accompanied her on the Crimean Mission. An excerpt from a work of one of the world's greatest poets is illustrative of the spiritual heritage Nightingale left to the nurses who would follow in her footsteps.

Santa Filomena

Thus thought I as by night I read
of the great army of the dead,
The trenches cold and damp,
The starved and frozen camp.
The wounded from the battle plain,
In dreary hospitals of pain,

The cheerless corridors,
The cold and stony floors.
Lo, in that house of misery,
A lady with a lamp I see
pass through the glimmering gloom
and flit from room to room.
And slow, as in a dream of bliss,
the speechless sufferer turns to kiss
her shadow as it falls,
upon the darkening walls.

HENRY WADSWORTH LONGFELLOW
(1857, p. 23)

The latter stanza of Longfellow's poem was based on factual reports from wounded soldiers in the Scutari hospital. The young Englishmen described in letters the peace they felt in simply seeing the "Lady with the Lamp"; her shadow falling across one's cot, it was said, brought comfort and relief.*

Contemporary nursing literature reflects a renewed interest in the spirituality of Florence Nightingale, one recent example being the 1995 article by Janet Macrae entitled "Nightingale's Spiritual Philosophy and Its Significance for Modern Nursing." In the piece, Macrae reported, "For Nightingale, spirituality is intrinsic to human nature and is our deepest and most potent resource for healing" (p. 8). Macrae also noted Florence Nightingale's attraction to mysticism, particularly the writings of Francis of Assisi and John of the Cross. She cited an excerpt from the preface to Nightingale's own unpublished book on mysticism. "Where shall I find God; In myself. That is the true mystical doctrine. But then I myself must be in a state for Him to come and dwell in me. This is the whole aim of the mystical life" (as cited in Macrae, 1995, p. 10). Ultimately, Macrae argued, Nightingale's spiritual philosophy, which views "spirituality as intrinsic to human nature and compatible with science," may provide important direction for the current and future development of nursing theory and practice (p. 8). Florence Nightingale's spiritual legacy is also advanced for current practitioners of nursing by Ann Bradshaw (1996) who asserted that holistic

---

*Longfellow's poem, although entitled "Santa Filomena," has long been considered to have been written for Florence Nightingale; thus her identification throughout history as "the lady with the lamp." Benet (1948) offered an explanation: "Longfellow called Florence Nightingale, 'Saint Filomena,' not only because 'Filomena' resembles the Latin word for 'nightingale,' but also because the Saint, in Sabatelli's picture, is represented as hovering over a group of the sick and maimed, healed by her intervention" (p. 970).

nursing must include attention to the spiritual needs and concerns of both patient and family as envisioned by Nightingale (p. 42).

Five smaller nursing communities of Catholic religious women founded 4, 75, 105, 140, and 171 years, respectively, after Florence Nightingale's birth are the Sisters of Bon Secours (1824), the Servants for Relief of Incurable Cancer (1895), the Medical Mission Sisters (1925), the Missionaries of Charity (1960), and the Sisters of Life (1991). These communities included care of the sick as a primary ministry of the early Sisters and continue to serve the sick poor in contemporary society, both in the United States and abroad.

Sisters of Bon Secours

The Congregation of Bon Secours was founded in 1824 in Paris. The Sisters' mission was to visit and care for the sick poor in their homes. The French words *bon secours* mean "good or compassionate help"; the contemporary community asserts, "Our purpose was [historically] and is to bring compassionate care to the sick and the dying" (Sisters of Bon Secours USA, 1997). Walsh (1929) reported that the community's ministry began with a group of 12 young French women living together to carry out the work of nursing the sick. The leader of the small community, Sister Marie Joseph (Josephine Potel), and her Sisters responded to the needs of 19th-century France, where health care generally was still unavailable for many people. The Sisters went out to the homes of those in need and "if the condition required extended care, the Sisters remained in the homes of the ill, often for long periods of time, always risking criticism from a public uncomfortable with such unconventional practices by religious women at that time" (O'Sullivan, 1995, p. 4). The early ministry of the Bon Secours Sisters was described by historian Walsh (1929) as follows:

> The Sisters of Bon Secours devote themselves only to the care of the sick in their own homes. They have no fixed charge, the poor give nothing, the rich offer what they will. . . . They make excellent nurses, and their patients learn to love them very dearly and are very much encouraged and consoled by their presence. (p. 266)

Some 57 years after their founding in Paris, the Sisters of Bon Secours arrived in Baltimore, Maryland, where they also visited and nursed the sick poor in their homes. In the early days after their arrival, there were many requests for trained nurses to minister to the sick in their homes. "For those living in poverty, the 'sickroom' was their hospital, and their home, the place where they had to recover and learn again to live healthfully" (Stepsis &

Liptak, 1989, p. 112). Stepsis and Liptak also reported that "the sisters were identified by the black bags they carried, filled with all sorts of food, medicines and tonics for the comfort of the sick" (p. 112).

The present work of the Bon Secours Sisters is identified as encompassing both a "healing and a spiritual ministry." The mission is carried out through "personal and corporate works, and especially through the facilities [the Sisters] operate: hospitals, hospices, long term care and rehabilitation facilities, community medical and wellness centers," among others (O'Sullivan, 1995, p. 1).

Some time elapsed following the founding of the Sisters of Bon Secours, an international community, before the creation of any American communities of women dedicated to nursing the sick. One of the earliest U.S. groups was the community of nursing sisters founded by the daughter of Nathaniel Hawthorne, whose mission was care of the terminally ill.

Servants for Relief of Incurable Cancer

Around the year 1895, the American Roman Catholic Nursing community, the Servants for Relief of Incurable Cancer, was founded in New York by Rose Hawthorne Lathrop (1851–1926). According to the accounts of her life, Rose Hawthorne had both a good friend and an employee who were afflicted by cancer, resulting in painful and prolonged deaths. Following these experiences, Rose determined to study nursing and to commit her life to caring for the victims of cancer who, in her era, were stigmatized outcasts. After a brief period of training, she and another friend, Alice Huber, opened a free house for those with incurable cancer in New York City (Joseph, 1965).

Robinson (1946) reported that "without distinction of race, or creed, or color or sex, there was only one passport to St. Rose's Free Home: poverty with Cancer" (p. 279). Gradually others came to join the two founders of St. Rose's Home, and Rose Hawthorne Lathrop became Mother Alphonsa, superior of a new community to care for those with incurable cancer. As Robinson (1946) observed, "Mother and the Sisters loved [the patients]; they were outcasts of society because of their terrible affliction, but they were honored guests in the home" (p. 280).

An important point about the work of the community, which also reflects the character of Mother Alphonsa, was made by historian Walsh (1929). "Until her death Mother Alphonsa made it a rule to assume her share of the duty of taking personal care of the patients" (p. 272); she also directed her Sisters to always take a "personal share" in the work of caring for the sick.

In a recent newsletter, the community of the Servants for Relief of Incurable Cancer (also referenced to as Hawthorne Dominicans) asserted again that "the congregation has one apostolate: to nurse incurable cancer patients, providing them with a free home" where they can end their days (Dominican Sisters, 1994, p. 1). The Dominican Sisters of Hawthorne currently administer seven free homes in six U.S. states.

Since the community's founding by Rose Hawthorne Lathrop, the Sisters have cared for more than 135,000 men, women, and children suffering from cancer. The community's current mission statement asserts, "Middle-class or poor, black or white, Christian or Jew, each finds a home with us where they can spend their precious final days in dignity. We see in each the image of Christ. We minister to each with the same tender care we give our beloved Savior" (Dominican Sisters, 1994, p. 1).

Nursing communities such as the Hawthorne Dominicans were founded with the purpose of caring for the sick poor in this country. As the U.S. economy stabilized to some degree, other American women interested in nursing as a vocation began to look to the needs of those living in less developed countries. Thus, the U.S. missionary nursing communities were born. One of these groups, whose primary identified ministry focuses on medical and nursing care, is the Medical Mission Sisters.

Medical Mission Sisters

Anna Maria Dengel (1892–1980) began her work with the sick poor in India after completing medical studies in England and Ireland. During her work in Rawalpindi, she realized that she could not accomplish much alone. "What was needed was a religious community of women, dedicated to serving those without access to health care" (Medical Mission Sisters "Celebrating the Gift," 1994, p. 1). Anna came to the United States to seek "recruits," and on September 30, 1925, she officially founded the community of Medical Mission Sisters in Pennsylvania (Medical Mission Sisters "Celebrating the Gift," 1994).

In a pamphlet entitled "Medical Mission Sisters: Committed to Health and Healing" (1994), it is reported, "Medical Mission Sisters have a specific call: to be present to life in the spirit of Jesus the healer" (p. 1). The call is lived out with "the poor, the sick, the neglected, the unjustly treated, and the oppressed" (p. 1).

In a Medical Mission Sisters newsletter, "Sisters in Mission" (1991), the healing ministry of the Sisters is poignantly summarized:

> It is a mission grounded in faith and lived out in love that says so simply, yet so profoundly, that each individual has a right to health and wholeness, that each individual should be cherished and held

dear. It is a mission of being an active presence of "Christ the healer" which all Medical Mission Sisters are privileged to live out. (p. 3)

Medical Mission Sisters currently serve as physicians, nurses, health educators, hospital chaplains, hospice volunteers, and in other health care-related activities. While a community such as the Medical Mission Sisters has many members engaged in professional medical and nursing care, Sisters in other communities provide nursing to the sick poor on a multiplicity of health care levels. One such group is the international community of the Missionaries of Charity.

Missionaries of Charity

One of the more contemporary Roman Catholic communities of religious women who engage in nursing the sick poor today are the Missionaries of Charity, distinguished by their habit, a blue and white Indian sari reflecting the country of their founding.

Mother Teresa of Calcutta, foundress of the Missionaries of Charity, heard a call to work with the poorest of the poor while missioned in India. The community, officially recognized in 1960, has now spread across the world. Although the majority of the Missionaries of Charity are not formally trained nurses, they are identified as a nursing community by nurse historian Josephine Dolan, who observed, "They [Missionaries of Charity] tend to the poor in the streets, in their homes, in the hospices which they have opened to care for children, the destitute, the dying and lepers" (1973, p. 315).

The Missionaries of Charity commit themselves as a community to caring for the poorest of the poor. To that end, a fourth vow is added to the usual three promises of poverty, chastity, and obedience. As Mother Teresa acknowledged, "We have a fourth vow where we profess to offer wholehearted and free service to the poorest of the poor" (Mother Teresa, 1984, p. 74). The Missionaries of Charity began with young women from Calcutta, many of whom had no training in nursing; they were taught, however, to care for the sick with love and compassion. A quotation of Mother Teresa's, which has become well known, reflects her attitude toward the work: "We can do no great things; only small things with great love!" (Mother Teresa, 1983, p. 45). She explained, "The Sisters are doing small things: helping the children, visiting the lonely, the sick, the unwanted. . . . When someone told me that the Sisters had not started any big work, that they were quietly doing small things, I said that even if they helped one person, that was enough. Jesus would have died for one person" (p. 45).

Mother Teresa's commitment to care for Christ in the person of the sick poor is reflected in an excerpt from her daily community prayer:

> Jesus my suffering Lord, grant that today and everyday I may see you in the person of your sick ones, and that in caring for them I may serve you. . . . (1982, p. 7).

Sisters of Life

Finally, a recently established Catholic religious community, the Sisters of Life, have the mission of providing services importantly related to nursing in a variety of areas. The Sisters of Life founded in 1991 by John Cardinal O'Connor, Archbishop of New York, is a contemplative-active community whose ministries include the care of vulnerable pregnant women, the frail elderly, and those who are terminally ill (Catholic News Publishing Co., 1998, p. B-91).

The Sisters' apostolate is focused on protecting and advancing the sacredness of human life, "beginning with the infant in the womb and extending to all those vulnerable to the threat of euthanasia" (Sisters of Life, 1991a, p. 1). The spiritual philosophy of the Sisters of Life is that articulated by John Cardinal O'Connor at the time of the community's founding. "Over the course of hundreds of years, Almighty God has inevitably raised up religious communities to meet the special needs of the day. I am convinced that the crucial need of our day is to restore to all society a sense of the sacredness of human life. Basic to the worst evils of *our* day is surely the widespread contempt for human life. My reading of the 'signs of the times' impels me to believe that the Holy Spirit, 'brooding over the bent world,' wants to inspire a religious community whose charism would be uniquely the protection and enhancement of a sense of the sacredness of human life itself" (1991, p. 1).

As well as the three promises of poverty, chastity, and obedience, the Sisters of Life make an additional vow to support the sacredness of human life. Some of the Sisters' activities include prayer, retreat work, spiritual counseling, and material assistance for those in need. A group of special concern is women facing unexpected pregnancies. The Sisters operate a residence for vulnerable pregnant women, Sacred Heart of Jesus Convent and Home for Mothers. In their apostolate of promoting the sanctity of life, the Sisters also direct the Dr. Joseph R. Stanton Human Life Issues Library and Resource Center.

Ultimately, it is stated in the community's constitutions that the heart of a Sister of Life's vocation is "the call to love as Christ loves" (Sisters of Life,

1991b, p. 4). The Sisters' charism is to understand that all are included in Christ's love and ministry; this concept is lived out through contemplative prayer and apostolic activity. The contemporary founding of a community such as the Sisters of Life lends continuity and credence to the 2,000-year-old message of Jesus that a "cup of cold water" be given in His name to all who thirst, either physically or spiritually.

As American society moves into this time of potential health care reform, the magnificent examples of caring and commitment of pre-Christian and Christian forebears, presented in this chapter, can serve to strengthen the contemporary nurse's sensitivity to the needs of those who are ill, especially the poor and disadvantaged. In such an atmosphere of care for brothers and sisters in need, the spiritual history of the profession will take on new and treasured meaning for those who strive to live a nursing commitment of compassion and love.

REFERENCES

Armstrong, R. J., & Brady, I. C. (1982). *Francis and Clare: The complete works.* New York: Paulist Press.

Austin, A. L. (1957). *History of nursing sourcebook.* New York: C. P. Putnam's Sons.

Baly, M. (Ed.). (1991). *As Miss Nightingale said . . . Florence Nightingale through her sayings—A Victorian perspective.* London: Scutari Press.

Benet, W. R. (Ed.). (1948). *The reader's encyclopedia.* New York: Thomas Y. Crowell.

Bowie, P., & Davies, O. (1992). *Hildegard of Bingen: Mystical writings.* New York: Crossroad.

Bradshaw, A. (1996). The legacy of Nightingale. *Nursing Times, 92*(6), 42–43.

Bullough, V. L., & Bullough, B. (1969). *The emergence of modern nursing* (2nd ed.). New York: Macmillan.

Bullough, V. L., & Bullough, B. (1987). Our roots: What we should know about nursing's Christian pioneers. *Journal of Christian Nursing, 4*(1), 10–14.

Catholic News Publishing Company. (1998). *A guide to religious ministries for Catholic men and women.* New Rochelle, NY: Author.

Daughters of Charity. (1993). *Daughters of Charity Vocation Program* (Video). Emmitsburg, MD: Author.

Daughters of Charity. (1995). *Reflection of the apostolic works of the province.* Emmitsburg, MD: Author.

Daughters of Charity National Health Services (DCNHS). (1994, September). *Audit Services Newsletter, 4.* Washington, DC: Author.

Deloughery, G. L. (1977). *History and trends of professional nursing.* St. Louis, MO: C. V. Mosby.

Dennis, M., Nangle, J., Moe-Lobeda, C., & Taylor, S. (1993). *St. Francis and the foolishness of God.* Maryknoll, NY: Orbis Books.

Dietz, L. D., & Lehozky, A. R. (1967). *History and modern nursing* (2nd ed.). Philadelphia: F. A. Davis.

Dock, L. L., & Stewart, I. M. (1920). *A short history of nursing.* New York: G. P. Putnam's Sons.

Dolan, J. A. (1973). *Nursing in society: A historical perspective.* Philadelphia: W. B. Saunders.

Dolan, J. A., Fitzpatrick, H. L., & Herrmann, E. K. (1983). *Nursing in society: A historical perspective.* Philadelphia: W. B. Saunders.

Dominican Sisters of Hawthorne. (1994, Fall). *Hawthorne happenings*, 1. Hawthorne, NY: Author.

Donahue, M. P. (1985). *Nursing: The finest art, an illustrated history.* St. Louis, MO: C. V. Mosby.

Foster Family Care in Gheel. (1991). *Flanders: The Magazine of the Flemish Community*, No. 9, (pp. 15–17). Antwerp, Belgium.

Fox, M. (1987). *Hildegard of Bingen's book of divine works.* Santa Fe, NM: Bear & Company.

Frank, C. M. (1959). *Foundations of nursing.* Philadelphia: W. B. Saunders.

Goodnow, M. (1916). *Outlines of nursing history.* Philadelphia: W. B. Saunders.

Gorman, M. R. (1917). *The nurse in Greek life.* Unpublished doctoral dissertation. Washington, DC: The Catholic Sisters College of The Catholic University of America.

Green, J. (1987). *God's fool: The life and times of Francis of Assisi.* San Francisco: Harper San Francisco.

Grippando, G. (1986). *Nursing perspectives and issues* (3rd ed.). Albany, NY: Delmar.

Jensen, D. M., Spaulding, J. F., & Cady, E. L. (1959). *History and trends of professional nursing.* St. Louis, MO: C. V. Mosby.

Joseph, Sr. M. (1965). *Out of many hearts: Mother M. Alphonsa Lathrop and her work.* Hawthorne, NY: The Servants for Relief of Incurable Cancer.

Just what is a deaconess? (1994). *Deaconess Beacon: A Student Publication of the Deaconess Program, 8*(2), 3–4. Riverforest, IL: Concordia University. Available at: http://tcmnet.com/ncc/lcms/deaconess/html (1997, July).

Kalisch, P. A., & Kalisch, B. J. (1995). *The advance of American nursing.* Philadelphia: J. B. Lippincott.

Lachman, B. (1993). *The journal of Hildegard of Bingen.* New York: Bell Tower.

Livingstone, E. A. (Ed.). (1990). *The concise Oxford dictionary of the Christian church.* New York: Oxford University Press.

Longfellow, H. W. (1857, November). Santa Filomena. *Atlantic Monthly, 1,* 22–23.

Macrae, J. (1995). Nightingale's spiritual philosophy and its significance for modern nursing. *Image, 27*(1), 8–10.

Maher, P. (2006). Reclaiming spirituality in nursing. In L. Andrist, P. Nicholas, and K. Wolf (Eds.), *A history of nursing ideas* (pp. 417–420). Sudbury, MA: Jones and Bartlett Publishers.

Maloney, R. P. (1992). *The way of Vincent de Paul: A contemporary spirituality in the service of the poor.* New Rochelle, NY: New City Press.

Matheussen, H., Morren, P., & Seyers, J. (1975, January). *The state psychiatric hospital: A center for family care in Gheel.* Gheel, Belgium (paper obtained from the Belgian Embassy, Washington, DC).

Maynard, T. (1948). *Richest of the poor: The life of St. Francis of Assisi.* New York: Doubleday.

Medical Mission Sisters. (1991). *Sisters in Mission, 21*(3). Philadelphia: Author.

Medical Mission Sisters. (1994). *Celebrating the gift of Mother Anna Dengel.* Philadelphia: Author.

Medical Mission Sisters. (1994). *Medical Mission Sisters: Committed to Health and Healing.* Philadelphia: Author.

Mother Teresa. (1982). *The love of Christ: Spiritual counsels.* San Francisco: Harper & Row.

Mother Teresa. (1983). *Life in the spirit: Reflections, meditations, and prayers.* San Francisco: Harper & Row.

Mother Teresa. (1984). *One heart full of love.* Ann Arbor, MI: Servant Publications.

Nutting, M. A., & Dock, L. L. (1935). *A history of nursing* (Vols. 1–2). New York: G. P. Putnam's Sons.

O'Brien, M. E. (2003). Navy nurse: A call to lay down my life. *Journal of Christian Nursing, 20*(4), 32–33.

O'Connor, John Cardinal. (1991). *The way of life.* Unpublished document.

Olson, J. E. (1992). *One ministry many roles: Deacons and deaconesses through the centuries.* St. Louis, MO: Concordia.

O'Sullivan, M. C. (1995). *Sisters of Bon Secours in the U.S., 1881–1991: Caring for God's sake.* Marriottsville, MD: Sisters of Bon Secours, USA.

Pavey, A. E. (1952). *The story of the growth of nursing.* Philadelphia: J. B. Lippincott.

Raymond of Capua. (1853). *Life of St. Catherine of Siena.* (Ladies of the Sacred Heart, Trans.). New York: J. P. Kenedy & Sons.

Robinson, V. (1946). *White caps: The story of nursing.* Philadelphia: J. B. Lippincott.

Sabatier, P. (1894). *Life of St. Francis.* New York: Charles Scribner's and Son.

Selanders, L. C. (1993). *Florence Nightingale: An environmental adaptation theory.* Newburg Park, NY: Sage.

Sellew, G., & Nuesse, C. J. (1946). *A history of nursing.* St. Louis, MO: C. V. Mosby.

Seymer, L. R. (1949). *A general history of nursing.* New York: Macmillan.

Sisters of Bon Secours USA. (1997). *A gift to heal.* Marriottsville, MD: Author.

Sisters of Life. (1991a). *Sisters of life.* New York: Author.

Sisters of Life. (1991b). *Sisters of life.* New York: Author.

Sisters of Mercy of the Americas. (1995). *Mercy health care.* Silver Spring, MD: Author.

Sisters of Mercy of the Americas. (1995). *Sisters of Mercy founded by Catherine McAuley.* Silver Spring, MD: Author.

Stepsis, M., & Liptak, D. A. (1989). *Pioneer healers: The history of women religious in American health care.* New York: Crossroad.

Sullivan, L. (1997). *Vincentian mission in health care.* Emmitsburg, MD: Daughters of Charity National Health System.

Swaffield, L. (1988, September 14). Religious roots. *Nursing Times, 84*(37), 28–30.

Swinburne, A. (1911). *The poems of Algernon Charles Swinburne.* London: Chatto and Windus.

Walsh, J. J. (1929). *The history of nursing.* New York: J. P. Kenedy & Sons.

Widerquist, J. G. (1992). The spirituality of Florence Nightingale. *Nursing Research, 41*(1), 49–55.

Woolsey, A. H. (1950). *A century of nursing.* New York: G. P. Putnam's Sons.

Zetterlund, J. (1997). Kaiserswerth revisited: Putting the care back into health care. *Journal of Christian Nursing, 14*(2), 10–13.

3 ❈ Nursing Assessment of Spiritual Needs

The healer has to keep striving for . . . the space . . . in which healer and patient can reach out to each other as travelers sharing the same broken human condition.

HENRI J. M. NOUWEN, *Reaching Out* (1986, p. 93)

The first step in planning spiritual care for one who is ill is conducting a needs assessment; this may be done formally in the context of nursing research, or informally through interaction with the patient and family. The ill individual's level of spiritual development and religious tradition and practice are important variables to be explored. In this chapter, tools to assess spiritual and religious beliefs and needs are presented; these tools were developed through nursing research with persons living with a variety of illness conditions. Nursing diagnoses related to alterations in spirituality, derived from patient assessment, are examined, and selected nursing studies in which patients' spiritual and religious beliefs and needs were identified are described.

NURSING ASSESSMENT

During the past few decades, nursing assessment of hospitalized patients' problems and needs has become increasingly more sophisticated. Assessment tools vary depending on the care setting, for example, intensive care versus a general care unit; nevertheless, today's nursing assessment instruments are much more detailed than the medical-model-oriented database forms of the past. Although it is admitted that some nurses may feel uncomfortable or unprepared to discuss spiritual or religious topics with patients (Brush & Daly, 2000; Ameling & Povilonis, 2001), a systematic approach to assessing spiritual well-being is recommended (Govier, 2000). In addition to assessing physiological parameters, caregivers also assess psychological and sociological factors that may impact patients' illness conditions. A significant weakness, however, among many contemporary nursing assessment tools is the lack of evaluation of a patient's spiritual needs. Frequently, the spiritual assessment is reflected in a single question asking the religious affiliation of the individual. The assumption is that the patient's spiritual care can then be turned over to a hospital chaplain assigned to minister to persons of that religious tradition.

Although the important role of the hospital chaplain is in no way devalued, the nurse, if he or she is to provide holistic care, should have firsthand knowledge of the spiritual practices and needs of a patient. If no detailed spiritual assessment is carried out, such information, even if revealed during a chaplain's visit, might never be communicated to the nursing staff. A patient may, however, reveal a spiritual problem or concern in some depth to the primary nurse during an assessment at the bedside. In health care facilities with well-functioning departments of spiritual ministry, excellent communication often takes place between pastoral caregivers and nursing staff. This is the ideal. In such situations, chaplains attend nursing care conferences and share in holistic health planning for patients. If the nursing staff has performed a spiritual assessment, this information, combined with the chaplain's insight and advice, can serve to round out the spiritual dimension of the holistic health care plan.

In the contemporary era of home health care, assessment of a patient's spiritual beliefs and needs is also critical to developing a holistic home nursing care plan. Frequently the home care patient experiencing or recuperating from illness is isolated from sources of spiritual support such as attendance at worship services and interaction with other members of a church or faith group. In such a case, the home health care nurse may be able to assist the patient in verbalizing his or her spiritual or religious needs; the nurse can then offer creative strategies for meeting those needs. The nurse may also provide a bridge between the patient and family and their church, recommending counseling from an ordained pastoral caregiver if this seems warranted.

JCAHO MANDATE ON ASSESSMENT OF SPIRITUAL NEEDS

During the past decade, the Joint Commission for Accreditation of Healthcare Organizations (JCAHO) has recognized the importance of spiritual and religious beliefs and traditions for persons who are ill or disabled. This concern is reflected in the JCAHO standards relating to spiritual assessment and spiritual care both for those who are hospitalized (Standard R1.1.3.5) and those living in nursing homes (Standard PE1.1.5.1) (Joint

Commission for Accreditation of Healthcare Organizations, 2003). The JCAHO's standards "reflect the need to recognize and meet the spiritual needs of patients" (Sanders, 2002, p. 107).

The JCAHO Web site suggests that assessment of patients' spiritual needs should be carried out not only to determine religious denomination, but also to identify spiritual and religious beliefs and practices, especially as related to coping with illness or disability. Some questions to be included in a spiritual assessment include: "Who or what provides the patient with strength and hope?"; "Does the patient use prayer in (his/her) life?"; "What type of spiritual/religious support does the patient desire?"; "What does dying mean to the patient?"; "Is there a role of church/synagogue in the patient's life?"; and "How does faith help the patient cope with illness?" (JCAHO, April 17, 2003).

SPIRITUAL DEVELOPMENT

Central to assessing a patient's spirituality is a basic knowledge of the spiritual development of the human person. A number of theories attempt to track spiritual development; significant among these is James Fowler's paradigm set forth in his book *Stages of Faith Development* (1981). Fowler's theory, encompassing seven stages of faith development, emerged from data generated from research with persons across the life span from 3½ to 84 years of age.

Fowler (1981) described faith as "not always religious in its content or context" (p. 4). He explained that faith has to do with one's finding coherence in life, with seeing oneself in relation to others "against a background of shared meaning and purpose" (p. 4). Faith is viewed as deeper and more personal than organized religion, as relating to one's transcendent values and relationship with a higher power, or God. Although Fowler admitted that more research needs to be done, his work demonstrated a preliminary pattern of relationships between the stages of faith development and chronological age. Fowler's seven faith stages and their approximate corresponding age categories are as follows:

> **Undifferentiated Faith** is a "prestage" (infancy) in which the seeds of trust, courage, hope, and love are joined to combat such issues as possible "inconsistency and abandonment in the infant's environment" (p. 121). This faith stage has particular relevance for the maternal–infant nurse concerned with issues of parental–infant bonding.

Intuitive–Projective Faith (3–6 years) is an imitative "fantasy-filled" period in which a young child is strongly influenced by "examples, moods, actions and stories of the visible faith of primarily related adults" (p. 133). Pediatric nurses, especially those working with chronically or terminally ill children, will find guidance for dealing with the child's spiritual and emotional needs from Fowler's conceptualization of this stage.

Mythic–Literal Faith (7–12 years) is described as the time when the child begins to internalize "stories, beliefs and observances that symbolize belonging to his or her own faith community" (p. 149). In working with slightly older pediatric patients, the concept of mythic–literal faith can help the nurse to support the child's participation in rites, rituals, and/or worship services of his or her tradition, which may provide support and comfort in illness.

Synthetic–Conventional Faith (13–20 years) describes the adolescent's experiences outside the family unit: at school, at work, with peers, and from the media and religion. Faith provides a "basis for identity and outlook" (p. 172). Fowler's definition of this faith stage provides an understanding of how the ill adolescent may relate to both internal (family) and external (peer) support and interaction during a crisis situation.

Individuative–Reflective Faith (21–30 years) identifies a period during which the young adult begins to claim a faith identity no longer defined by "the composite of one's roles or meanings to others" (p. 182). This is a time of personal creativity and individualism that has important implications for the nurse, including patient autonomy in planning care for the ill young adult patient.

Conjunctive Faith (31–40 years) is a time of opening to the voices of one's "deeper self" and the development of one's social conscience (p. 198). Nurses caring for patients in this faith stage must be sensitive to the adult's more mature spirituality, especially in relation to finding meaning in his or her illness.

Universalizing Faith (40 years and above) is described by Fowler as a culmination of the work of all of the previous faith stages, a time of relating to the "imperatives of absolute love and justice" toward all humankind (p. 200). Nurses need to be aware that patients may vary significantly in terms of degree of accomplishing the imperatives of this final stage. Assessing approximately where the mature adult patient is, related to such faith, will help in understanding both the patient's response to an illness condition and his or her need for external support in coping with the crisis.

Although a nurse may not be able to identify every patient's stage of faith development chronologically, Fowler's theory with its approximate age-associated categorization does present some guidelines to assist in broadly estimating a patient's level of spiritual development.

NURSING ASSESSMENT OF SPIRITUAL NEEDS

The Spiritual Assessment Scale

In their 1993 fundamentals of nursing text, Taylor, Lillis, and LeMone asserted that assessment of a patient's spirituality should be considered part of any "comprehensive nursing history" because, they reasoned, "a person's spirituality and religious beliefs have the potential to influence every aspect of being" (p. 1173). Although an initial spiritual assessment or history can provide baseline information regarding a patient's spirituality, it is important to remember that spiritual needs may change, or new spiritual concerns may arise during an illness experience. And, because a patient may find it difficult to discuss spiritual problems, the nurse is advised to look for signs of possible spiritual distress such as "sudden changes in spiritual practices [rejection, neglect, fanatical devotion]; mood changes [frequent crying, depression, apathy, anger]; sudden interest in spiritual matters [reading religious books or watching religious programs on television, visits to clergy]; and disturbed sleep" (Taylor, Lillis, & LeMone, 1993, p. 1174).

One set of questions describing a patient's spirituality that may be included as part of a nursing history are those contained in the spiritual history guide developed by Ruth Stoll (1979). The guide is divided into four subsections or "areas of concern": "The person's concept of God or deity; the person's source of strength and hope; the significance of religious practices and rituals to the person; and the person's perceived relationship between his spiritual beliefs and his state of health" (p. 1574). Some more recently developed standardized spiritual assessment tools created by nurses include the Spiritual Perspective Scale, which measures adult spiritual views (Reed, 1991); Kerrigan and Harkulich's Spiritual Assessment Tool, developed to identify the spiritual needs of nursing home residents (1993); and the JAREL Spiritual Well-Being Scale, a tool to assess the spiritual attitudes of older adults (Hungelmann, Kenkel-Rossi, Klassen, & Stollenwerk, 1996); Puchalski's

"Spiritual History," which includes four domains: "Faith, Importance, Community, and Address" (2000, p. 129); the multidimensional "Spiritual Needs Survey," which includes seven major constructs: "belonging, meaning, hope, the sacred, morality, beauty, and acceptance of dying" (Galek, Flannelly, Vane, & Galek, 2005, p. 62); and the spiritual assessment model, including focus on one's "spiritual belief system, personal spirituality, integration/involvement in a spiritual community, ritualized practices and restrictions, implications for care and terminal events planned (advanced directives)" (Dameron, 2005, p. 16).

The author's original standardized instrument to assess adult, cognitively aware individuals' spiritual beliefs and practices, entitled the "Spiritual Assessment Guide," was initially developed and published in 1982 (O'Brien, 1982a, pp. 99–102). The 53-item tool contained six subscales: General Spiritual Beliefs, Personal Spiritual Beliefs, Identification with Institutionalized Religion, Spiritual/Religious Support Systems, Spiritual/ Religious Rituals, and Spiritual Deficit/Distress. Items contained in the instrument were derived from content analysis of qualitative data generated in interviews with 126 chronically ill hemodialysis patients. The patients had been asked to discuss their spiritual beliefs, practices, concerns, and needs in relation to living with a long-term life-threatening illness. It was admitted at the time of construction that this early version of the tool, which contains a mix of both closed- and open-ended questions, was more detailed than appropriate for nursing use in short-term care but could prove valuable in nursing research on the spiritual beliefs and behaviors of the chronically ill patient.

During the past decade, the Spiritual Assessment Guide was revised several times and selected items were used in research with such populations as nursing home residents (O'Brien, 1989), persons living with HIV and AIDS (O'Brien, 1992, 1995; O'Brien & Pheifer, 1993), and the homebound elderly (Brennan, 1994).

The Spiritual Assessment Guide has recently been significantly revised again and retitled the Spiritual Assessment Scale (SAS). The standardized instrument, which measures the construct of Spiritual Well-Being, now contains 21 items organized into three subscales: Personal Faith (PF), seven items; Religious Practice (RP), seven items; and Spiritual Contentment (SC), seven items. In its newly abbreviated form, the SAS, which takes approximately three to four minutes to complete, can be used by practicing nurses in the health care setting, as well as being employed as a research instrument. The tool, as revised, will provide nursing staff and nurse researchers with a broad overview of a patient's personal faith beliefs, the type of spiritual support he or she receives from religious practices, and the type and degree of spiritual contentment/distress the patient is currently experiencing. The 21-item scale is organized with Likert-type scale response categories (SA—Strongly Agree, A—Agree, U—Uncertain, D—Disagree, SD—Strongly Disagree) following each item to facilitate administration; the appropriate categories may be checked by the patient or read aloud and marked by the nurse if a patient is unable to write.*

Validity and Reliability of the SAS

The construct measured by the SAS, Spiritual Well-Being, includes the dimensions of both spirituality and religiousness, or "religiosity," operationally defined in terms of three discrete concepts: Personal Faith, Religious Practice, and Spiritual Contentment.

Spiritual Well-Being

The term *spiritual well-being* is described historically as having emerged following a 1971 White House Conference on Aging. Sociologist of Religion David Moberg (1979) identified spiritual well-being as relating to the "wellness or health of the totality of the inner resources of people, the ultimate concerns around which all other values are focused, the central philosophy of life that guides conduct, and the meaning-giving center of human life which influences all individual and social behavior" (p. 2). The concept of hope is central to a number of definitions of spiritual well-being. In a discussion of holistic nursing care, spiritual well-being is described as "an integrating aspect of human wholeness, characterized by meaning and hope" (Clark, Cross, Deane, & Lowry, 1991, p. 68). Lindberg, Hunter, and Kruszewski (1994) included "the need to feel hopeful about one's destiny" (p. 110) in a litany of patient needs related to spiritual well-being; and Droege (1991), in discussing the "faith factor" in healing, suggested that when an individual does not experience spiritual well-being, serious "spiritual maladies" may occur, such as "depression, loneliness, existential anxiety and meaninglessness" (p. 13).

Most notions of spiritual well-being also contain some reference to philosophy of life and transcendence. Blaikie and Kelson (1979) described spiritual well-being as "that type of existential well being which incorporates some reference to the supernatural, the sacred or the transcendental"

---

*The Spiritual Assessment Scale does assume belief in a Supreme Being, or God.

(p. 137); and Barker observed that spiritual well-being is "to be in communication, in communion with that which goes beyond oneself in order to be whole in oneself" (1979, p. 154). For the Christian, spiritual well-being is identified as "a right relationship of the person to God, and, following that, a right relationship to neighbor and self" (Christy & Lyon, 1979, p. 98).

Spirituality is generally identified as being related to issues of transcendence and ultimate life goals. Nurse theorist Barbara Dossey (1989) explained spirituality as encompassing "values, meanings, and purpose" in life; it includes belief in the existence of a "higher authority"; and it may or may not involve "organized religion" (p. 24). O'Brien (1989), in reporting on research with the chronically ill, suggested spirituality is a broad concept relating to transcendence [God]; to the "non-material forces or elements within man [or woman]; spirituality is that which inspires in one the desire to transcend the realm of the material" (p. 88).

Religiousness, or "religiosity," as it is sometimes identified in the sociological literature, refers to religious affiliation and/or practice. Kaufman (1979) described religiousness as "the degree to which religious beliefs, attitudes and behaviors permeate the life of an individual" (p. 237). In their classic work of 1968, Stark and Glock identified five primary elements of religiousness: belief, religious practice (ritual, devotional), religious experience, religious knowledge, and consequence of religious practice on day-to-day living.

The "spirituality" dimension of spiritual well-being is measured in terms of the concepts of Personal Faith and Spiritual Contentment; the "religiousness" element of the construct is reflected in the concept of Religious Practice.

Personal Faith. Personal faith, as a component concept of the spiritual well-being construct, has been described as "a personal relationship with God on whose strength and sureness one can literally stake one's life" (Fatula, 1993, p. 379). Personal faith is a reflection of an individual's transcendent values and philosophy of life.

Religious Practice. Religious practice is primarily operationalized in terms of religious rituals such as attendance at formal group worship services, private prayer and meditation, reading of spiritual books and articles, and/or the carrying out of such activities as volunteer work or almsgiving.

Spiritual Contentment. Spiritual contentment, the opposite of spiritual distress, is likened to spiritual peace (Johnson, 1992), a concept whose correlates include "living in the now of God's love," "accepting the ultimate strength of God," knowledge that all are "children of God," knowing that

"God is in control," and "finding peace in God's love and forgiveness" (pp. 12–13). When an individual reports minimal to no notable spiritual distress, he or she may be considered to be in a state of "spiritual contentment."

Construct Validity of the SAS

In research with young adults, David Moberg (1979) identified eight corre-lates or characteristics of spiritual well-being: Peace with God (PG), Inner Peace (IP), Faith in Christ (God) (FG), Good Morals (GM), Faith in People (FP), Helping Others (HO), Good Health (GH), and Being Successful (BS) (p. 8). Moberg reported that study participants placed greatest importance on the concepts Peace with God, Inner Peace, and Faith in Christ. The majority of respondents believed that Good Health and Being Successful were not crit-ical elements to spiritual well-being. Those persons, however, who did not seem to possess spiritual well-being were reported as being "more likely to interpret these [health and success] as essential or most likely to be present" with overall spiritual well-being (Moberg, 1979, p. 9).

The SAS, developed to assess spiritual well-being, was constructed to broadly reflect Moberg's eight correlates. In some cases a liberal interpreta-tion of the characteristic was accepted; for example, Faith in Christ is un-derstood also as Faith in God, to include the tradition of the non-Christian believer; Good Health, which Moberg described as physical, may also in-clude good mental health, for the person whose body is suffering the ravages of illness; and Being Successful may relate to an individual's positive feeling about self related to the strength of his or her spiritual beliefs.

The SAS items relate to Moberg's conceptualization of spiritual well-being as follows: Peace with God—item 2; Inner Peace—items 13, 14; Faith in God/Christ—items 1, 3, 5, 6; Good Morals—items 8, 9; Faith in People—items 7 (also GH), 11, 12; Helping Others—item 10; Good Health—item 7 (also FP); Being Successful—item 4.*

Construct validity of the SAS is also derived, in part, from the associa-tion of individual items with James Fowler's conceptualization of the stages of faith development (1981, p. 113), proceeding from the prestage, infancy (Undifferentiated Faith), to the late adult stage (Universalizing Faith):

---

*SAS items 15–21, assessing spiritual contentment/spiritual distress, explore negative *or* lack of negative experiences associated with Moberg's correlates of Inner Peace and Faith in God.

Prestage (trust, courage, hope, and love): items 3, 6

Stage 1 (child learns examples of faith from related adults): items 11, 12

Stage 2 (internalization of stories of one's own faith community): items 1, 4

Stages 3 and 4 (religious faith as a basis for identity and world outlook): items 2, 5

Stage 5 (conjunctive faith): items 7, 13, 14

Stage 6 (universalizing faith; one recognizes imperatives of love and justice toward all humankind): items 8, 9, 10[†]

Content Validity of the SAS

Content validity of the SAS was established through submission of the revised items to a panel of experts in the area of spirituality and health/illness. Following the expert judges' review, certain tool items were modified and/or reworded.

Reliability of the SAS

Reliability of the newly revised 21-item SAS was determined through administration to a sample population of 179 chronically ill persons who agreed to respond to the tool items for the purpose of statistical analysis.

The sample group, employed for the purpose of establishing instrument reliability, consisted of 36 men and 143 women. One hundred thirty-eight members of the group (76 percent) were Roman Catholic; 34 were Protestant; 3 were Jewish; and 4 identified no specific religious belief system. Sixty-three persons attended church services weekly; 26 individuals attended daily church services; and 6 persons reported never going to church or synagogue. The mean age of the sample group was 49 years, with ages ranging from 19 to 89. Seventy-seven persons were single; 79 individuals were married. The participants were well educated, with 70.3 percent reporting some level of college education; the range was from 16.2 percent with two years of college or A.A. degrees to 5 percent who had achieved an M.D. or Ph.D.

[†]SAS items 15–21 assessing *spiritual* contentment/spiritual distress explore negative *or* lack of negative experiences associated with Fowler's stages of faith development; focus is placed especially on internalization of trust and hope (stage 1) and the development of one's personal reflective faith (stage 5).

Selected occupations of the sample group members included physician, nurse, teacher, social worker, secretary, pastoral minister, nursing aide, counselor, engineer, chaplain, and speech pathologist. Some examples of the chronic illnesses reported by the study population, as categorized by body system, included gastrointestinal—ulcer, GERD (gastroesophageal reflux disease), colitis, esophageal cancer, colorectal cancer; genitourinary—ESRD (end-stage renal disease), nephritis, polycystic kidneys; cardiovascular—hypertension, rheumatic heart disease, prolapsed mitral valve, pernicious anemia; respiratory—COPD (chronic obstructive pulmonary disease), asthma, lung cancer, emphysema; neurological—brain cancer, epilepsy; musculoskeletal—osteoarthritis, osteoporosis, arthritis, multiple sclerosis; gynecological—uterine cancer, breast cancer, ovarian tumors, herpes; psychiatric—chronic depression, bipolar disease, transient amnesia, bulimia/anorexia.

Statistical reliability was calculated for a sample of 171 cases (11 cases were deleted because of missing data). Items 15–21, comprising a subscale measuring the degree of spiritual distress, were recoded in the opposite direction to reflect the concept of Spiritual Contentment.

Cronbach's Alpha coefficients for the overall SAS and the subscales Personal Faith (PF), Religious Practice (RP), and Spiritual Contentment (SC) demonstrated statistically significant reliability for the instrument, both in regard to the overall tool and its subscales as examined individually:

Spiritual Assessment Scale (SAS)—21 items
   Alpha coefficient = 0.92

Personal Faith (PF)—7 items
   Alpha coefficient = 0.89

Religious Practice (RP)—7 items
   Alpha coefficient = 0.89

Spiritual Contentment (SC)—7 items
   Alpha coefficient = 0.76

Mean total scale and subscale scores reflected a sample population with a strongly positive sense of spiritual well-being. The overall mean SAS score was 91.7, out of a possible total scale score of 105. The subscales reflected a similar pattern with a PF subscale mean of 32.2 (possible total subscale score of 35); and RP and SC subscale means of 29.7 and 29.6, respectively (possible total scores of 35 for each subscale).

Spiritual Assessment Scale

Instructions: Please check the response category which best identifies your personal belief about the item (response categories: SA—Strongly Agree; A—Agree; U—Uncertain; D—Disagree; SD—Strongly Disagree).

A. Personal Faith

1. There is a Supreme Being, or God, who created humankind and who cares for all creatures.
   SA _____ A _____ U _____ D _____ SD _____
2. I am at peace with God.
   SA _____ A _____ U _____ D _____ SD _____
3. I feel confident that God is watching over me.
   SA _____ A _____ U _____ D _____ SD _____
4. I receive strength and comfort from my spiritual beliefs.
   SA _____ A _____ U _____ D _____ SD _____
5. I believe that God is interested in all the activities of my life.
   SA _____ A _____ U _____ D _____ SD _____
6. I trust that God will take care of the future.
   SA _____ A _____ U _____ D _____ SD _____
7. My spiritual beliefs support a positive image of myself and of others, as members of God's family.
   SA _____ A _____ U _____ D _____ SD _____

B. Religious Practice

8. Belonging to a church or faith group is an important part of my life.
   SA _____ A _____ U _____ D _____ SD _____
9. I am strengthened by participation in religious worship services.
   SA _____ A _____ U _____ D _____ SD _____
10. I find satisfaction in religiously motivated activities other than attending worship services, for example, volunteer work or being kind to others.
    SA _____ A _____ U _____ D _____ SD _____
11. I am supported by relationships with friends or family members who share my religious beliefs.
    SA _____ A _____ U _____ D _____ SD _____
12. I receive comfort and support from a spiritual companion, for example, a pastoral caregiver or friend.
    SA _____ A _____ U _____ D _____ SD _____
13. My relationship with God is strengthened by personal prayer.
    SA _____ A _____ U _____ D _____ SD _____

14. I am helped to communicate with God by reading or thinking about religious or spiritual things.

    SA _____ A _____ U _____ D _____ SD _____

C. Spiritual Contentment

15. I experience pain associated with my spiritual beliefs.

    SA _____ A _____ U _____ D _____ SD _____

16. I feel "far away" from God.

    SA _____ A _____ U _____ D _____ SD _____

17. I am afraid that God might not take care of my needs.

    SA _____ A _____ U _____ D _____ SD _____

18. I have done some things for which I fear God may not forgive me.

    SA _____ A _____ U _____ D _____ SD _____

19. I get angry at God for allowing "bad things" to happen to me, or to people I care about.

    SA _____ A _____ U _____ D _____ SD _____

20. I feel that I have lost God's love.

    SA _____ A _____ U _____ D _____ SD _____

21. I believe that there is no hope of obtaining God's love.

    SA _____ A _____ U _____ D _____ SD _____

NURSING DIAGNOSES: ALTERATIONS IN SPIRITUAL INTEGRITY

Nursing diagnoses are currently used in a number of health care facilities to label those patient conditions whose treatment falls within the purview of the nurse. From early in the nursing diagnosis movement, spiritual issues have been addressed with such diagnoses as "alterations in faith" (Gebbie, 1976; Gebbie & Lavin, 1975) and "nursing diagnoses related to spiritual distress" (Campbell, 1978). This concern for the identification of patients' spiritual needs and deficits has continued among contemporary theorists of nursing diagnosis. The nursing diagnosis "high risk for spiritual distress related to confrontation with the unknown" was described by Holloway in 1993. Two other diagnoses related to faith beliefs, "potential for spiritual well-being" and "spiritual distress," were identified in 1994 by the North American Nursing Diagnosis Association (Brennan, 1994, p. 852). The potential for spiritual well-being is associated with "the process of an individual's developing an un-folding of mystery through harmonious interconnections that spring from inner strength"; "spiritual distress is a disruption of the life principle that per-vades a person's entire being and that integrates and transcends one's bio-logical and physiological nature" (Brennan, 1994, p. 852). A recently advanced nursing diagnosis for human response in the domain of spirituality is that of "enhanced spirituality" (Cavendish et al., 2000).

As contemporary nurses become more involved with diagnosis and intervention in the spiritual arena, some basic knowledge of the beliefs and behaviors associated with the major religious cultures is essential (Engebretson, 1996). This information will allow nurses to accurately identify and address significant spiritual needs and problems exhibited or reported by their patients.

Seven nursing diagnoses related to "alterations in spiritual integrity," which were identified from the author's research (1982a) on spirituality and life-threatening illness, include:

> "**Spiritual Pain**, as evidenced by expressions of discomfort or suffering relative to one's relationship with God; verbalization of feelings of having a void or lack of spiritual fulfillment, and/or a lack of peace in terms of one's relationship to one's creator" (O'Brien, 1982a, p. 106). A terminally ill patient, experiencing such "spiritual pain," may verbalize a fear that he or she has not lived "according to God's will"; this concern is exacerbated as the possibility of imminent death approaches.

> "**Spiritual Alienation**, as evidenced by expressions of loneliness, or the feeling that God seems very far away and remote from one's everyday life; verbalization that one has to depend upon oneself in times of trial or need; and/or a negative attitude toward receiving any comfort or help from God" (O'Brien, 1982a, p. 106). Often, a chronically ill person expresses frustration in terms of closeness to God during sickness; the comment may be heard: "Where is God when I need Him most?"

> "**Spiritual Anxiety**, as evidenced by an expression of fear of God's wrath and punishment; fear that God might not take care of one, either immediately or in the future; and/or worry that God is displeased with one's behavior" (O'Brien, 1982a, p. 106). Some cultural groups entertain a concept, although not held by all members of the culture, that illness may be a "punishment" from God for real or imagined faults or failures.

> "**Spiritual Guilt**, as evidenced by expressions suggesting that one has failed to do the things which he or she should have done in life, and/or done things which were not pleasing to God; articulation of

concerns about the 'kind' of life one has lived" (O'Brien, 1982a, p. 106). Certain individuals, especially those schooled in more fundamentalist religious traditions, experience "guilt" related to their perceived failure to follow God's will, as they understand it. This "guilt" frequently is exacerbated during times of physical or psychological illness.

"**Spiritual Anger**, as evidenced by expressions of frustration, anguish or outrage at God for having allowed illness or other trials; comments about the 'unfairness' of God; and/or negative remarks about institutionalized religion and its ministers or spiritual caregivers" (O'Brien, 1982a, p. 107). Family members of those who are ill may express anger at God for allowing a loved one to suffer.

"**Spiritual Loss**, as evidenced by expression of feelings of having temporarily lost or terminated the love of God; fear that one's relationship with God has been threatened; and/or a feeling of emptiness with regard to spiritual things" (O'Brien, 1982a, p. 107). A sense of "spiritual loss" may frequently be associated with psychological depression; for an individual who feels useless and powerless, there may also be a resultant feeling of alienation from anything or any person perceived as good, such as God.

"**Spiritual Despair**, as evidenced by expressions suggesting that there is no hope of ever having a relationship with God, or of pleasing Him; and/or a feeling that God no longer can or does care for one" (O'Brien, 1982a, p. 107). Although spiritual despair is generally rare among believers, such a diagnosis may be associated with serious psychiatric disorders. If such thoughts or feeling are expressed by a patient, the nurse needs to be alerted, also, to the potential for suicidal ideation or possible behavior.

Of the seven nursing diagnoses related to alterations in spiritual integrity, the one that occurred most pervasively in patient data was that of spiritual pain (O'Brien, 1982a, p. 104).

A STUDY OF SPIRITUAL PAIN

Spiritual pain, or pain of the soul, is a concept that has been, and continues to be, discussed at length in the spiritual and theological literature. From the classic work of John of the Cross, *Dark Night of the Soul*, to contemporary writers, spiritual pain has been identified, described, and analyzed. Michael Kearney (1990) suggested that spiritual pain can be "recognized by the questions the patient is asking, and in the feelings he is experiencing and expressing,"—questions such as "why me," and feelings "such as hopelessness, despair, fear, and guilt" (p. 50). Kearney observed, "after meeting an individual in spiritual pain I find that terms like 'suffering,' 'anguish' or 'deep restlessness' most aptly describe the experience" (p. 50). In discussing the spiritual needs of hospice patients, Lamont Satterly observed that "in addition to physical, social and psychological pain, religious or spiritual pain can add to the struggles of many patients" (2001, p. 30). Satterly explained, "Religious pain is rooted in guilt leading towards punishment and experienced as fear. . . . Spiritual pain is rooted in shame leading a patient to abandon hope in God's love" (p. 30).

In seeking to identify spiritual pain, however, one must also attempt to distinguish the concept from psychological or emotional pain. Following the general theses that pain may be described as an individual's personal perception of hurt, or that pain is "what the patient says it is" (McCaffrey, 1972; Sternback, 1968), an empirical exploration of the understanding of spiritual pain was undertaken. The author asked a group of nurses, pastoral caregivers, and patients to describe, in their own words, what spiritual pain meant to them. Some of the responses follow.

> **Spiritual Pain:** is thinking about failing God, who loves you so much, by selfishness and sinfulness; it occurs whenever one sees evil in the world; I experience spiritual pain when I am not able to say what I have to say; perhaps spiritual pain is the same as psychological pain in all ways except the source; I equate it with loving deeply; spiritual pain can occur when a person has fallen away from his religion and is not reconciled with God; it is experienced by a person who is denied the blessings of his church; I feel it when I think about my faults and failings before God; it's a feeling of loss, a void; spiritual pain is a separation from God; it is suffering that results from a lack of spiritual fulfillment; spiritual pain is an internal aching due to a disquieted self, an unsettled self; it's having an ideal, someone you look up to who doesn't live up to your expectations; it's a sense of discomfort or unease that is very deep within oneself related to one's relationship to God or to others in a spiritual sense; spiritual pain is a loneliness of spirit, a loneliness for God; it is when one's sense of self as a person, that part of the person that is spirit, is violated. (O'Brien, 1982a, pp. 104–105)

Six dominant themes emerged from content analysis of the above comments and those of a number of other patients and health and spiritual caregivers:

> Spiritual pain is the loss of or separation from God and/or institutionalized religion; the experience of evil or disillusionment; a sense of failing God; the recognition of one's own sinfulness; lack of reconciliation with God; and/or a perceived loneliness of spirit. (O'Brien, 1982a, p. 105)

Ultimately, spiritual pain was defined as

> An individual's perception of hurt or suffering associated with that part of his or her person that seeks to transcend the realm of the material; it is manifested by a deep sense of hurt stemming from feelings of loss or separation from one's God or deity, a sense of personal inadequacy or sinfulness before God and man; or a pervasive condition of loneliness of spirit. (O'Brien, 1982a, p. 105)

SPIRITUALITY AND NURSING RESEARCH

Although clinical nursing research efforts in the area of spirituality and nursing practice have not been extensive, some nurse investigators have addressed the spiritual needs of particular patient groups. Examples include Soeken and Carson (1987), "Responding to the Spiritual Needs of the Chronically Ill"; Clifford and Gruca (1987), "Facilitating Spiritual Care in the Rehabilitation Setting"; Reed (1991), "Preferences for Spiritually Related Nursing Interventions among Terminally Ill and Non-terminally Ill Hospitalized Adults and Well Adults"; Toth (1992), "Faith in Recovery: Spiritual Support after an Acute M.I."; Highfield (1992), "Spiritual Health of Oncology Patients"; Mickley, Soeken, and Belcher (1992), "Spiritual Well-Being, Religiousness, and Hope among Women with Breast Cancer"; Harris et al. (1995), "The Role of Religion in Heart-Transplant Recipients' Long-Term Health and Well-Being"; Smith (1995), "Power and Spirituality in Polio Survivors: A Study Based on Roger's Science"; Twibell, Wieseke, Marine, and Schoger (1996), "Spiritual and Coping Needs of Critically Ill Patients: Validation of Nursing Diagnoses"; and Post-White et al. (1996), "Hope, Spirituality, Sense of Coherence, and Quality of Life in Patients with Cancer."

Nursing studies, especially those in the arena of chronic illness, have frequently included the concepts of spirituality, religion, and/or religiosity (religious practice) as key variables in a larger matrix. Some examples include the author's research with chronic renal failure patients, migrant farmworkers, nursing home residents, and persons living with HIV infection and AIDS. One other study consisted of a qualitative exploration of the spiritual care attitudes and experiences of contemporary nurses. Brief examples of the methods and findings, as well as the spirituality instruments used in these studies, are described here; more detailed qualitative data elicited in the research are included in later chapters to illustrate instances of spiritual need and spiritual care. The methodology and findings of a recent study of the spiritual needs of three groups of older adults—active elders living with chronic illness, homebound elders, and nursing home residents—are presented in chapter 9.

Study Title: Religious Faith and Adaptation to Maintenance Hemodialysis

The purpose of this study was to examine the relationship between religious faith and adaptation to chronic renal failure (CRF) and its treatment regimen of maintenance hemodialysis. The religious faith question represented one variable in a multivariate study of adaptation to renal disease and dialysis. The study subjects consisted of 126 adult hemodialysis patients who were interviewed first to obtain baseline data and again in a three-year follow-up, when 63 of the original sample were identified. Among the initial population, 87 were Protestant, 25 were Catholics, and 8 were Jewish; 6 persons reported no religious affiliation. At the time of the follow-up interviews, 50 patients were Protestant, 10 were Catholic, 3 were Jewish, and none reported having no religious affiliation. Data were collected by means of both quantitative and qualitative interviews. Selected findings describe the patients' perception of the importance of religious faith in coping with renal failure and dialysis.

Quantitative Data Reflecting CRF Patients' Perceptions of the Import of Religious Faith

At initial interview, 33 hemodialysis patients reported that religious beliefs were "never" relevant in relation to coping with chronic renal failure, 27 responded that religion was "sometimes" important, 31 stated "usually," and 35 patients asserted that their religious faith was "always" a mediating factor in adapting to renal failure and hemodialysis. In fact, then, 93 renal dialysis patients, or 73.8 percent of the original population, believed that their religious beliefs were supportive of adaptation to their disease and to the hemodialysis regimen; data obtained at follow-up interviews demonstrated a similar pattern (O'Brien, 1982c, p. 75).

Qualitative Data Reflecting CRF Patients' Perceptions of the Import of Religious Faith

One hemodialysis patient asserted that he had "found the Lord" through his illness. He reported that during three cardiac arrests and numerous surgeries, he had prayed and noted, "Each time I knew everything would be alright because I asked God to carry me through; I know that He's got His arms around me." A dialysis patient who had stated at his initial interview that "the church didn't help" and "religion does not influence me," explained three years later, "without religion I would have no faith in dialysis or the people working with me; I'm just beginning to accept religion." A third patient, whose response to the question of the import of religious faith at the first interview was a blunt "none," later stated, "Oh, yes. A lot of people couldn't have gone through what I went through without faith in God." A chronic renal patient who had been undergoing hemodialysis for almost six years joyfully asserted, "I have grown a lot closer to God, through this experience with renal failure" (O'Brien, 1982c, p. 76).

Research Instruments

Within the context of a standardized interview schedule exploring adaptation to renal failure and dialysis, two quantitative items elicited data on religious affiliation (i.e., Protestant, Catholic, Jewish, Muslim, other, or none) and religiosity (i.e., frequency of attendance at church or religious worship services of one's tradition). The patients' perception of the importance of religious faith in adjusting specifically to renal failure and to the hemodialysis treatment regimen were evaluated by two additional measures. The first was a quantitative item that stated, "Religious faith is important in helping me adjust to renal failure and dialysis," with response choices of Always, Usually, Sometimes, or Never. The second item consisted of a qualitative, open-ended question, "Could you describe the importance of religious faith in helping you adjust to renal failure and hemodialysis"; the patient's response to this item was "probed" by the interviewer to expand the qualitative data on religious faith and chronic renal failure.

Study Title: Spirituality and Health Beliefs and Practices of Migrant Farmworkers

The research consisted of an exploratory descriptive qualitative study of the overall health attitudes and behaviors of a sample group of Mexican American migrant farmworkers. Central to the study was an examination of the spirituality and religious beliefs of the population, as related to health/illness beliefs and practices. The methods of data collection were observation and focused interview. During the three-month data collection phase of the study, the investigator attended many of the group's religious services and rituals, including weekly Spanish Masses, evening Mass in migrant camps, Baptisms, First Communion services, a Mass of departure as the migrants moved from one work setting to another, and a "coming of age" religious service for a teenage girl. The author visited several Mexican American religious shrines and interviewed three practitioners of folk religion/medicine. Focused interviews were also conducted with 125 adult migrant workers in three midwestern states.

Selected Findings

The population studied was close to 98 percent Roman Catholic in terms of identified religious affiliation; many of the group's Catholic religious beliefs and practices, however, were culturally modified according to ethnic tradition. For example, some migrants admitted to belief in more than one Virgin Mary: La Virgin de Guadalupe, La Virgin de San Juan de Los Lagos, and others, whom they considered as cousins. The Christ Child was venerated by many as Santo Niño de Atocha, a religious personage of Spanish descent first identified by the Atocha Indians in Mexico. Both the Virgins and Santo Niño were important religious persons to whom one prayed in times of illness or injury. The Mexican American migrants' Catholicism was also often juxtaposed with a multiplicity of folk religious/health care beliefs and practices that were part of a family's cultural tradition. Thus, a patient, while adhering to prescriptions of the Catholic faith, might also support such folk beliefs as the existence of *susto* or *espanto*, that is, fear or anxiety; *castiga*, illness viewed as a punishment from God; or *mal de ojo*, the evil eye as a cause of illness. These conditions were thought not to respond to usual religious prayer or medical intervention, but fell within the purview of the traditional folk healer, or *curandera*, who could prescribe magical religious remedies to heal the patient. The three curanderas interviewed all reported that they believed their power to heal was a gift from God; thus, a strong link was observed between religion and medicine in the migrant's folk tradition. The association was also found between health/illness and religion, in relation to the group's Roman Catholic tradition. Personal faith in Jesus Christ, as central to one's life and health, was identified among most migrants. Pilgrimages to shrines of Our Lady, where candles were lighted to ask for healing, were important in times of injury or sickness; and medals and holy pictures were carried to alleviate or ward off illness (O'Brien, 1982b, 1991).

Research Instrument

An overall Observation/Interview Guide related to health beliefs and practices of Mexican American migrant farmworkers was developed; within this tool, a subset of items was created to focus discussions on the relationship between religion and spirituality, and health.

Religion and Spirituality Interview Guide

1. Do you believe in God, or a Supreme Being, who cares for you in times of health and sickness? Please explain.
2. Can you tell me about your church or religious denomination? How often do you attend worship services?
3. How helpful is your church or church members in times of sickness?
4. How often do you pray to Jesus or to God about your or your family's health or illness? Please explain.
5. Do you ever read about religious things that help you in times of illness? If so, what does that mean to you?
6. What kinds of religious practices do you use if you get sick, or to keep good health (for example, religious pictures, religious medals, visiting religious shrines, lighting religious candles, singing or listening to religious music)?
7. Do your family members and friends have similar religious beliefs and practices as you do, especially in regard to health and sickness?
8. Do you have a priest or minister who supports you and your family when you are ill?
9. Do you ever feel hurt or pain related to your religious beliefs and practices? Please explain.

Study Title: Spiritual Beliefs and Behaviors of the Institutionalized Elderly

The purpose of this exploratory case study, conducted over a two-year period, was to examine and describe the overall institutional nursing home setting, as well as the patterns of attitude and behavior exhibited by the residents, family members, medical and nursing caregivers, and ancillary staff. A key variable of interest was spirituality, or the spiritual perceptions, attitudes, behaviors, and needs of the residents. The nursing home studied was a 230-bed residential facility that provided three levels of care: skilled, semiskilled, and domiciliary. The author collected data by means of direct and participant observation, as well as through focused interviews with staff, family members, and 71 alert and cognitively aware residents (62 women and 9 men). Variables of particular interest related to the spiritual/religious attitudes, experiences, and practices of the residents. Selected data on religion and spirituality are presented as excerpted from verbatim interview transcripts.

The Residents

Female resident, 90 years old, said, "My belief in God means everything to me. It is so lovely to have the chapel in this building. We don't have to go outside in any weather. We have Mass in the chapel. During Lent now we have the Rosary and then we have Benediction. So the day goes along very well. I have an awful lot to be thankful to God for." Female resident, 82 years old, said, "The hereafter is pleasant to think about. I have been brought up a Christian, and my belief is a great support to me now." Female resident, 88 years old, said, "I don't like to sound 'preachy,' but the ability to have that chapel and go to daily Mass after you have worked in the world for 52 years like I did, and didn't have time, except to rush to Mass on Sunday, then you appreciate the chapel" (O'Brien, 1989, p. 47).

The Nursing Staff

A head nurse in the nursing home observed, "I don't think I ever realized the importance of religion until I came here. . . . The patients seem to have the feeling that God is going to take care of them. . . . They feel at peace" (O'Brien, 1989, p. 109).

Research Instruments

A subsection of the Nursing Home Residents Discussion Guide was labeled "Religion and Spirituality"; one item relating to spirituality was included also in both the Family Interview Guide and the Nursing Home Environment Observation Guide. Examples of discussion items include:

1. What are the resident's religious beliefs and behaviors?
2. In what way are the resident's spiritual faith interests supported?
3. What Church provides religious support to the resident?
4. Can the resident select his or her own pastoral caregiver?
5. How important is religion and/or personal faith in the resident's life? What religious practices does the resident engage in?

Study Title: Religious Faith and Living with HIV Infection

Personal faith beliefs, as well as the support of an individual's church group or religious denomination, were examined in a study of Coping Response in HIV Infection. The overall aim of the longitudinal project was to establish a database of physical, psychosocial, and spiritual needs associated with HIV infection, from which appropriate caregiving strategies could be derived. The study population consisted initially of 133 men and 3 women, all of whom were categorized within the CDC IV classification: "Constitutional Disease, Secondary Infections, Secondary Cancers, or Other Conditions Related to HIV Infection." A number had diagnoses of AIDS. A subgroup of 41 men with HIV/AIDS was followed over a five-year period, as long-term survivors of the infection. Data were collected by both quantitative (interview schedule) and qualitative (tape-recorded focused interview) measures. Data on the relationship of religion and spirituality revealed the importance of personal faith beliefs and church affiliation in coping with HIV (O'Brien, 1992, 1995).

Demographic Profile: Religious Affiliation

Data on both current religious affiliation and religious heritage for the original population of 133 men revealed a significant number of study participants (31, or 23 percent) who did not identify membership in any religious denomination; of that subgroup, however, 22 percent admitted having a religious heritage. For the remainder of the group, 26 were Roman Catholic, 64 were Protestant, and 2 were Jewish; 10 persons categorized religious beliefs as "personal faith." Of the 41 long-term survivors of HIV, 4 percent fewer individuals reported having no specific religious affiliation when compared with the larger study group.

Religious Faith and Coping with the HIV Diagnosis

Selected comments from HIV-positive study participants in the early phase of the research revealed the importance of religion and personal faith in coping with the HIV diagnosis.

Peter—at the time, a 27-year-old, eight-year survivor of HIV—described his personal faith:

> I don't think I'm living in a fantasy world. I don't think I have rose-colored glasses on. I may get sick. I may die from AIDS, and even still, I'm not worried about it. Even in death I know that there's a life

after and I believe that I will be in Heaven or whatever it is God in-
tends for me. (O'Brien, 1992, p. 46)

Alain, a 30-year-old who was a five-year survivor of HIV, explained how
his beliefs had changed since his diagnosis:

I was not prepared for the news that I was HIV-positive. And, I felt
very small and scared and alone. And I didn't have much use for
churches, but I looked up to help me find that greater something to
help me and to carry me through. You know, the "Footprints in the
Sand" thing. And I found faith. (O'Brien, 1992, p. 47)

Religious Faith and Long-Term Survival with HIV

Comments of long-term survivors of the HIV diagnosis reflect the importance of faith beliefs in coping with their condition over time.

Sean, who had been HIV-positive for more than five years, reminisced
about his early days with the diagnosis and described the support of his faith:

Well, when I found out that I was HIV-positive, I did really get angry
at God. I got very angry and I distinctly remember praying. I mean
falling down on my knees at the foot of my bed and praying out loud,
crying out for this to be lifted from me. I prayed my way through it
with God. (O'Brien, 1995, p. 140)

Jon Michael, now HIV-positive for more than six years, spoke about
how spirituality supported his survival with the virus:

Christ is my role model, and even if I stray, I have that constant with
which I credit my life. . . . I say my prayers every day, every night. It
is very much a part of my life. That's the strength of my making it so
long with this disease. (O'Brien, 1995, p. 137)

Research Instrument

The following nine-item instrument was developed to guide interviews on the
relationship between religion/spirituality and coping with HIV infection.

HIV Infection Interview Guide: Religion and Spirituality

1. Do you believe in God or a Supreme Being; if so, could you tell me
   about that?

2. In what way do you picture God as involved with your day-to-day activities in coping with HIV?
3. How does your church or religious group provide support in your coping with HIV?
4. What do worship services or other religious practices mean in your life since the HIV diagnosis?
5. In what ways does prayer play a part in your coping with HIV?
6. How much support do you receive in dealing with your diagnosis from a pastoral caregiver (e.g., priest, minister, rabbi, or other)?
7. Do family and friends support your faith beliefs? If so, does their spirituality help or strengthen you in coping with HIV?
8. Do you ever experience spiritual pain or distress associated with your faith or religion vis-à-vis your HIV diagnosis?
9. What role does your personal faith play in helping you cope with your HIV diagnosis?

Study Title: Spirituality and Nursing Practice

The concept of spirituality as related to nursing practice—that is, the nurse–patient relationship—was examined in a qualitative exploratory descriptive study of 66 nurse administrators, educators, researchers, and practitioners. An overview of the method and findings, the latter summarized in a construct labeled "The Nurse: The Anonymous Minister," is presented in chapter 4. To direct the open-ended interviews, a focused interview guide was developed; the tool contains 12 items related to spirituality and the practice of nursing.

Research Instrument

Spirituality and Nursing Interview Guide

1. Would you briefly describe your personal spiritual beliefs; that is, do you believe in a "higher power" or Supreme Being whom many call "God"? If so, how does your relationship with God support your nursing activities?
2. How does your religious affiliation or tradition impact your nursing activities?
3. How does your personal faith help you cope with the stresses of nursing (e.g., questions related to the "why" of suffering)?
4. How does your church or religious community support your nursing activities?

5. Do you engage in any "religious rituals" that support your nursing activities, for example, attendance at church services, retreats, spiritual reading, meditation, prayer, or others? Please explain.

6. Describe some instance(s) of providing spiritual care for patients, for example, praying with a patient (and/or family), praying for a patient (and/or family), reading to a patient (Scripture or some other spiritual reading), listening to a patient talk about his or her pain, being with a dying patient (and/or family), or any other activity(ies) you consider to fall within the realm of spiritual care.

7. Do you ever use touch in providing spiritual care to patients, either formally in the "laying on of hands" (healing touch) or informally, such as a caring touch to indicate empathy and concern? Please describe.

8. Do you feel that patients seek spiritual care from nurses? If so, how is the desire usually manifested?

9. Would you comment on use of the nursing diagnosis, alteration in spiritual integrity?

10. Do you ever discuss patients' spiritual needs/care with nursing colleagues, physicians, or pastoral care staff? Please explain.

11. Did you experience much emphasis on spiritual care for patients and families in your own nursing education, either in basic nursing curricula or through ongoing continuing education? Please explain.

12. Is there anything else you would like to share related to your perceptions or experiences with spirituality and nursing practice?

Although not all nurses may or must feel comfortable in providing spiritual care, the assessment of a patient's spiritual needs is a professional responsibility. Contemporary holistic health care mandates attention to the problems and concerns of the spirit as well as to those of the body and mind. In carrying out an assessment of the patient's spiritual well-being, a nurse may glean information important to supporting the medical and nursing therapies planned for the ill person. Following a spiritual assessment, appropriate spiritual or religious interventions may be provided either by the nurse or through referral to a designated pastoral caregiver.

REFERENCES

Ameling, A. & Povilonis, M. (2001). Spirituality, meaning, mental health and nursing. *Journal of Psychosocial Nursing & Mental Health Services, 39*(4), 15–20.

Barker, E. (1979). Whose service is perfect freedom. In D. O. Moberg (Ed.), *Spiritual well-being: Sociological perspectives* (pp. 153–171). Washington, DC: University of America Press.

Blaikie, N. W., & Kelson, G. P. (1979). Locating self and giving meaning to existence. In D. O. Moberg (Ed.), *Spiritual well-being: Sociological perspectives* (pp. 133–151). Washington, DC: University of America Press.

Brennan, M. R. (1994). *Spirituality in the homebound elderly.* Doctoral dissertation, The Catholic University of America. Ann Arbor, MI: UMI.

Brush, B. L. & Daly, P. R. (2000). Assessing spirituality in primary care practice: Is there time? *Clinical Excellence for Nurse Practitioners, 4*(2), 67–71.

Campbell, C. (1978). *Nursing diagnosis and intervention in nursing practice.* New York: Wiley.

Cavendish, R., Luise, B. K., Horne, K., Bauer, M., Medefindt, J., Gallo, M. A., Calvino, C., & Kutza, T. (2000). Opportunities for enhanced spirituality relevant to well adults. *Nursing Diagnosis, 11*(4), 151–163.

Christy, R. D., & Lyon, D. (1979). Sociological perspectives on personhood. In D. O. Moberg (Ed.), *Spiritual well-being: Sociological perspectives* (pp. 91–98). Washington, DC: University of America Press.

Clark, C. C., Cross, J. R., Deane, D. M., & Lowry, L. W. (1991). Spirituality: Integral to quality care. *Holistic Nursing Process, 3*(1), 67–76.

Clifford, M., & Gruca, J. (1987). Facilitating spiritual care in the rehabilitation setting. *Rehabilitation Nursing, 12*(6), 331–333.

Dameron, C. (2005). Spiritual assessment made easy . . . with acronyms. *Journal of Christian Nursing, 22*(1), 14–15.

Dossey, B. M. (1989). The transpersonal self and states of consciousness. In B. M. Dossey, L. Keegan, L. G. Kolkmeier, & C. E. Guzzetta (Eds.), *Holistic health promotion* (pp. 23–35). Rockville, MD: Aspen.

Droege, T. (1991). *The faith factor in healing.* Philadelphia: Trinity Press International.

Engebretson, J. (1996). Considerations in diagnosing in the spiritual domain. *Nursing Diagnosis, 7*(3), 100–107.

Fatula, M. A. (1993). Faith. In M. Downey (Ed.), *The new dictionary of Catholic spirituality* (pp. 379–390). Collegeville, MN: The Liturgical Press.

Fowler, J. W. (1981). *Stages of faith development.* New York: HarperCollins.

Galek, K., Flannelly, K., Vane, A., & Galek, R. (2005). Assessing a patient's spiritual needs: A comprehensive instrument. *Holistic Nursing Practice, 19*(2), 62–69.

Gebbie, K. M. (1976). *Summary of the second national conference, classification of nursing diagnoses.* St. Louis, MO: C. V. Mosby.

Gebbie, K. M., & Lavin, M. A. (1975). *Classification of nursing diagnoses, proceeds of the first national conference.* St. Louis, MO: C. V. Mosby.

Govier, I. (2000). Spiritual care in nursing: A systematic approach. *Nursing Standard, 14*(17), 32–36.

Harris, R. C., Dew, M. A., Lee, A., Amaya, M., Bushes, L., Rettz, D., & Coleman, G. (1995). The role of religion in heart-transplant recipients' long-term health and well-being. *Journal of Religion and Health, 34*(1), 17–32.

Highfield, M. (1992). Spiritual health of oncology patients. *Cancer Nursing, 15*(1), 1–8.

Holloway, N. M. (1993). *Medical surgical care planning* (2nd ed.). Springhouse, PA: Springhouse Corporation.

Hungelmann, J., Kenkel-Rossi, E., Klassen, L., & Stollenwerk, R. (1996). Focus on spiritual well-being: Harmonious interconnectedness of mind-body-spirit—Use of the JAREL spiritual well-being scale. *Geriatric Nursing, 17*(6), 262–266.

Johnson, R. P. (1992). *Body, mind, spirit: Trapping the healing power within you.* Liguori, MO: Liguori.

Joint Commission for Accreditation of Healthcare Organizations (2003). Spiritual assessment. www.jcaho.org/accredited+organizations/hospitals/standards/hospital+faqs/assessment. 4/17/2003.

Joint Commission for Accreditation of Healthcare Organizations (2003). *Comprehensive accreditation annual for hospitals: The official handbook.* Oakbrook Terrace, IL: JCAHO.

Kaufman, J. H. (1979). Social correlates of spiritual maturity among North American Mennonites. In D. O. Moberg (Ed.), *Spiritual well-being: Sociological perspectives* (pp. 237–254). Washington, DC: University of America Press.

Kearney, M. (1990). Spiritual pain. *The Way, 30*(1), 47–54.

Kerrigan, R., & Harkulich, J. T. (1993). A spiritual tool. *Health Progress, 74*(5), 46–49.

Lindberg, J. B., Hunter, M. L., & Kruszewski, A. Z. (1994). *Introduction to nursing: Concepts, issues and opportunities.* Philadelphia: J. B. Lippincott.

McCaffrey, M. (1972). *Nursing management of the patient with pain.* Philadelphia: J. B. Lippincott.

Mickley, J., Soeken, K., & Belcher, A. (1992). Spiritual well-being, religiousness and hope among women with breast cancer. *Image, 24*(4), 267–272.

Moberg, D. O. (1979). The development of social indicators of spiritual well-being and quality of life. In D. O. Moberg (Ed.), *Spiritual well-being: Sociological perspectives* (pp. 1–13). Washington, DC: University of America Press.

North American Nursing Diagnosis Association (NANDA). (1994). *NANDA, nursing diagnoses: Definitions and classification, 1995–1996.* Philadelphia: Author.

Nouwen, H. J. M. (1986). *Reaching out.* New York: Doubleday.

O'Brien, M. E. (1982a). The need for spiritual integrity. In H. Yura & M. Walsh (Eds.), *Human needs and the nursing process* (Vol. 2, pp. 82–115). Norwalk, CT: Appleton Century Crofts.

O'Brien, M. E. (1982b, April). Pragmatic survivalism: Behavior patterns affecting low level wellness among minority group members. *Advances in Nursing Science, 4*(3), 13–26.

O'Brien, M. E. (1982c). Religious faith and adjustment to long-term hemodialysis. *Journal of Religion and Health, 21*(1), 68–80.

O'Brien, M. E. (1983). *The courage to survive: The life career of the chronic dialysis patient.* New York: Grune & Stratton.

O'Brien, M. E. (1989). *Anatomy of a nursing home: A new view of resident life.* Owings Mills, MD: National Health Publishing.

O'Brien, M. E. (1991). Reaching the migrant worker. In B. W. Spradley (Ed.), *Readings in community health nursing* (pp. 564–568). Philadelphia: J. B. Lippincott.

O'Brien, M. E. (1992). *Living with HIV: Experiment in courage.* Westport, CT: Auburn House.

O'Brien, M. E. (1995). *The AIDS challenge: Breaking through the boundaries.* Westport, CT: Auburn House.

O'Brien, M. E., & Pheifer, W. G. (1993). Nursing care of persons infected with HIV. In M. Maas, K. Buckwalter, & M. Titler (Eds.), *Nursing clinics of North America, 23*(2), 303–315.

Post-White, J., Ceronsky, C., Kreitzer, M. J., Nickelson, K., Drew, D., Mackey, K. W., Koopmeiners, L., & Gutknecht, S. (1996). Hope, spirituality, sense of coherence, and quality of life in patients with cancer. *Oncology Nursing Forum, 23*(10), 1571–1579.

Puchalski, C. (2000). Taking a spiritual history allows clinicians to understand patients more fully. *Journal of Palliative Medicine, 3*(1), 129–137.

Reed, P. G. (1991). Preferences for spiritually-related nursing interventions among terminally ill and non-terminally ill hospitalized adults and well adults. *Applied Nursing Research, 4*(3), 122–128.

Sanders, C. (2002). Challenges for spiritual care-giving in the millennium. *Contemporary Nurse, 12*(2), 107.

Satterly, L. (2001). Guilt, shame and religious and spiritual pain. *Holistic Nursing Practice, 15*(2), 30–39.

Smith, D. W. (1995). Power and spirituality in polio survivors: A study based on Roger's science. *Nursing Science Quarterly, 8*(3), 133–139.

Soeken, K., & Carson, V. B. (1987). Responding to the spiritual needs of the chronically ill. *Nursing Clinics of North America, 22*(3), 603–611.

Stark, R., & Glock, C. (1968). *American piety: The nature of religious commitment.* Berkeley, CA: University of California Press.

Sternback, R. A. (1968). *Pain: A psychophysiological analysis.* New York: Academic.

Stoll, R. I. (1979). Guidelines for spiritual assessment. *American Journal of Nursing, 79*(9), 1574–1577.

Taylor, C., Lillis, C., & LeMone, P. (1993). *Fundamentals of nursing: The art and science of nursing care* (2nd ed., pp. 1163–1186). Philadelphia: J. B. Lippincott.

Toth, J. C. (1992). Faith in recovery: Spiritual support after an acute M.I. *Journal of Christian Nursing, 9*(4), 28–31.

Twibell, R. S., Wieseke, A. W., Marine, M., & Schoger, J. (1996). Spiritual and coping needs of critically ill patients: Validation of nursing diagnoses. *Dimensions of Critical Care Nursing, 15*(5), 245–253.

4 ✦ A Middle-Range Theory of Spiritual Well-Being in Illness

For everything there is a season, and a time for every matter under heaven:
a time to be born and a time to die; a time to plant and a time to pluck up
what is planted.

ECCLESIASTES 3:1

N
ursing theorists, as the author of the Book of Ecclesiastes, recognize that in their world of caring for the sick there is indeed "a time to be born and a time to die"; a time for planting and a time to harvest what has been planted. They know that in their patients' lives there is "a time for every matter under heaven." Thus, the early "grand theorists" of nursing developed conceptual schemas that attempted to address, in some way, all of a patient's possible "seasons" of life.

More recently, however, nurse metatheorists, also sensitive to the varied and unique seasons of patients' lives, have encouraged the development of theories of the middle range. That is, those theories that address specific health- and illness-related phenomena of concern to practicing nurses.

To respond to the call for such theories, a middle-range theory of *spiritual well-being in illness* was developed based on the author's many years of clinical nursing research with persons experiencing chronic and life-threatening illnesses.*

A BRIEF HISTORY OF THEORY DEVELOPMENT IN NURSING

During the decades of the 1970s and 1980s, especially, both academicians and practicing nurses began to incorporate theories of nursing into their research and practice. The majority of these early nursing models fell into the

*Major sections of this chapter have been taken from Chapter 5, "Conceptual Models of Parish Nursing Practice: A Middle-Range Theory of Spiritual Well-Being in Illness" in *Parish Nursing: Healthcare Ministry Within the Church*, 2003, Jones and Bartlett Publishers. Used with permission of the publisher.

category of "grand theories" of nursing, or those conceptual frameworks that attempted to present a way of describing and understanding the overall discipline of professional nursing practice. Each model contained some exploration of the concepts: person, health, nursing, and environment. There were a number of nursing theory conferences organized to analyze and discuss the logical adequacy and practicality of these theories for use in research and practice. The meetings often included presentations by key nursing theorists of the day, such as Dorothea Orem, Callista Roy, Martha Rogers, and Betty Neuman. Some of the most frequently cited conceptual frameworks were Orem's self-care model for nursing, the Roy adaptation model, the Neuman systems model, and Rogers' model of unitary person. Despite focus on the work of the theorists of the late 20th century, as contemporaries of that era, most nurse metatheorists, however, acknowledged and still acknowledge Florence Nightingale as the first nursing theorist; this accolade is based on Nightingale's exploration and understanding of the need for a framework for nursing practice as described in her 1859 book *Notes on Nursing.*

While some nurse researchers have attempted to use grand theories of nursing to undergird their studies, the breadth of these models makes such efforts difficult. Usually, the grand theory is dissected by an investigator, a portion of the model being employed to provide the framework for research. While the grand theories of nursing provide valuable parameters to delineate and explain the practice of professional nursing, metatheorists have called for and continue to advocate the development of middle-range nursing theories, or those theories that strive to explain more discrete phenomena of interest to practicing nurses.

Distinct from the grand theories of nursing, which attempt to incorporate myriad concepts representing a broad range of phenomena within the discipline, a number of middle-range theories have begun to emerge in the professional literature. Some of these include frameworks dealing with such issues as pain control, chronic sorrow, end of life, uncertainty of the illness experience, and skill acquisition. The concept of "middle-range theory" was introduced in the sociological literature by Robert Merton in 1957 (p. 9); midrange theories were viewed as bodies of knowledge that would encompass a more limited number of variables than grand theories and could be empirically tested. Middle-range nursing theories cluster "around a concept of interest" (Chinn & Kramer, 1995, p. 40), such as those identified previously. They are also described as "theories that focus on specific nursing phenomena that reflect clinical practice" (Meleis, 1997, p. 18); "not covering the full range of phenomena that are of concern within the discipline" (Chinn & Jacobs, 1987, p. 205); sharing "some of the conceptual economy of grand theories but also [providing] the specificity needed for usefulness in research and practice" (Walker & Avant, 1995, p. 11); and "made up of a limited number of concepts and propositions that are written at a relatively concrete . . . level" (Fawcett, 1992, p. 5). As middle-range theories address a specific phenomenon, their goal is thus to "describe, explain or predict phenomena" (Fawcett, 1992, p. 5). In sum, middle-range theories fall somewhere between the more abstract or grand theories/conceptual models and circumscribed practice theories.

A MIDDLE-RANGE THEORY OF SPIRITUAL WELL-BEING IN ILLNESS

A middle-range theory of spiritual well-being in illness can be useful in orienting the practice of any nurse carrying out holistic health care, which includes attention to the needs of body, mind, and spirit. Such a theoretical orientation is especially important for nurses caring for those experiencing long-term chronic illness, life-threatening and terminal illness, as well as any illness or injury that affects an individual's personal and/or professional life goals. In such cases, patients frequently struggle mightily to find some reason that can help them find meaning in the illness or disability. Regardless of religious affiliation or its lack, individuals coping with life-altering conditions generally strive to make some sense of the state in which they find themselves. Or, this seeming impossible, most patients try to achieve a sense of acceptance, and even peace, in the midst of their suffering.

A middle-range theory of spiritual well-being in illness can help both nurse practitioners and nurse researchers working with seriously ill persons to assess and evaluate their patients' spiritual needs and, if warranted, to institute appropriate spiritual care interventions.

DEVELOPMENT OF THE THEORY OF SPIRITUAL WELL-BEING IN ILLNESS

The nursing literature suggests that "middle-range theories generally emerge from combining research and practice, and building on the work of others" (McEwen, 2002, p. 207). The latter point is validated by nurse theorists who assert that middle-range theories may be derived or deduced from grand theories or conceptual frameworks (Ruland & Moore, 1998, p. 170) or from established clinical guidelines (Good, 1998, p. 120). The midrange nursing theory of spiritual well-being in illness was derived from earlier conceptualizations in the area of spiritual well-being and also from the nursing model conceived by Joyce Travelbee, in which a central focus of the framework is the concept of finding meaning in an illness experience.

The core component of the nursing theory of spiritual well-being in illness is the concept of finding *spiritual* meaning in the experience of illness. While Travelbee (1971) indeed introduced the importance of spiritual concerns—"the spiritual values a person holds will determine to a great extent his [sic] perception of illness" (p. 16)—she never explicitly described the concept of "spiritual well-being" in her model. Rather, Travelbee developed an interactional framework based on "human-to-human," nurse–patient relationships, viewing the nurse's role as assisting "the ill patient to experience hope as a means of coping with illness and suffering" (Chinn & Kramer, 1995, p. 176); illness was envisioned as a "spiritual, emotional and physical" experience that might be defined both "subjectively and objectively" (Chinn & Jacobs, 1987, p. 188).

For Travelbee, one's definitions of illness and suffering depended very much on "the symbolic meaning attached to these concepts by the individual" (Thibodeau, 1983, p. 90); she further postulated that "a person's attitude toward suffering ultimately determines how effectively he [sic] copes with illness" (Meleis, 1997, p. 361). Finally, Joyce Travelbee (1971) taught that "the professional nurse practitioner must be prepared to assist individuals and families not just to cope with illness and suffering but to find meaning in these experiences" (p. 13). "This is the difficult task of professional nursing," she admitted, (but) "it must not be evaded" (p. 13).

Joyce Travelbee, a psychiatric nurse practitioner and educator, died at age 47 just as she was beginning doctoral study; thus, we do not know how she might have expanded her beginning conceptual model for nursing practice. Travelbee has been described as a deeply spiritual woman, whose human-to-human vision of nursing practice was importantly influenced by her early educational experience at Charity Hospital in New Orleans, by the work of the great psychotherapist Viktor Frankl, and by the writings of nurse theorist Ida Orlando. Although Joyce Travelbee did not live to further explain and validate her interaction model, her groundbreaking work on the concept of a sick person finding meaning in the experiences of illness and suffering provides a solid and scholarly basis for the development of a midrange-level theory exploring and describing the spiritual meaning of illness and suffering: a nursing theory of spiritual well-being in illness.

As noted, the middle-range theory of spiritual well-being in illness was also inductively derived and concretized through a number of nursing studies exploring the importance of spiritual well-being in coping with chronic illness and disability. Overwhelmingly positive associations, both quantitatively and qualitatively, were found between spiritual well-being and quality of life. That is, those persons who reported a higher degree of personal faith, spiritual contentment, and religious practice were much more positive about and satisfied with other aspects of their lives and had greater hope for the future, despite sometimes painful and debilitating illnesses. Several case examples are those of Mr. Jones, a 62-year-old Methodist parishioner who was suffering from leukemia; Mrs. Manley, an 82-year-old Lutheran parishioner with a multiplicity of disease conditions, including osteoporosis, congestive heart failure, and diabetes; and 75-year-old Mrs. McDermott, a Roman Catholic parishioner who was disabled with rheumatoid arthritis, among other diagnoses. In completing the Spiritual Assessment Scale (chapter 3), which measures spiritual well-being, all three scored very positively on the items measuring faith, religious practice, and spiritual contentment or lack of spiritual distress. Similarly, all three study participants were most positive in their responses related to quality of life: hope for the future, for example, being positive about life, being able to get through difficulties, and feeling loved; and life satisfaction, for example, agreeing that they are "just as happy as when younger" (O'Brien, 2001). In looking back, they agreed they were "fairly well satisfied" with their lives (O'Brien, 2001).

Philosophy and Key Concepts

Every theory must have a philosophical basis undergirding the concepts and relationships articulated in the framework. The middle-range theory of spiritual well-being in illness is grounded in the belief that the human person, as well as being possessed of a physical and psychosocial nature, is also a spiritual being capable of transcending and/or accepting such experiences as pain and suffering in the light of his or her higher nature. Over and over, clinical nurses have witnessed ill or disabled patients rise above constraining physical or psychosocial deficits to live extraordinarily positive and productive lives. This ability to accept, and in some cases even embrace, illness and suffering is primarily a function of the patients' personal spiritual resources. It is for the purpose of identifying, supporting, and strengthening the influence of these spiritual resources, in relation to sickness or disability, that the nursing theory of spiritual well-being in illness has been developed.

The key concept of the middle-range theory of spiritual well-being in illness is, of course, that of spiritual well-being itself. In the conceptual model (Figure 4.1), an ill individual is presented as having the ability to find spiritual meaning in the experience of illness, which can ultimately lead to an outcome of spiritual well-being for the sick person. The capacity to find spiritual

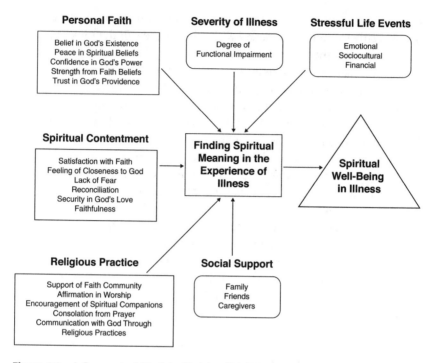

Figure 4.1   A Conceptual Model of Spiritual Well-Being in Illness

meaning in an occasion of illness or suffering is influenced by a number of factors. First and foremost, an individual's perception of the spiritual meaning of an illness experience is influenced by personal spiritual and religious attitudes and behaviors. These attitudes and behaviors include variables related to *personal faith*: belief in God, peace in spiritual and religious beliefs, confidence in God's power, strength received from personal faith beliefs, and trust in God's providence; *spiritual contentment*: satisfaction with faith, feeling of closeness to God, lack of fear, reconciliation, security in God's love, and faithfulness; and *religious practice*: support of a faith community, affirmation in worship, encouragement of spiritual companions, consolation from prayer, and communication with God through religious practices.

The impact of these spiritual and religious attitudes and behaviors on one's finding spiritual meaning in illness may also be mediated by such potentially intervening variables as *severity of illness*: degree of functional impairment; *social support*: support of family, friends, and/or caregivers; and current *stressful life events*: emotional, sociocultural, and/or financial.

The first step in developing a middle-range theory is to conduct an analysis of the core concepts in the model. Nurse metatheorists Walker and

Avant (1995) identify a series of "steps" to be included in a "concept analysis," which include (among others) determining the "aims of the analysis," identifying "uses of the concept," and "defin[ing] empirical referents" (p. 39). The aim of exploring the concept of spiritual well-being is to identify and describe its meaning in terms of contemporary usage, especially in relation to experiences of illness and suffering. The usage and empirical referents of the concept have been examined from the extant literature as well as nursing practice and nursing research. The concept of spiritual well-being was explored in both the nursing and sociological literature in the process of developing the earlier referenced Spiritual Assessment Scale (SAS) (see chapter 3).

Based on prior nursing practice and nursing research, I envision the concept of spiritual well-being as consisting of two dimensions: that of spirituality or one's personal relationship with God or the Transcendent; and religiosity or religiousness, reflecting an individual's practice of his or her faith beliefs (this dimension of spiritual well-being may or may not involve participation in an organized religious tradition). Thus, empirical referents of spiritual well-being are conceptualized in terms of *personal faith* and *spiritual contentment* (spirituality) and *religious practice* (religiosity or religiousness).

The definitions of the three empirical referents of spiritual well-being are also included in chapter 3.

Theory Synthesis

Theory synthesis is defined as "a strategy aimed at constructing theory, an interrelated system of ideas, from empirical evidence" (Walker & Avant, 1995, p. 155). In theory synthesis "a theorist pulls together available information about a phenomenon. Concepts and statements are organized into a network or whole, a synthesized theory" (Walker & Avant, 1995, p. 155). In the preceding discussion, a diagrammatic model of the theory of spiritual well-being in illness is presented (Figure 4.1) to identify the relationships between key concepts and potentially mediating variables relevant to the framework. A sick or disabled individual's ability to find spiritual meaning in an experience of illness or suffering is perceived as being influenced by his or her spiritual and religious attitudes, beliefs, and practices, including those reflecting the concepts of *personal faith, spiritual contentment,* and *religious practice.*

An ill person's personal faith—not only whether or not he or she believes in the existence of God, but also his or her trust in the power and the goodness of God's care, sense of peacefulness about these beliefs, and courage and strength derived from them—is critical to whether the individual will be able to identify and/or accept an illness experience as having a spiritual dimension. If one believes in God, yet does not truly trust in or feel at peace in accepting His loving providence, an illness experience may be considered an unwarranted and unfair burden at best, or a punishment for some perceived past indiscretion at worst. In terms of the concept of *spiritual contentment*, an ill person may indeed *believe* in God's existence, His power, His care for all of humankind, and yet not personally feel close to the Lord; his or her faith may be based on a relationship that incorporates fear of God's judgment rather than security in His love. In such a situation, again, it may be very difficult for the individual to perceive an experience of illness or suffering as anything more than a possible retaliation or punishment for past sins.

While *religious practice*, in the formal sense of attending church services, may not be necessary for one to find a spiritual meaning in illness or disability, coping with illness can be greatly facilitated if a sick person has the support of such devotions as prayer or spiritual reading. The encouragement of a faith community with whom one may occasionally share worship or whose members pray for sick parishioners during communal worship services and/or the guidance of a pastor or spiritual companion can also be very comforting spiritual supports in times of illness and suffering.

A practicing nurse can provide important nursing intervention in helping an ill patient who may be struggling with a number of spiritual issues. Very often, as will be seen in the many empirical examples presented throughout this book, nurses facilitate either the enhancement of, or in some cases the return to, religious practices that may have waned or even been abandoned by a patient during the onset of an illness experience.

Also, as demonstrated in the diagrammatic model presented in Figure 4.1, there are a number of potentially confounding variables that may interfere with a sick person's ability to achieve a sense of spiritual well-being in his or her illness. A nurse may have the opportunity to intervene in relation to a number of these factors hindering the ability to find meaning in the illness experience. For example, a nurse may be able to serve as a referral agent assisting sick persons in finding some relief for a functional impairment. For instance, if an ill individual is hard of hearing, the nurse may recommend audiology testing if this has not been done and/or may assist the individual in obtaining a hearing aid if necessary.

A nurse may also serve as a "bridge" facilitating communication with family and friends if these relationships have become strained due to illness or disability. Finally, through the various roles of educator, referral agent, counselor, and patient advocate, the nurse may have the opportunity to guide, advise, teach, or support an ill patient in regard to a variety of emotional, sociocultural, and even financial concerns that may interfere with the individual achieving a sense of spiritual well-being in the illness experience.

Hypotheses Derived from the Theory

Based on the middle-range theory of spiritual well-being in illness, as described, several hypotheses might be derived related to the association between spiritual well-being and quality of life for those dealing with illness and/or disability. First, it can be proposed that there will be a significant relationship between the degree of a sick person's personal faith and his or her perceived quality of life in an illness experience. Second, there will be a significant relationship between the activity of a sick person's religious practice and his or her perceived quality of life in an illness experience. Third, there will be a significant relationship between the degree of a sick person's feeling of spiritual contentment and his or her perceived quality of life in an illness experience. An overall hypothesis might be stated as follows: there will be a significant relationship between spiritual well-being (personal faith, spiritual contentment, and religious practice) and quality of life among sick persons experiencing illness or disability, controlling for the variables of severity of illness, social support, and stressful life events.

Empirical Testing

As presented in chapter 11, testing of the preceding relationships has already begun. Empirical findings support both the subhypotheses and the overall hypothesis, correlating spiritual well-being (as a total concept and in its subcomponents: personal faith, spiritual contentment, and religious practice) with quality of life. The research was conducted among chronically ill adults at the end of life experiencing myriad illness conditions; study participants belonged to a variety of religious traditions and faith communities. It is anticipated that future nursing studies might be carried out with other patient populations experiencing both similar and different illness conditions and disabilities. Such research would greatly assist in validating the importance of the nursing role of spiritual caregiving; positive findings would strengthen and potentially expand the spiritual care role of the nurse while also supporting the health care dimension of the nursing ministry.

It is suggested that, as in the studies presented in this book, nursing research to test the middle-range theory of spiritual well-being in illness

employ methodological triangulation; that is, the collecting of both quantitative and qualitative data to explore the relationship of spiritual well-being
to coping with illness and disability. While the quantitative data would provide a strong statistical basis for the relationship, the qualitative data elicited
in focused conversational interviews with ill persons could provide the detailed narrative examples from which guidelines for the nurse's role of integrator of faith and health could be further expanded and clarified.

REFERENCES

Chinn, P. L., & Jacobs, M. K. (1987). *Theory and nursing: A systematic approach* (2nd ed.). St. Louis, MO: C. V. Mosby.

Chinn, P. L., & Kramer, M. K. (1995). *Theory and nursing: A systematic approach* (4th ed.). St. Louis, MO: C. V. Mosby.

Fawcett, J. (1992). *The relationship of theory and research* (3rd ed.). Philadelphia: F. A. Davis.

Good, M. (1998). A middle-range theory of acute pain management: Use in re-search. *Nursing Outlook, 46*(3), 120–124.

McEwen, M. (2002). Middle-range nursing theories. In M. McEwen & E. M. Wills (Eds.), *Theoretical basis for nursing* (pp. 202–225). Philadelphia: Lippincott, Williams & Wilkins.

Meleis, A. I. (1997). *Theoretical nursing: Development and progress* (3rd ed.). Philadelphia: Lippincott.

O'Brien, M. E. (2001). *Spiritual well-being in chronic illness.* Unpublished study report, Catholic University of America, Washington, DC.

O'Brien, M. E. (2003). *Parish nursing: Healthcare ministry within the church.* Sudbury, MA: Jones and Bartlett.

Ruland, C. M., & Moore, S. M. (1998). Theory construction based on standards of care: A proposed theory of the peaceful end of life. *Nursing Outlook, 46*(4), 169–175.

Thibodeau, J. A. (1983). *Nursing models: Analysis and evaluation.* Monterey, CA: Wadsworth Health Sciences Division.

Travelbee, J. (1971). *Interpersonal aspects of nursing.* Philadelphia: F. A. Davis.

Walker, L. O., & Avant, K. C. (1995). *Strategies for theory construction in nursing* (3rd ed.). Norwalk, CT: Appleton & Lange.

5 ✸ The Nurse–Patient Relationship: A Sacred Covenant

I have made a Covenant with my Chosen One.

PSALM 89, Verse 3

For centuries, the nurse–patient relationship has been unique and individualized. Both patient and nurse bring into the partnership a multiplicity of personal life variables, including such factors as demographics (age, gender, marital status, ethnicity, religion, and socioeconomic status), family history, illness experience, and spiritual orientation. All of the characteristics associated with these variables may affect how the nurse–patient relationship is played out during the course of an interaction. The research data in this chapter poignantly describe the covenantal spiritual dimension of the nurse–patient relationship as identified by a cadre of contemporary nurses. The nurses' own words are employed to label concepts in a paradigm of interaction that reveals the nurse as an *anonymous minister*. In this ministerial role the nurse enters into a sacred covenant of caring for the sick.

THE NURSE–PATIENT COVENANT

One critical and constant dimension of the nurse–patient relationship relates to the degree of trust engendered between the interacting parties. The element of trust is lived out in most nurse–patient partnerships in terms of a covenant relationship. Although not always formally articulated as such, the presence of an understood covenant between a patient and nurse not only supports the concept of trust between the partners, but also sets up parameters for appropriate *role* behaviors and attitudes. This covenant can be viewed as sacred given the nature of the intimacy, indeed the holiness, of the nurse–patient relationship, as demonstrated in this chapter. Examining the term *covenant* from a spiritual/theological perspective also supports an understanding of the concept of nursing practice as involving a sacred covenant.

The word *covenant* is derived "from the Hebrew word *berith*, which means 'a binding agreement or pact' " (Senior, 1993, p. 237). The concept of covenant is "one of the Bible's most pervasive means of describing the relationship between God and the community of faith" (Senior, 1993, p. 237). Examples of covenant abound in the Scriptures, beginning with God's covenant with Abraham in the Old Testament (Genesis 12:1–3). In the Old Testament theology, Yahweh's covenant with Israel "established bonds of loyalty and responsibility between God and humanity" (Boadt, 1984, p. 547). The New Testament covenant relates to Jesus Christ, as the "Son of David and fulfillment of the Messianic prophecies," as depicted in Luke 22:20 (Nowell, 1990, p. 245). Livingstone (1990) observed that in New Testament theology the "life and death of Christ is the perfect covenant between God and man," man's imperfect "righteousness" becoming perfected through the divine grace of the Incarnation (pp. 133–134). The concepts of contract and covenant are differentiated, a contract being viewed as an agreement that may cease if one partner fails to keep the commitment. A covenant, however, as envisioned by Henri Nouwen (1991), underlies the spiritual care relationship, "In the covenant there is no condition put on faithfulness. It is the unconditional commitment to be of service" (p. 56).

Many of the covenant-related concepts cited from the theological and pastoral literature have relevance for the nurse–patient relationship:

> **Bonds of Loyalty and Responsibility**—the nurse's commitment to employ all of his or her knowledge and skill to provide the best possible care for the patient; and, in turn, the patient's responsibility to comply, to the best of his or her ability, with the prescribed treatment regimen.
>
> **Mutual Obligations**—the mutual obligations, on the part of both patient and nurse, to respect and seek to understand the other's attitudes and role behaviors in the context of the nurse–patient relationship.
>
> **No Conditions Put on Faithfulness**—the nurse will not cease to care lovingly for the patient, regardless of attitudes such as apathy, anger, or even outright noncompliance on the part of a patient.
>
> **Not Expecting a Return for Good Services**—the degree of the nurse's care and compassion cannot be predicated on the patient's, or fam-

ily's, gratitude; for physical or emotional reasons, or perhaps both, such thanks may not always be demonstrated.

Isaiah 49:15 provides a moving example of God's covenantal constancy. "Can a mother forget her infant, be without tenderness for the child of her womb, even should she forget, I will never forget you."

Thus, for the nurse called to a ministry of service, whether in nursing practice, nursing education, nursing administration, or nursing research, the theological concept of covenant serves to teach, guide, strengthen, and inspire. The concept of the personal covenantal relationship of God to His people provides a powerful model for the caring and supportive nurse–patient relationships that reflect the art as well as the science of nursing.

SPIRITUALITY AND THE NURSE

In discussing nurses' spiritual needs, Philip Burnard (1988) posed a number of questions that may help a nursing practitioner explore his or her own spirituality in relation to caregiving. These questions focus on such topics as understanding the term *spiritual*, religious education, the importance of spirituality to the nurse, feelings about spiritual beliefs different from one's own, the potential for changing personal spiritual beliefs, feelings regarding talking about spiritual beliefs with other nurses, and the perception of how one's own spiritual beliefs affect patient care (p. 36). For seasoned nurses, these questions may have been well explored in the course of their own faith development; for the newer clinician, exploring spiritual beliefs can be a valuable and growth-producing faith experience. Ultimately, responses to Burnard's questions may have an important impact on the nurse–patient covenantal relationship.

Although the author's interviews with practicing nurses described in the following pages did address the nurses' own spiritual needs, only a modest amount of data was elicited on the topic. Nurses who participated in the study were clearly more interested in talking about the spiritual concerns and needs of their patients, how they had attempted to meet these, and how they might better practice spiritual care in the future. Nursing has historically been a discipline of service to others; the concern with one's personal well-being, spiritual or otherwise, was secondary to meeting the needs of the ill. The study nurses who did speak about their own spirituality, however, described the importance of such religious activities as prayer and Scripture reading in providing support for their practice.

Ellie, a pediatric oncology nurse practitioner who had worked with terminally ill children for more than 15 years, explained the significance of her personal spirituality:

> In this job, in this work I do with little ones, some of them are so, so sick. It hurts a lot to watch them get sicker and sicker; they are so brave, some of them. And the parents! It can get to you. Some days you just want to run away and say "no more!" I can't keep doing this job. You want to forget that babies are dying. . . . I truly do believe it's my faith in God, in the Lord Jesus, that holds me up. I try to pray every morning while I'm getting myself together for work. And when I can steal a few minutes I read some Scripture or something like Henri Nouwen; I love his books. And my church, they're a big, big support. I guess I could say that it is the spiritual that keeps me in oncology nursing.

THE NURSE: THE ANONYMOUS MINISTER

In addition to the nurse's personal spirituality, a number of other factors are relevant to the spiritual dimension of nurse–patient interactions, including the nurse's comfort level in discussing spiritual issues with patients; the degree of spiritual support provided in the care setting, i.e., support for both patients' and caregivers' spiritual needs; and the emphasis or lack of emphasis on providing spiritual care to patients in the course of professional nursing education. In order to explore, empirically, these questions and issues regarding spirituality and the covenantal nurse–patient relationship, the author conducted focused interviews with 66 contemporary nurses employed in two East Coast metropolitan areas, soliciting individual experiences, attitudes, and behaviors regarding the relationship between spirituality and nursing practice. The nursing cadre was purposely chosen to include a broad range of experience and education. The 6 men and 60 women comprising the population of nurses reported the following religious affiliations: 39 Roman Catholics; 25 Protestants (4 Baptists, 3 born-again Christians, 2 Methodists, 2 Episcopalians, 2 Presbyterians, 1 Lutheran, 1 "Christian," and 10 persons who described themselves broadly as "Protestant"); one Jewish nurse; and one nurse who reported having no religious affiliation.

Two members of the group were licensed practical nurses, five were diploma registered nurses, and one had an associate in arts nursing degree. Eleven individuals had baccalaureate degrees in nursing, 25 had masters in nursing degrees, 14 had doctorates in nursing science, and 8 were registered nurses with doctorates in the biological or behavioral sciences.

The largest subgroup of 38 nurses identified a history of 16 to 25 years of nursing experience; 19 had been nurses for 26 to 40 years; and only 9 had practiced nursing for less than 15 years. Thirty-three percent of the group described their specialty area as medical–surgical nursing. Seven nurses worked in the area of psychiatric–mental health, and seven worked in pediatrics. Five critical care nurses and five cardiovascular nurses were included in the group; there was one oncology nurse, as well as three hospice and five gerontological nurses. Three nurses worked in the area of maternal–child health, and two each represented the areas of community health, emergency room, and operating room nursing. Three of the study nurses worked with the mentally retarded/developmentally disabled, and three worked in home health care nursing; one of the latter group of nurses was primarily involved with the health care of homeless persons.

Sixteen of the study nurses were employed at military health care facilities; 10 were faculty members in schools of nursing. Ten nurses were employed by medical centers, 7 by research institutions, 12 by private religiously affiliated hospitals, 3 by hospice facilities, 7 by city-run health care facilities, and 1 nurse worked for an HMO. More than half of the group were identified as working in the area of nursing practice; 10 were nurse educators, 10 were nurse administrators, and 4 were employed as nurse researchers.

Interviews with the nursing group explored experiences and attitudes associated with nursing and spirituality, focusing on such topics as nurse–patient interactions related to patients' spiritual needs and/or spiritual care, the nurse's personal spirituality and/or spiritual needs, spiritual support provided in the health care setting, and the inclusion or lack of inclusion of spiritual concepts in the nurse's educational program. Discussions were tape-recorded to preserve the nurses' attitudes, perceptions, and experiences in their own words. Confidentiality was assured to the nurses participating in the interviews; wherever naming is warranted, pseudonyms are used. (The Spirituality and Nursing Interview Guide employed to focus discussions with nurse respondents is presented in chapter 3.)

Tape-recorded interviews were transcribed and content analyzed to identify dominant themes related to nursing and spirituality. A multiplicity of concepts emerged associated with such broad areas as nurses' attitudes toward spirituality and spiritual care, the identification of patients' spiritual needs, nursing behaviors regarding the spiritual care of patients, and nurses' perceptions of their roles in ministering to patients' spiritual needs.

TABLE 5.1   The Nurse: The Anonymous Minister

A Sacred Calling	*Nonverbalized Theology*	*Nursing Liturgy*
A Sense of Mission	United in Suffering	Healing Rituals
Messengers of Good Faith	Proddings of the Holy Spirit	Experiencing the Divine
The Almost Sacred	The Day the Lord Has Made	Touching the Core
Touching the Hand of God	Crying for More	Being Present
Sensing the Vibrations	Needing Ventilation	Midwifing the Dying
A Healing Ministry	Praying a Lot	Privileged Moments

All dominant themes and related concepts are derived from the practicing nurses' own words.*

Study Findings

Ultimately, an overall construct describing the association between spirituality and the nurse–patient relationship emerged from analysis of the interview data and was labeled "The Nurse: The Anonymous Minister."

This construct, which identifies the nurse's frequently unrecognized role in spiritual ministry, consists of three dominant themes: A Sacred Calling, Nonverbalized Theology, and Nursing Liturgy. Each theme incorporates six key concepts reflective of the category's content and orientation (see Table 5.1).

A Sacred Calling

The first concept of the empirically derived construct, The Nurse: The Anonymous Minister, is reflected in a dominant theme derived from the nurses' interviews and labeled A Sacred Calling. This theme relates to a perceived professional nursing role in ministering to the spiritual needs of patients. A majority of the nurse practitioners, educators, administrators, and

---

*The nurses who participated in the Nursing and Spirituality interviews were identified through informal sampling. The author requested key nurses, in the various types of health care facilities described, to approach members of their staff who might be willing to meet and discuss the topic of spirituality. No criteria regarding the nurses' religious affiliations were specified. As demonstrated in the demographic profile, 64 of the overall group of 66 nurses who agreed to participate in the project identified themselves as Christian. Thus, many of the themes and concepts relating to spirituality and the nurse–patient relationship presented in this chapter are undergirded by Christian theology and spirituality. It is expected, however, that the reader affiliated with another religious tradition will be able to appreciate the universal themes of love, caring, compassion, and ministry to those in need.

researchers interviewed described nursing as being a vocation or calling, reflecting a spiritual element incorporated within their profession.

Peg, a master's-prepared psychiatric–mental health nurse with eight years of experience in the field, observed:

> When I was 16 I felt a "calling" to be a nurse; it's like a sacred calling. Over time you develop a devotion. I can't imagine doing anything else.

And Catherine, a doctorally prepared medical–surgical practitioner with 25 years of experience, perceived nursing as a calling from early on in her education:

> I went to school because I felt called to be a nurse. I see nursing as a spiritual vocation. It's much more than work; I find it a way of serving.

The term *vocation*, which is derived from the Latin word *vocare*, "to call," has been identified as a key theme "in both Hebrew and Christian scriptures" (O'Connell, 1993). "[V]ocation is central to understanding the relationship between Divine initiative and human response" (O'Connell, 1993, p. 1009). The concept of vocation is broadly understood as defining an individual's felt call to a particular ministry or work. In theological terminology the word *vocation* generally refers to "a Divine call to undertake a particular activity or embrace a particular 'stage of life' on behalf of God or the community" (Holland, 1990, p. 1087).

One of the younger study discussants, Amy, a 24-year-old baccalaureate-prepared nurse with one year of experience in the pediatric intensive care unit, asserted that although it had been a real "challenge" to master the health care technology used in the care of critically ill children, it was the spiritual dimension of nursing that appealed to her: "When the day comes that I don't minister spiritually to that child or the family, then I need to get out. This is why I felt called to go into nursing; I don't just want to be a technician."

Supportive of envisioning nursing as a vocation, also, is the recent resurgence of interest among nurse researchers and educators in the relationship of moral belief to the practice of nursing. Ray (1994) observed that nurse theorist Jean Watson "illuminated caring as the moral ideal in nursing where protection, preservation, and enhancement of human dignity are the mandates for the nurse" (p. 106).

The theme of vocation, or a sacred calling, may be further explained in terms of six key concepts derived from the data elicited in the Nursing and Spirituality discussions. These include A Sense of Mission, Messengers of

Good Faith, The Almost Sacred, Touching the Hand of God, Sensing the Vibrations, and A Healing Ministry.

A Sense of Mission

A number of nurses described their perceptions of and experiences with spiritual care in terms of a call to mission or ministry. For Christians, all are called to ministry as pointed out in the New Testament:

> Then the king will say to those at his right hand, "Come you that are blessed by my Father, inherit the kingdom prepared for you from the foundation of the world; for I was hungry and you gave me food, I was thirsty and you gave me something to drink, I was a stranger and you welcomed me, I was naked and you gave me clothing, I was sick and you took care of me, I was in prison and you visited me . . . I tell you, just as you did it to one of the least of these . . . you did it to me. (Matthew 25:34–36; 40)

Although several terms are used to indicate the concept of ministry in the New Testament, interestingly, one used at least 20 times is the word *therapeu*, which means "to care for," "attend," "serve," "treat," especially by a physician, hence, "to heal" (Rademacher, 1991, pp. 39–40). Rademacher pointed out as well that "since the Jews, unlike some of the Greeks, did not divide the person into body and soul, we must assume the word describes a holistic healing of the total person" (p. 40). Most practicing nurses used the terms *ministry* and *mission* interchangeably; they also linked the concept of holistic nursing assessment and nursing care with a sense of ministering to the "whole" person, which they perceived as including the patient's spiritual needs.

Sarah, a baccalaureate-prepared nurse with 12 years of experience in hospice care and pediatric oncology, explained that, although she did need to work for financial reasons, she would not have chosen nursing if it were not for the ministry aspect, "I feel a real 'sense of mission' in nursing. It's a spiritual ministry. If I didn't feel that, I wouldn't be here." She added:

> I really depend on God to direct me. Every morning I try to spend some time in prayer and reading Bible verses to give myself strength. I try, when I have time off, to be alone and have a sense of God's presence. I know that I can't heal the children, but to just be there, that helps, and I pray that Jesus will work through me, to use my hands to in some way comfort or do the right thing for the patients.

A doctorally prepared pediatric nurse educator with 14 years of experience in practice described a strong sense of congruence between nursing and ministry:

> My nursing is my service to God. I believe that this is what I am supposed to be doing; this is my ministry. For me nursing and spirituality are intertwined. I deal with people in their hour of greatest need; whether it's rocking a dying child or helping to support a family. People need more than physical care; they need love and acceptance. And this is when your mission, your ministry, can be a healing presence.

Paula, a master's-prepared medical–surgical nurse, perceived ministry as a key role in nursing practice:

> We are ministering when we sit and counsel with patients; you are ministering to them when you are talking spiritual beliefs. This is part of our mission; we nurses wear so many different hats. We go from teacher, to being ministers, to doing the technical things of our trade like catheters and IVs. But the ministry part is a special gift; it is central to caring and to nursing.

And Martha, a critical care nurse, described how she learned the importance of spiritual ministry to those living with HIV/AIDS:

> I've found that ministering to [people with HIV], to be open, to listen to them, has led to some very humbling experiences for me, and [they] have also been some of my most rewarding experiences. Once I learned that it was OK to cry with the patients; to scream with them. It was OK to just sit there and say nothing because I just didn't know what to say. I learned to just sit there and hold their hand; they will let you know if they want to talk. They don't want anything a lot of times. All they want is a touch or just to know that you are there; they don't want anything else.

Finally, Shannon, in describing her ministry to intensive care unit (ICU) patients, spoke about her approach to critical care, which included a reluctance to impose her personal faith beliefs on patients:

> I try to figure out where a patient or their family is in terms of spirituality, and if there are needs there and they don't know how to bring

it up. So, when something good comes up in a conversation, I'll say something like, "Well, you really have been blessed, haven't you?" And about 98 percent of the time that gives them the permission to let me know about their spirituality. I discovered that this way I can get to their spiritual side without being real threatening; it's just a word choice. . . . I've always been real sensitive to the fact that I have no right to impose my faith on anybody else, but to give folks a chance to articulate their own. If they're not clear on what they believe, sometimes just talking it out with a caring listener puts those issues in perspective. . . . There have been a number of times when folks have asked for a prayer after a conversation like that.

In sum, the spiritual mission of nursing might well be encapsulated in the challenge of Brother Roger of Taize (1991) who asked, "Who will give the best of their creative gifts so that suffering throughout the world may be alleviated, in places where there is sickness, or hunger, or appalling housing conditions?" (p. 13). Brother Roger advised, "Perhaps you could place these Gospel words on the wall of your home; they come straight from the heart of Christ: 'Whatever you do to the least of my brothers and sisters, you are doing to me,' Matthew 25:40" (p. 13).

Messengers of Good Faith

A baccalaureate-prepared pediatric oncology nurse, Maria, described her perceived nursing vocation as related to the comments of a priest–chaplain at her hospital orientation. Maria explained:

In our orientation Fr. O'Connor told us that we were "messengers of good faith." I really feel that is right but don't always see it happening on the units. The advanced technology has taken us somewhat away from the patients. But this is the kind of nurse I want to be, a nurse with a sense of vocation, of "good faith." . . . The spirituality, the strength of these children and their families amazes me; going through chemo and all that really affects their lives. I, being Catholic, attribute that strength to God. I need to support them with my faith.

Anna, a long-term hospice nurse, also spoke about the importance of spiritually supporting patients and families without imposing one's own beliefs:

The idea of spiritual care is particularly important in the hospice setting. The spiritual component is just as important to hospice personnel as the physical component is. At every team meeting the spirituality of the patients is discussed; it is very holistic. . . . But we can't just go in and force our spirituality or our belief system on any patient. We need to meet patients wherever they are.

In their roles as messengers of good faith, nurses walk "among the hurting" attempting to "heal" and to "comfort"; they need to proclaim the love of God for His people. In her deeply moving book *May I Have This Dance?*, Joyce Rupp (1992) reminded us that "[t]he Spirit of God dances among us, calls us to appreciate and enjoy life, and invites us to participate in the Divine Song that makes melody in the heart of all of creation" (p. 95).

No one is ignored; no one is excluded from the call to loving participation in the "Divine Song."

The Almost Sacred

The term *sacred* is defined variously as relating to "the service or worship of a deity"; "a thing worthy of religious veneration, or Holy"; or "something associated with religion or the religious" (*Webster's Seventh New Collegiate Dictionary*, 1976, p. 757). A number of practicing nurses who shared spiritual thoughts or experiences used the word *sacred* in relating to some dimension of their interaction with patients. This is exemplified in the comments of Anne Marie and Karen.

A master's-prepared psychiatric–mental health nurse presently working at a research institution, Anne Marie noted that her choice of nursing had been strongly motivated by an "idealistic desire to help people." She reported:

I considered other careers along the way but nursing gives you an opportunity to make a difference in people's lives. In nursing you deal with the "almost sacred." I know that sounds like strong words but nursing almost touches on the religious. Our work with patients is a real gift. The deep experiences and talks I have had with patients are the closest thing to a spiritual experience. These are the times when you make these deeper connections with people that are spiritual; that is Christ within. Although you don't always recognize it or define it as God's presence within. I have been personally touched by those times.

And Karen, a doctorally prepared medical–surgical nurse, spoke about her approach to patient spiritual care as being a sacred trust:

> I try to look and see if there is a way that patients are signaling me that they need spiritual support. I look to see if maybe they have a Bible laying out and if they're in pain or not sleeping, and I say, "I see you have your Bible here; is there a favorite passage you'd like me to read?" I might also ask, "What kinds of things are important to you?" to see if they might want to go to church or to talk to a chaplain. . . .
>
> I know that my calling as a Christian is to share the Gospel, the good news of Christ; this is a sacred trust. But also, the patient is a captive there and I struggle with getting the balance of "OK, how much am I injecting my values?" So that's why I look for clues to see what's important in their lives; so if it's meditation or listening to music, or whatever, I can pick up on that but if they do mention something to do with the Lord then I can either talk about Scripture or call a chaplain without hitting the person over the head with denominational religion. . . . We have to separate religion and spirituality. Religion is a lot different from spirituality and may be tied up with a lot of rules and prejudices and judgments, but spirituality is about how God reaches out to us and how we respond to that.

Frequently, practicing nurses noted that, although they might not be affiliated with the same religious denomination as a patient, there was, nevertheless, a common sense of spirituality to which they could relate. This provided a starting point from which the nurse could then assess the patient's spiritual needs or concerns.

Touching the Hand of God

The sacredness of a nurse's spiritual ministry was recognized clearly in instances of care for those facing life-threatening illness. In discussing ministry to the terminally ill, Niklas and Stefanics (1975) admitted that this may represent a time when the patient, faced with the reality of his or her own mortality, is open to the presence and the love of God. They suggested that the one ministering actually "walks with the dying person through the valley of the shadow of death" (p. 115). Thus, ministers need to be secure in their own relationship with God and in the understanding of their role in spiritual care.

Christian, a doctorally prepared nurse with 18 years of experience in hospice care, which had recently included a significant amount of care for those with HIV or AIDS, related his nursing vocation to work in the area of death and dying:

> In nursing we have many opportunities to minister but we some-times miss the opportunity to do this. But when facing death you really face the concept of spirituality, your own and your patients'. AIDS patients really articulate their spirituality in their coping. When you work with people who are dying, you touch the hand of God. . . . Spirituality is an area of nursing that would provide a really won-derful expanded role; for me, [spirituality] is primary.

Peg, a master's-prepared medical–surgical nurse with more than 20 years of experience, also described such a perception of closeness to God in caring for seriously ill patients:

> I remember working with some really critically ill patients, and really sensing the presence of God and their spiritual closeness. And es-pecially at night when the hospital is quieter and more lonely, I felt that they [the patients] just wanted me to be there and to under-stand what they were going through. They may have only a few days to live but I could hold their hand and give them that presence of God's love and caring.

Sensing the Vibrations

Joyce, a master's-prepared nursing administrator with approximately 24 years of experience in medical–surgical and intensive care nursing, un-derstood the concept of nursing as a sacred calling. She commented, "Spir-ituality, for me, is to allow both nurses and patients to self-actualize; to love, that is what brings about healing. That is what makes nursing, caring." Joyce observed that when she entered a nursing unit, she considered that part of her role as a clinical nursing administrator was in sensing the vibrations:

> When I walk on a ward, I can sense the vibrations, whether there's a lot of sickness, whether there's a lot of anxiety, a "darkness," and I think that those vibrations are part of spirituality. And I think that the more we love the more we send out our own vibrations of peace and we can lower the anxiety. As we love people we can bring them light; we can make them feel "lighter" and happier. I think that nurses need to do this to their stressful environments, to promote a whole-some, healthy, healing environment. . . . We are all connected in God.

A Healing Ministry

Jesus taught about the concept of ministry through His example of preaching, teaching, and especially of healing the ill and infirm. McGonigle (1993) pointed out that "Jesus sealed the truth of His ministry by the total gift of Himself for the Salvation of all those whom He came to serve" (p. 658). Many Christian health caregivers feel most appropriate in envisioning their work as a spiritual ministry when they relate their activities to Jesus' healing ministry.

This is well exemplified in the comments of Emily, a master's-prepared critical care nurse with 15 years of experience:

> Nurses, I believe, minister to patients, just as I believe that certified clergy do, as Christ did in his healing ministry. I look at the person in totality, the holistic approach. Sometimes it's just by being there, by listening. We talk about God and the love of God, and that He looks at the whole person, not just the last things you did. I have had many patients ask me to pray with them. . . . Nursing is a calling, a healing ministry. You can read and study but it has to be something that is within you, something you are called to do spiritually. . . . Especially in working with dying or critically ill patients you call on your spirituality. Sometimes if someone is suffering a lot you even pray that they will die but it's OK because of faith in God. We say, "I see an angel on the foot of the bed.". . . "Growing up" in critical care you can become focused on the technology but you need to go beyond that. You can cry with the family; I have cried with so many patients and families.

Finally, Emily observed that there was a "definite need for staff nurses to 'marry-up' with chaplains and begin to talk about their spiritual experiences."

The comments from the Spirituality and Nursing study group represent only a few selected examples of the nurses' perceptions of their chosen profession as representing a sacred calling. As observed earlier, virtually all of the group members viewed some dimension of vocation or spiritual ministry as integral to their profession. Although this perception might be articulated through different concepts or anecdotes, the essential theme of nursing as a sacred calling pervaded the discussions.

Nonverbalized Theology

The second concept supporting the construct of the nurse as anonymous minister is described as Nonverbalized Theology. Repeatedly, discussions revealed individual nurses' "God-relationships" and "God-understanding" as being supported by such practices as the reading of Scripture, attendance at formal religious worship services, and personal prayer and meditation. None of the group, however, reported having formally studied theology, although several nurses suggested that it was something they had thought about and might consider doing in the future.

For Christians, theology is the study of "Divinely revealed religious truths. Its theme is the being and nature of God and His creatures and the whole complex of the Divine dispensation from the fall of Adam to the Redemption through Christ" (Livingstone, 1990, p. 509). Gerald O'Collins (1981), in his classic text *Fundamental Theology*, noted that the common understanding of the theological discipline is "faith seeking understanding" (p. 5). Although O'Collins accepted that we must come to the study of theology from a position of personal faith, he posited that the discipline "can help believers to describe, explain, interpret, and account for their faith" (p. 10). O'Collins added, "[Christians] know that they believe in the God revealed in Jesus Christ. Theology makes it easier or even possible to say just what it is they believe. With this help they can state their faith to both themselves and others" (p. 11).

Most of the nurses interviewed were articulate in describing their own faith beliefs, especially in terms of the Christian admonition to care for brothers and sisters in need. Many, however, admitted that they generally did not spend a lot of time speaking or consciously thinking about the dimension of spiritual ministry incorporated into their nursing practice; it was simply considered part of the caring activity central to the profession.

The concept of Nonverbalized Theology was suggested by Paula, a doctorally prepared medical–surgical nurse administrator with 22 years of experience. Paula asserted that nurses "minister" spiritually throughout their professional careers, although the underlying theology may never be verbalized:

> Ministry is not a discreet function; a separate task. It is embedded in the careful giving of the meds, the wiping of the brow, the asking of the right questions, the acknowledgment of the patients' humanness, and what they are experiencing in their sickness. I can be there, to be a person of the love of God. You want to alleviate suffering, convey hope, bring love. It is in giving your care in a caring way; but there is no theology being verbalized; it's a nonverbalized theology. It's in our nursing that we recognize the spiritual side of ourselves and others.

Judith, a doctorally prepared cardiovascular nurse, supported the position:

> I believe that nurses have been doing, and still do, spiritual care a whole lot but we just haven't called it that. . . . Before we didn't verbalize our theology or spirituality but now at least we have an official "nursing diagnosis" for "spiritual distress." I think that gives us a big opening for spiritual assessment of our patients. . . .
>
> Nursing is a ministry but you don't have to speak Scriptures every time you see a patient. When you do spiritual care it can be like Jesus; He just didn't go in and do teaching; He went in and took care of the needs of people first. He fed them and healed them. So when you go in to a patient, take care of their physical needs before you do spiritual care; I believe that nursing is a combination between the art of caring and science. . . . We need to be sensitive. You can turn somebody off by coming on too strong; but you never turn them off by loving them. You always draw them to the Lord; by letting His love flow through you to them. That is the "Cup of Cold Water"; "you did it unto me."

Peter, a master's-prepared psychiatric–mental health nurse with 25 years of experience, also envisioned the concept of Nonverbalized Theology as supporting his clinical nursing practice:

> We are oriented to look at patients holistically, as having a biological, psychological, and spiritual dimension. So, if you're dealing holistically with a patient, and if your underlying theology is that man is made in the image and likeness of God, and you have the perspective of an Incarnational theology, then this is how you approach the patient, even if not on a conscious or verbal level. I am an instrument through which God is present to this person, and in this person is the suffering, or the joyful, Christ. Christ is always present to the other person through you and you encounter Christ in that patient. So even if this theology is not always spoken, or conscious in your mind, but is your underlying theology, then, in holistic nursing, you are relating to the patient's spiritual needs as well as his physiological and psychological; you can't compartmentalize man.

In content analyzing the discussion data, six key concepts articulated by the nurses were identified as being reflective of the overall theme of

Nonverbalized Theology: United in Suffering, Proddings of the Holy Spirit, The Day the Lord Has Made, Crying for More, Needing Ventilation, and Praying a Lot.

United in Suffering

Frequently during the discussions, nurse practitioners movingly demonstrated a nonverbalized theological concept of community by revealing a deep sense of empathy with and understanding of their patients' pain. Without sharing specific details, some of the nurses reported that personal experiences of pain and suffering had helped them become more sensitive caregivers; their interpretation was that having "been there" helped them better identify, at least broadly, with the concerns and anxieties of their patients. This is supported by Henri Nouwen's concept of the wounded healer, which he explained this way: "Making one's own wounds a source of healing . . . does not call for a sharing of superficial personal pains but a constant willingness to see one's own pain and suffering as rising from the depth of the human condition which all men share" (1979, p. 88).

Sharon, a doctorally prepared gerontological nurse with 19 years of experience, observed:

> The older I get, the more confident I feel in sharing spiritual issues with my patients; we are all united in suffering, all children of God. I may not talk about my own pain, my own theology, a lot but I feel comfortable praying with my patients or assisting with a person's rituals. I understand where they're coming from if they're hurting. At this point in my career I am secure in my spirituality. . . . Some nurses are afraid of saying the wrong thing. I think it is a fear of confronting their own spirituality in dealing with patients. . . . Spirituality is that sense of community where God is most, through the presence of other people; Grace in our lives comes through other people.

The concept that we are all united in suffering is well reflected in 1 Corinthians 12:12–26:

> As a body is one though it has many parts, and all the parts of the body though many, are one body, so also Christ. For in one Spirit we were all baptized into one body, whether Jews or Greeks, slaves or free persons, and we were all given to drink of one Spirit; . . . The eye cannot say to the hand, "I do not need you," nor again the head to

the feet, "I do not need you." Indeed the parts of the body that seem to be weaker are all the more necessary, and those parts of the body that we consider less honorable, we surround with greater honor and our less presentable parts are treated with great propriety. . . . But God has so constructed the body . . . that the parts may have the same concern for one another. If one part suffers, all the parts suffer with it.

Proddings of the Holy Spirit

In Christian theology the Holy Spirit is understood as "the Third Person of the Trinity, distinct from, but consubstantial, co-equal and co-eternal with the Father and the Son, and in the fullest sense God" (Livingstone, 1990, p. 245). Farrelly (1993) suggested that in the early Church the "dynamism of Christian life" was ascribed to the Holy Spirit as the vehicle of God's love given to His people (p. 496). In John's Gospel, the "personal character" of the Holy Spirit is demonstrated. " 'I will ask the Father and He will give you another advocate to be with you always, the Spirit of Truth'; John 14:16–17" (Farrelly, 1993, p. 499). A number of the nurse respondents spoke of the importance of the Holy Spirit's guidance in their work with patients, staff, or students. Maggie, a nursing administrator for over 11 years, who described herself as a Southern Baptist and born-again Christian, noted that, although she would never impose her spirituality on a patient, she was "comfortable discussing her own beliefs," if this seemed warranted. Maggie believed that there was definitely a "spiritual care" role for nurses "if you take the time to go a little deeper." She advised that the nurse has to observe and listen carefully to what a patient may be seeking, prior to any spiritual intervention, however. Her suggestion was, "Be attuned to the proddings of the Holy Spirit." Maggie reported, "I have prayed with patients. The times I have felt good about a spiritual interaction [with a patient], I knew I was ministering."

Maggie described a specific instance in which she recognized the guidance of the Holy Spirit in her nursing ministry:

I was working with a mom whose little girl was having some diagnostic tests and they didn't know what was going on and she was really worried. And when they were getting ready to transfer her, the mom came to me and said, "Are you a Christian?" And I said, "Yes, I am," and she said, "I thought you were. And I wanted you to know that you were an answer to prayer; because I prayed for a guardian angel during this hospital experience, because we didn't know what was going on and you were there for me, from the first day to the last."

Maggie concluded, "In those types of experiences I give credit to God; to the Holy Spirit. It was not me; I was just His instrument."

In commenting on the characterization of the Holy Spirit in St. John's Gospel (chapters 14–15), the ecumenical community of the Brothers of Taize (Taize Community, 1992) explained that we are not expected to actually see or experience the Spirit who dwells in us. "What is asked . . . is that we believe in the Holy Spirit, that we trust in Him, that we abandon ourselves to Him. Far from being another demand made on us, this call to faith sets us free" (p. 75).

The Day the Lord Has Made

Several nurses spoke of their gratitude for the spiritual ministry involved in their nursing practice. They saw it as a gift from God to whom they now gave thanks, as directed in Psalm 118:

> Give thanks to the Lord for He is good; His mercy endures forever. . . . The Lord is with me; He is my helper. . . . The Lord is my strength and my song. . . . This is the day the Lord has made; let us rejoice and be glad in it.

Margaret, a practical nurse with 16 years of experience who worked more recently with HIV and AIDS patients, asserted strongly:

> I may not discuss religion a lot but I couldn't do this work without my faith. I ask God to help me and then I can be calm. Prayer is important to me and seeing God in the smallest of things; in the miracles of flowers and birds. To deal with AIDS I have to do this. . . . I am so grateful to God for all that He has given me. I look at the trees in the morning and say, "this is the day the Lord has made." That's what will get you through.

Evelyn, an LPN with extensive experience working with mentally and physically challenged adults, also described her perception that each day was a day to give thanks for serving the Lord. "There is no separation of my day-to-day nursing and my spirituality. I live with it 24 hours a day; prayer in the morning, prayer at night. Each day is a gift of God. I'm not always conscious of it. I think it's like living prayer. It's all the time." Evelyn related her conscious awareness of the spiritual dimension of nursing to when she did hands-on care:

> I don't get to do as much "hands on" as I would like but when I do it's such a gift. I'm so grateful. There is something so holy. You say, "This person is completely dependent upon my hands and my compassion to be cared for." It's seeing Christ there.

Crying for More

Repeatedly, nurses' comments reflected their perceptions of patients' spiritual hunger for God, their need for spiritual care and healing, even if not articulated in theological terminology. In his classic book *Reaching Out* (1975), Henri Nouwen observed that increased sophistication of the healing professions has resulted in depersonalizing the "interpersonal aspects" of the work (p. 92). Caregivers often are forced, by the demands of their jobs, to "keep some emotional distance to prevent over-involvement with . . . patients" (p. 73). Thus, Nouwen advised that "the healer has to keep striving for a spirituality . . . by which the space can be created in which healer and patient can reach out to each other as fellow travelers sharing the same broken human condition" (p. 93).

Anna, a doctorally prepared nurse educator who has worked with students in the clinical medical–surgical area for more than 28 years, expressed concern about patients' spiritual needs not being met:

> People have psychological and emotional needs, but deep down they have real spiritual needs; they are crying for more. . . . I think it's a real gap in our nursing practice; we get so caught up with the technology, there's no time for theology. There are times in life, especially when you're ill, when you really need spiritual support. . . . I try to get the students to see the whole person. They often don't get to that; especially the values, beliefs, religion. If we're going to look at the whole person, you have to include spirituality.

In the preface to her classic spiritual allegory *Hinds' Feet on High Places*, Hannah Hurnard (1975) reminded us that, as the Song of Songs expresses, there is in each human heart a cry for more, a desire for a deeper union with God. "He has made us for Himself, and our hearts can never know rest and perfect satisfaction until they find it in Him" (p. 11).

Needing Ventilation

Related to the concept of patients' spiritual "cry for more," is that of a need to verbalize spiritual and theological concerns and anxieties in the presence of a caring and supportive listener. Allowing a patient to tell his or her story was a concept that emerged frequently in discussions. Emotional pain, often long held at arm's length, may emerge vividly when the physiological component of one's persona has been wounded. Defenses may be at an all-time low; this is a time when important healing can begin. Nouwen (1992) asserted that old wounds can only be healed by allowing them out of the dark corners of "forgetfulness." Caregivers must "offer the space in which the wounding memories of the past can be reached and brought back into the light without fear" (p. 23).

Karen, an ICU nurse with 30 years of experience, spoke at length about her intensive care unit patients' need to talk about their old anxieties and fears, especially related to the topics of illness and death. She recounted that when physicians suggest the administration of tranquilizing medication to calm patient anxieties, she reminds the staff that the patients "need ventilation, not sedation!" Karen, as ICU head nurse, directs her staff nurses to "sit down and hold their patients' hands: Be open to listen; it's a humbling and rewarding experience." Karen advises, "It's OK to say nothing!" And she encourages the staff to do continual assessments of their patients' spiritual needs. She also teaches that "It's OK to cry with patients; crying is not a weakness. This may validate the patient's legitimacy in ventilating anxiety through tears."

During periods of illness or physical debilitation, a patient's latent emotional stresses may surface, generating responses such as anxiety and feelings of loneliness and alienation. It is important, as demonstrated by the nurses' anecdotes, that these stress responses be ventilated.

Praying a Lot

Prayer is as unique as the individual who prays. Whether one's prayer is of petition, adoration, reparation, or thanksgiving, both the form and the content may vary greatly. A few generalizations about prayer, however, can be offered.

The term *prayer* means "a petition or request": "Although the word may be used to mean a petition made to anyone at all, its customary use is ... more particular, made to God or some holy person reigning with God" (Wright, 1993, p. 764). Some methods of prayer identified by Jesuit John Wright (1993) include "vocal prayer," which employs a specific word formula; "mental prayer," which is more of a conversation with God; "discursive prayer," which is led by one's reason; "affective prayer," in which love, joy, or other emotions may predominate; "meditation," in which one considers different aspects of God's activity; "contemplation," which involves a "simple gazing" lovingly upon God; "centering prayer," in which one contemplates God at the center of one's being; "mystical prayer," which is led by God's grace; and finally, "private" and "communal prayer," the latter consisting of a group of worshippers praying together (pp. 773–775).

In relation to the theme of Nonverbalized Theology, the majority of practicing nurses admitted that prayer, in some form, was an important part of their lives. Mark, a baccalaureate-prepared eight-year nursing veteran working with HIV/AIDS patients, reported that his personal faith was critical to his nursing practice:

> I have strong faith. I truly believe that God puts you where He wants you. God tests us as Christians and as nurses. You become friends with your patients; it hurts to lose them. I pray a lot; I can't do what I do without a lot of prayer. . . . Some AIDS patients feel guilty and not worthy of healing; they are afraid that God won't hear their prayers. I tell them that God does not punish illness. I tell them to pray.

And a long-term critical care nurse spoke about prayer in the midst of technology:

> Critical care nurses have to deal with a lot of technology; but the beauty of technology is that after a while it becomes so rote that you can do it without thinking. Once you've got the moves down, I think it is quite possible for you, in the midst of a "Code," while you are pulling up drugs, to pray for that patient, to pray for whoever is making the decisions, to pray for the families who have to cope with whatever happens.

Although most of the nurses interviewed admitted that they did not often speak about theology or spirituality with nursing colleagues, it was definitely an underlying theme related to their practice. Frequently, at the end of the discussions, nurses offered such comments as, "At first, I didn't think I had much to say, but I really enjoyed talking about these spiritual things"; or "I do give spiritual care but I don't often take the time to think about it, or talk about it." The latter seems an excellent reflection of the overall theme of Nonverbalized Theology.

Nursing Liturgy

The third and final concept supporting the research-derived construct of the nurse as an anonymous minister is labeled Nursing Liturgy. Anecdotes describing creative nursing behaviors involving worship related to spiritual care of patients and families abound in the transcripts of the Spirituality and Nursing discussions. The term *liturgy* is broadly understood as relating to rites or rituals associated with public worship; the word *liturgy* is derived from the Greek, *leitourgia,* meaning "the work of the people" (The Liturgy Documents, 1991, p. xiv). In its early pre-Christian use, the term was understood to mean any public activities undertaken to promote communal well-being (Collins, 1990, p. 592). Christian usage focused the word's meaning on "the public worship of the Church" (p. 592).

Nursing Liturgy is conceptualized here as consisting of communal, worship-related, spiritual care activities carried out by nurses in the context of their professional practice. In its broadest meaning, the term *communal* may include worshipful interactions of the nurse–patient dyad only; that is, a nurse and patient praying together. The latter activity constitutes liturgy, for, as noted in Scripture, "Wherever two or three come together in My Name, I am there among them" (Matthew 18:20). Key concepts reflective of the Nursing Liturgy theme include Healing Rituals, Experiencing the Divine, Touching the Core, Being Present, Midwifing the Dying, and Privileged Moments.

Healing Rituals

The term *ritual* is derived from the Latin word *ritus,* meaning "structure." "Ritual is understood as a social, symbolic process which has the potential for communicating, creating, criticizing, and even transforming meaning" (Kelleher, 1990, p. 906). Madigan (1993) noted that "Religious rituals, like social rituals, are intended to be formative and expressive of personal and communal identity" (p. 832). Madigan asserted that, essentially, "Religious rituals are symbolic actions that unify the doer with the sacred" (p. 832).

In relating instances of what they perceived to be "spiritual care," many nurses described poignant worship-associated "rituals" that provided healing to both patients and caregivers; several discussants labeled these "graced moments."

Cathy, a pediatric nurse clinician with 15 years of experience, much of it in the area of pediatric critical care, told a touching story of the "liturgy" that she and two other staff members created to mark the passing of an anencephalic newborn.

The baby, a "preemie," had lived for a couple of weeks, but there were so many congenital anomalies that there was no hope; so the family signed the papers to terminate life support. The parents just couldn't be there, though, so we decided to plan something. It was a very young neonatologist, it was really hard on him, and myself, and the peds ICU head nurse. We came into the NICU [neonatal intensive care unit] at about 5 A.M. on a Saturday, when there weren't a lot of staff around. We took the baby into a separate little isolation room and discontinued the vent and the IVs, all the life support systems. And then we prayed and we sang hymns and we just held her and loved her until she died. It was her special ritual to go to God, and we shared it with her; that baby gave a lot to us too.

Julia, a master's-prepared nurse educator with 22 years of experience in medical–surgical and ICU nursing, described a nursing ritual she had created for her students on completion of their clinical experience:

At the end of the semester I wanted to do something special for the students, to acknowledge their gifts and their talents in caring for patients. It was to provide some type of rite of passage that they were finished with their clinical. I called it an "anointing of the hands"; it was a "blessing with oil." I would explain that oil is healing and say something specific to each student about her gifts as I rubbed the oil on her hands. As I was massaging the oil into the palms of their hands, I would describe their giftedness and their talents in terms of who they were. I would bless them in the name of the Lord. After I had been with them for 15 weeks, I could make the prayer specific to each one. It was acknowledging the sacredness within them. Some students would cry.

Megan, a doctorally prepared nursing administrator with 27 years of experience in hospital care, described what she labeled a "para-liturgical" service, during which she also conducted an "anointing of the hands." In this liturgy she anointed and blessed with oil the hands of her hospital's medical interns at their closing assembly of the year. Megan prayed over each young physician as she did the anointing. She reported that many were close to tears during the experience.

The symbol of anointing has always had a special place in the care of the sick. Oil is used sacramentally as a sign of healing and provides comfort for those who are ill and their loved ones. The concept of anointing the sick is found repeatedly in Scripture, for example, Mark 6:13. "And they cast out many demons, and anointed with oil many that were sick and healed them." Cunningham (1990) suggested that any "anointing" of a person may result in "a change in the person physically [health, strength, fertility] or in the relationship one has with the community" (p. 21).

Several of the nurse educators teaching in schools of nursing reported that they began their classes with a ritual of prayer or spiritual meditation. Frequently these rituals were nondenominational in order to include all of the students present. One nursing faculty member explained, "At the beginning of each class I give about a two-minute spiritual reflection. One day, when we started into some questions about an exam without doing it, the students stopped me and said, 'Aren't we going to pray today?'"

Experiencing the Divine

The majority of practicing nurses indicated having at some time experienced God through interactions with their patients. For some the experience was conscious and ongoing; for others "critical incidents" highlighted a sense of experiencing the divine in a patient. This varied to some degree according to age and nursing experience, with more than a few nurses explaining that the longer they practiced their profession, the more "tuned in" they became to the presence of God within; this occurred in regard to both themselves and their patients. One nurse observed, "I feel like this kind of caring, this kind of experiencing and caring for God in your patients, is like going to church; it's a worship experience."

Julia, with her 22 years of experience in nursing practice, commented, "Nurses are always involved in spiritual care but they don't talk about it; they don't put a label on it" (as reflected in the theme Nonverbalized Theology). She went on to identify some nursing encounters that she perceived as reflecting spiritual experiences in nurse–patient interactions:

> I remember the first time that I ever experienced the divine in another person, in the woundedness of an individual. It just happened. It was an unattractive little old man who was drooling and unable to feed himself. His name was Tom. He seemed repulsive to me. He wasn't pleasant to look at and couldn't even respond to you. But I was caring for him and all of a sudden I thought, "Oh, this is what is meant by Christ within. Christ is present within this man who I initially saw as repulsive." . . . This was a graced moment for me. It was like a quiet kind of awakening; it was parallel to a faith experience!

Touching the Core

As a dimension of the dominant theme of Nursing Liturgy, several nurses spoke about the unique nature of the relationships developed in providing spiritual care for those who are ill. This was true whether the interactions consisted of formal spiritually oriented rites or rituals or more informal types of behaviors, such as praying with patients or discussing spiritual needs or concerns. Repeatedly the concept of depth in nurse–patient interactions related to spirituality emerged from discussion data; nurses spoke of the special opportunity to relate to patients intimately at a time when they are particularly open and vulnerable. This was perceived as a rewarding experience for the caregiver as well as for the patient.

Kinast (1990) asserted that in spiritual ministry to the sick "the deepest and richest human experiences are those which are shared between persons" (p. 9); that is, those in which the minister is able to touch the heart of another person.

Barbara, a doctorally prepared nurse educator with 23 years of experience in the area of pediatrics, commented that "Nursing is much more important than what you are doing [technically] to people; healing takes place just by being with people, by touching their spirituality. A gift to us as nurses is to be able to touch the core of someone."

Barbara's concept of touching the (spiritual) core, or holy place, of another is supported by a description of ministry to those living with HIV infection, in which a caregiver labeled his patient interactions "holy places we share when we have time together" (p. 99). The caregiver continued, "There is an incredible sweetness in being with these persons [with HIV], even when they are very ill and death is imminent; it gives one the incredible sense of 'holding a sacredness'" (O'Brien, 1992, p. 99).

Being Present

Barbara also spoke about the concept of being present, which she perceived as "integral to the spirituality of the nurse–patient relationship." Barbara described being present as the idea of "listening with a loving heart." She affirmed, "I don't know how you can relate to somebody, to be with them in their loneliness, without that dimension."

Holst (1992) highlighted the loneliness of being ill in his discussion of the hospital as "paradox." Although, he noted, privacy is rare, "there can be an eerie loneliness in the midst of all those human contacts" (p. 6). This is, in part, related to the fact that, although advanced technology is devoted to carefully monitoring disease, the person experiencing the disease may be neglected. Technology, Holst (1992) observed, makes us "more preoccupied with the heart as a pump, than with the heart as the seat of emotions" (p. 7).

This paradox is also addressed by James Nelson (1976) who asserted that fundamental to a patient's healing process is the presence of caring persons in the health care facility. "Caring," Nelson added, "is an active attitude which genuinely conveys to the other person that he or she really does matter. It is different from wanting to care for another in the sense of making that person dependent on us. Rather it involves a profound respect for the otherness of the other" (p. 63). To take the concepts of presence and caring a step further, Henri Nouwen (1991) observed that the basis of caring ministry, the point at which ministry and spirituality touch each other, is compassion (p. 33). "Compassion," Nouwen continued, "is hard because it requires the inner disposition to go with others to the place where they are weak, vulnerable, lonely and broken" (p. 34). This, he added, is not our natural response to suffering; we generally either desire to flee from it or to find a "quick cure" (p. 34). In so doing, however, Nouwen argued "we ignore our greatest gift, which is our ability to enter into solidarity with those who suffer" (p. 34).

Many other project participants highlighted the importance of being present to patients in their suffering.

Pat, a baccalaureate-prepared critical care nurse with three years of experience, observed that in providing spiritual care "You have to have intuition beyond the psychological. We're the ones right there at the bedside. You can be the facilitator, find out what the patient and family need spiritually, just by being present."

Kathryn, a master's-prepared psychiatric–mental health nursing administrator with more than 30 years of experience in nursing, noted that "Taking care of the sick is a ministry in and of itself. The idea of ministering and really being present to people helps me to see them as whole individuals, and my own spirituality leads me to see the individual through the eyes of Christ."

And, Diane, a master's-prepared operating room nurse with 19 years of experience, described her conceptualization of being present to her OR patients by praying for them during surgery. "Especially when open-heart surgery patients are in the OR, on the 'Pump,' and we are literally touching their hearts; that's the time when I especially pray for that patient." Diane added, "I serve God through being present for my patients."

Midwifing the Dying

In his article "Religious Approaches to Dying," Anglican Father David Head (1994) reminded us that "Death is integrated as a concept into religious belief systems, and also the religious belief systems integrate death and life" (p. 306). For many "religious" people the beliefs surrounding death "may be comforting" (p. 305). Their tenets often include such concepts as "the transitory nature of the state of death" and "entry into an unknown mystery that is congruent to human experience" (p. 305).

In ministering to a dying person, the caregiver must understand not only the patients' beliefs and feelings about death, but his or her own as well. Niklas and Stefanics (1975) pointed out that if a caregiver is "not in tune with his feelings [about death], they become a weapon or a barrier preventing the dying person and his family from expressing their feelings, or cause him to lack appreciation of the feelings that are being expressed" (p. 114).

Although a number of nurses spoke about the importance of being present to their patients and their families during the death and dying experience, two actually described themselves as being like midwives helping their patients to be "born into a new life." One was Jan, a master's-prepared medical–surgical clinician with 21 years of nursing experience, a significant portion of which involved working with terminally ill patients. She observed, "I help patients to 'cross-over' in the last few days. Part of our job is being like midwives in assisting people in getting to that next state, to their new life in God. We are not only nurses and spiritual caregivers, we are family."

And Sarah, a peds oncology nurse with extensive experience in dealing with death and dying among children, related a special midwifing experience:

> I just got a letter at Christmastime from a family of a little boy who died about 5 years ago. And it was such a precious experience for me; how I bonded with him and with the family. When he was dying we picked him up and we held him and prayed with him and sang to him, and I felt like a midwife; that was really a gift. Being a midwife; it was like helping him to be born into eternal life. You feel so humbled and so privileged just being a part of it.

Sherrie, a master's-prepared critical care nurse with 15 years of experience, described her privileged experience in working with a family whose baby died shortly after birth:

> This was a gift for me and I hope I helped the family. We spent a lot of time with [the baby] in the three days before she died. We dressed her and held her and sang to her. I told the family, "We are all God's angels and some of us He wants back with Him sooner." . . . God had a special role for that baby. In the three days' time this baby gave

and received more love than you will ever know. . . . It's a gift to us to be with anyone who is so close to being with God, to be with them in this special time of transition from this life to a new life.

The spiritual and religious needs of dying adult patients and their families are discussed in chapter 12; the spiritual needs of dying children are discussed in chapter 9.

Privileged Moments

As noted earlier, gratitude for the opportunity for spiritual encounters with patients emerged frequently as a theme in the Nursing and Spirituality discussions. Our nurse project participants reported a multiplicity of privileged moments related to spiritual care interactions with patients. A number of these are evident in the comments and anecdotes already presented. Especially touching are those related by Mary, Daniel, and Sarah.

Mary, a master's-prepared community health nurse with approximately 16 years of experience, most of it in hospice care, described her perception of spiritual care:

> Nurses should never force their spiritual beliefs on patients. . . . Just sitting with a patient, especially one who is dying, I think that is very much spiritual care. . . . Being a hospice nurse is so humbling; it's such a privilege. As hospice nurses, people really take us into their hearts. We have the opportunity to be with people during that time of life transition. We are connecting with the very depth of a person who is facing death. And when they actually pass on, that is a very privileged moment to share with them.

Daniel, a 25-year nursing veteran, also spoke about the privilege of working with patients close to death:

> I have always felt so privileged to work with patients in the final chapter of their lives on earth because it is such a rewarding experience. It is the tremendous privilege of being there. You try to do things that the patient is comfortable with. I remember especially the time I was caring for Mark; he was terminal with AIDS and he wanted me to take him upstairs to the bathroom. So I got him up there and then I thought, "Now, how can I get him back down?"; getting him up had been challenging enough! And I just said, "Well, Mark, I think the

best thing is if you just get on my back." And I carried him that way, and it was really a privileged moment, like a mystical experience, I guess. It was like carrying Christ, a really powerful experience. . . . In situations like this you see yourself as merely an instrument through which God's love is present in the life of the suffering person. It's a mystery to us but it's through grace that I am here and can do what needs to be done in order to make God's love and compassion present to this person in his time of need. . . . We don't usually think of this consciously but there are times when it raises our consciousness, to be used by God, like when I carried Mark down the stairs.

Finally, Sarah related a poignant story which she described as a special and privileged moment with one of her small oncology patients:

Timmy was very disfigured with basel cell sarcoma and he hated to have his blood drawn. He usually screamed and his mom cried, so I'd started praying when I drew it; we prayed together. And so one day we prayed, and I got right in and got the blood, and Timmy was very happy. And it was the first time he had really made a connection with me. So he came into the utility room with me to help label the tubes, and he picked one up to put on the label and dropped it; and it shattered all over the floor. And I thought, "Oh God, how could you have let this happen after we all prayed?" But when I talked to the doctor he said that we could do without the blood that day. But Timmy felt really bad, and as a result, I spent a lot of time with him, and when they went to leave, I went over and hugged and kissed him; that was the first time that we really had connected like that. Since that time Timmy, when he comes in, always runs up and we hug and kiss. And, I realized that God was really working in our lives that day, except maybe not in the way I expected; that hug was much more important than the blood getting drawn. When God reveals something like that to you it is a very privileged moment.

THE MYSTICISM OF EVERYDAY NURSING

The comments of Mary, Daniel, and Sarah, like those of other nursing practitioners reported in the previous pages, exemplify a concept identified by theologian Karl Rahner as the "mysticism of everyday life." Rahner contended that "the human person is 'homo mysticus'—one who experiences

God because of an orientation to God rooted in the way God has made human nature" (Egan, 1989, p. 8). In Rahner's mind "everyone is at least an anonymous mystic" (p. 8). Egan observed that for Karl Rahner nothing about day-to-day life was "profane": "Wherever there is radical self-forgetting for the sake of the other . . . surrender to the mystery that embraces all life, there is . . . the mysticism of everyday life" (p. 8). Rahner's concept might appropriately be translated to read: the mysticism of everyday nursing.

Throughout this chapter members of the professional nursing community have, through their anecdotes and reflections, demonstrated themselves to be not only "anonymous ministers" but also "anonymous mystics." This is evidenced by the many reports of tender care and compassion provided for patients. Although contemporary nurses, whether practitioners, educators, administrators, or researchers, generally do not consciously think of themselves as either mystics or ministers, the data, as exemplified in their attitudes and behaviors, warrant the use of both labels. These findings indeed explain why at least one author has called nursing "the finest art" (Donahue, 1985), and why mysticism and ministry may truly be considered integral dimensions of everyday nursing.

REFERENCES

Boadt, L. (1984). *Reading the old testament: An introduction.* New York: Paulist Press.

Burnard, P. (1988). Search for meaning. *Nursing Times, 84*(37), 34–36.

Collins, M. (1990). Liturgy. In J. Komonchak, M. Collins, & D. Lane (Eds.), *The new dictionary of theology* (NDT) (pp. 591–601). Collegeville, MN: The Liturgical Press.

Cunningham, J. L. (1990). Anointing. In J. Komonchak, M. Collins, & D. Lane (Eds.), *The new dictionary of theology* (NDT) (pp. 21–23). Collegeville, MN: The Liturgical Press.

Donahue, M. P. (1985). *Nursing: The finest art, an illustrated history.* St. Louis, MO: C. V. Mosby.

Egan, H. D. (1989, February). The mysticism of everyday life. *Studies in Formative Spirituality, 10*(1), 7–25.

Farrelly, M. J. (1993). Holy Spirit. In M. Downey (Ed.), *The new dictionary of Catholic spirituality* (NDCS) (pp. 492–503). Collegeville, MN: The Liturgical Press.

Head, D. (1994). Religious approaches to dying. In I. Corless, B. Germino, & M. Pittman (Eds.), *Dying, death and bereavement* (pp. 229–314). Boston: Jones and Bartlett.

Holland, P. D. (1990). Vocation. In J. Komonchak, M. Collins, & D. Lane (Eds.), *The new dictionary of theology* (NDT) (pp. 1087–1092). Collegeville, MN: The Liturgical Press.

Holst, L. E. (1992). *Hospital ministry.* New York: Crossroad.

Hurnard, H. (1975). *Hind's feet on high places.* Wheaton, IL: Tyndale House.

Kelleher, M. M. (1990). Ritual. In J. Komonchak, M. Collins, & D. Lane (Eds.), *The new dictionary of theology* (NDT) (pp. 906–907). Collegeville, MN: The Liturgical Press.

Kinast, R. L. (1990). Caring for God's covenant of freedom: A theology of pastoral care. In H. Hayes & C. Van der Poel (Eds.), *Health care ministry* (pp. 7–21). New York: Paulist Press.

Livingstone, E. A. (1990). *The concise Oxford dictionary of the Christian church.* New York: Oxford University Press.

The liturgy documents: A parish resource. (1991). Chicago, IL: Liturgy Training Publications.

Madigan, S. (1993). Ritual. In M. Downey (Ed.), *The new dictionary of Catholic spirituality* (NDCS) (pp. 832–833). Collegeville, MN: The Liturgical Press.

McGonigle, T. (1993). Ministry. In M. Downey (Ed.), *The new dictionary of Catholic spirituality* (NDCS) (pp. 658–659). Collegeville, MN: The Liturgical Press.

Merriam-Webster's seventh new collegiate dictionary. (1976). Springfield, MA: Merriam-Webster.

Nelson, J. (1976). *Rediscovering the person in medical care.* Minneapolis, MN: Augsburg.

Niklas, G., & Stefanics, C. (1975). *Ministry to the hospitalized.* New York: Paulist Press.

Nouwen, H. J. M. (1975). *Reaching out.* New York: Doubleday.

Nouwen, H. J. M. (1979). *The wounded healer.* Garden City, NJ: Image Books.

Nouwen, H. J. M. (1991). *Creative ministry.* New York: Image Books.

Nouwen, H. J. M. (1992). *The living reminder: Service and prayer in memory of Jesus Christ.* New York: HarperCollins.

Nowell, I. (1990). Covenant. In J. Komonchak, M. Collins, & D. Lane (Eds.), *The new dictionary of theology* (NDT) (pp. 234–246). Collegeville, MN: The Liturgical Press.

O'Brien, M. E. (1992). *Living with HIV: Experiment in courage.* Westport, CT: Auburn House.

O'Collins, G. (1981). *Fundamental theology.* New York: Paulist Press.

O'Connell, L. J. (1993). Vocation. In M. Downey (Ed.), *The new dictionary of Catholic spirituality* (NDCS) (pp. 1009–1010). Collegeville, MN: The Liturgical Press.

Rademacher, W. (1991). *Lay ministry: A theological, spiritual and pastoral handbook.* New York: Crossroad.

Ray, M. A. (1994, May–June). Communal moral experience as the starting point for research in health care ethics. *Nursing Outlook, 43*(3), 104–109.

Roger of Taize. (1991). *No greater love.* Collegeville, MN: The Liturgical Press.

Rupp, J. (1992). *May I have this dance?* Notre Dame, IN: Ave Maria Press.

Senior, D. (1993). Covenant. In M. Downey (Ed.), *The new dictionary of Catholic spirituality* (NDCS) (pp. 237–238). Collegeville, MN: The Liturgical Press.

Taize Community. (1992). *Listening with the heart.* Collegeville, MN: The Liturgical Press.

Wright, J. H. (1993). Prayer. In M. Downey (Ed.), *The new dictionary of Catholic spirituality* (NDCS) (pp. 764–775). Collegeville, MN: The Liturgical Press.

6 ❋ Spiritual Care: The Nurse's Role

And remember every nurse should be one who is to be depended upon . . . she must have a respect for her own calling, because God's precious gift of life is often literally placed in her hands.

FLORENCE NIGHTINGALE, 1859

In years past, spiritual care was generally not considered a dimension of nursing therapeutics. With the advent of the holistic health movement, however, together with the notion of holistic nursing, assessment of an ill person's spiritual needs, and in some cases the practice of spiritual care, became recognized as legitimate activities within the domain of nursing. In light of the current interest in the nurse's role in patients' spiritual care, the present chapter explores the practice of spiritual care as nursing intervention; the attention given to patients' spiritual needs and concerns within the grand theories of nursing; some basic tenets of key Eastern and Western religious traditions; and the nurse's use of spiritual and religious resources such as prayer, Scripture, and sacred music. Referral to a formally designated pastoral caregiver is an acceptable option for the nurse not personally comfortable with the practice of spiritual care.

THE NURSE'S ROLE IN SPIRITUAL CARE

Clinical and research professionals sometimes question whether indeed the nurse has a relevant role in providing spiritual care to patients in his or her charge. The topic has been addressed briefly in chapter 3 in terms of nursing assessment of spiritual needs. The point bears repeating, however, that identification of the nurse's role in providing spiritual care is in no way meant to devalue the role of the hospital chaplain or the pastor ministering to the ill in the community. Rather, the nurse and pastoral care provider can work together to assess the spiritual needs of the ill person and support a comprehensive plan of spiritual care. Although not all nurses may feel comfortable providing spiritual care in all situations, the nurse should always be sensitive to the spiritual needs of his or her patients. With the advent of the holistic health care concept, it is suggested that the "nursing profession must expand its awareness and competence in the spiritual dimension" (Nelson, 1984, p. 26).

Contemporary nursing textbooks, particularly those addressing fundamentals of nursing and medical–surgical nursing, reveal that the nurse's role in both assessment of patients' spiritual needs and the provision of spiritual care is a significant component of overall nursing. Several fundamental texts contain chapters with titles such as "Spirituality," "Spiritual Health," and "Spirituality and Religion" (Kozier, Erb, Blais, & Wilkinson, 1995; Potter & Perry, 1997; Taylor, Lillis, & LeMone, 1997). These chapters include such topics as spiritual health, spiritual problems, assessment of patients' spiritual needs, religious practices, spirituality and family needs, spirituality and the nursing process, and nursing diagnosis of spiritual distress. Many current medical–surgical nursing texts also contain discussions of the nurse's role in spiritual care of the patient. Topics included are spirituality and nursing practice, spiritual care, assessment of patients' spiritual needs, nursing diagnoses, religious beliefs and practices, death-related spiritual beliefs, and spiritual beliefs in coping with acute and chronic illness (Black & Matassarin-Jacobs, 1997; Ignatavicius, Workman, & Mishler, 1995; Phipps, Cassmeyer, Sands, & Lehman, 1995; Smeltzer & Bare, 1996). In discussing the psychosocial dimensions of medical–surgical nursing, Edmision (1997) stated unequivocally that "meeting the spiritual needs of clients has become a recognized part of nursing care" (p. 68).

In the periodical nursing literature also, spiritual care is identified as a recognized element of holistic practice (Bruner, 1985; Labun, 1988; Sims, 1987) and is viewed as central to quality care (Clark, Cross, Dean, & Lowry, 1991; Simsen, 1988). A number of spiritual care models (Ceronsky, 1993; Karns, 1991) and creative approaches to spiritual care (Praill, 1995) have been advanced. Julia Lane (1987) suggested that the spiritual care of patients be addressed in three parts: first, by identifying the characteristics of spiritual care in relation to the essential nature of the human person; second, by identifying spiritual care interventions; and finally, by viewing nursing as a vocation (p. 332). Emblen and Halstead (1993) identified five spiritual care interventions appropriate to nursing: "listening to the patient express key concerns; praying with the patient; reading favorite portions of religious readings; spending time with the patient; and making a referral to a chaplain" (pp. 181–182). Dennis (1991), in a study of ten nurses who reported providing spiritual support from a nonreligious perspective, also found the concepts of listening and spending time with patients to be important components of spiritual care. Recent research has demonstrated that there is a need for educational strategies to prepare nurses for spiritual caregiving (Greenstreet, 1999); spiritual care infiltrates all aspects of nursing care (Carroll, 2001); there are cultural aspects involved in spiritual care (Sellers, 2001); and nurses themselves derive much satisfaction from providing spiritual care to their patients (Nolan, 2000; Narayanasamy & Owens, 2001; Treloar, 2001; Stephenson & Wilson, 2004; and Kumar, 2004). From a review of the literature, three key competencies of spiritual care were identified, including "awareness of the use of self; spiritual dimensions of the nursing process; and assurance and quality of expertise" (van Leeuwen & Cusveller, 2004, p. 234).

Chapter 1 introduced a nursing theology of caring on which a nurse may base his or her practice, including the practice of spiritual care. However, how can the nurse not grounded in a religious tradition or spiritual philosophy practice spiritual care? Should such a nurse attempt to intervene relative to the spiritual needs of an ill person? Ultimately the response must lie with the individual nurse.

As noted earlier, all nurses have the responsibility to be aware of and sensitive to their patients' spiritual needs as a dimension of holistic health care. The minimizing or neglect of this aspect of patient care may have serious implications for the overall illness adaptation. The nurse must consider spiritual needs as part of a comprehensive nursing assessment. What may vary, however, is the degree to which individual nurses carry out therapeutic intervention in response to spiritual needs. As demonstrated by the comments and anecdotes in chapter 4, many nurses do feel both comfortable and confident in engaging in such spiritual care activities as praying with patients, sharing the reading of Scripture passages, and listening to and counseling a patient about spiritual concerns. These activities may be appropriately carried out by a nurse if acceptable to the patient and family. For the nurse who does not feel adequately prepared to be involved in the practice of spiritual care, the appropriate course of action is referral to another nurse comfortable with providing spiritual intervention or to a formally trained pastoral caregiver.

Related to the nurse's role as anonymous minister, as described in chapter 4, the majority of spiritual care provided as a component of nursing activity is unrecognized and unacknowledged. Spiritual care is rarely documented on patients' charts (Broten, 1997, p. 29). Nevertheless, current nursing research and clinical evaluations continue to identify the value placed on the nurse's role in providing spiritual care, by both patients and families.

SPIRITUAL CARE AND RELIGIOUS TRADITION

In order to engage in the assessment of spiritual needs and the provision of spiritual care for patients whose personal spirituality is intimately inter-woven with religious beliefs and practices, the nurse should have some basic knowledge about the traditions of the major world religions. Obviously, the nurse may not herself subscribe to the religious tenets and practices of a particular patient; however, a broad understanding of the patient's religious culture will assist in identifying spiritual problems and in making referrals to an appropriate pastoral caregiver. The spiritual care of the atheist, who denies the existence of God, and the agnostic, who questions the existence of God, may consist of listening to and providing emotional support for the patient.

It is neither the intent nor within the scope of this book to present a comprehensive review of world religions. The following discussion is in-tended only as an overview of key tenets of the religious groups described. This delineation of selected spiritual and religious beliefs and practices may, however, provide the nurse with a starting point in interaction with patients of different faiths. The best strategy in conducting a spiritual assessment is to attempt to learn from the patient or a family member which religious be-liefs and practices are most important, especially those pertinent to health and illness issues.

Two major categories of religious tradition are generally considered to be Western spiritual philosophy and Eastern spirituality. The three key Western religions are Judaism, Christianity, and Islam; all are founded on a monotheistic theology. Major Eastern traditions include Buddhism, Hinduism, and Confucianism, the tenets of which differ, especially in re-gard to the worship of God or of a multiplicity of gods.

Native American religions, of which there are many, generally look to the earth and the spirits of nature for comfort, sustenance, and support. Most Native American religions share a common view of the cycle of life and death and use ritual ceremonies to mark life transitions (Taylor, Lillis, & LeMone, 1997).

Western Religious Traditions

Within the Western religions, Judaism, Christianity, and Islam, the one supreme being is named Yahweh, God, or Allah.

Judaism is described as one of the oldest religions "still practiced in western civilization" and "the foundation on which both Christianity and Islam were built" (Taylor, Lillis, & LeMone, 1997, p. 885). The major religious

Jewish groups are Orthodox, Conservative, and Reform; a more recently identified fourth Jewish tradition, which emerged out of a conservative mindset, is Reconstructionist Judaism (Pawlikowski, 1990, p. 543). The groups differ significantly in regard to religious beliefs and practices. Orthodox Jews follow the traditional religious practices, including careful observance of the Talmudic laws; the Conservative and Reform movements interpret the laws more broadly (Charnes & Moore, 1992). All Jewish traditions emphasize the practice of good deeds or *mitzvahs* each day (Nutkiewicz, 1993, p. 561). Although daily religious rituals are central to the faith of most Jewish persons, health is so valued that "almost all religious injunctions may be lifted to save a life or to relieve suffering" (Charnes & Moore, 1992, p. 66). Jewish people tend to believe that the occurrence of illness is not an accident but rather a time given one to reflect on life and the future (Beck & Goldberg, 1996, p. 16). The keeping of a kosher dietary regimen, if not injurious to health, is very important to many Jewish patients' coping with an illness experience (Fine, 1995), as is the keeping of *Shabbat* or Sabbath, which is observed from sunset on Friday evening to sunset on Saturday. Death, for the Jewish believer, is viewed as part of life; it is important to document the precise hour when death occurs in order to establish the time of mourning, *shiva*, and the annual "honoring of the dead, *Yahrzeit*" (Beck & Goldberg, 1996, p. 18).

Christianity, the largest of the world religions, consists of three main divisions: Roman Catholicism, Eastern Orthodox religions, and the Protestant faiths.

Roman Catholicism identifies that group of Christians who remain in communion with Rome, and who profess allegiance to the doctrines, traditions, philosophies, and practices supported by the pope, as religious leader of the Church. Roman Catholics are trinitarian in theology and place great importance on the seven sacraments: Baptism, Reconciliation (Confession), Holy Eucharist, Confirmation, Matrimony, Holy Orders, and Anointing of the Sick (formerly called "Extreme Unction"); participation in the holy sacrifice of the Mass is the central element of worship.

The Eastern Orthodox tradition, which represents a group of churches whose international leaders are located in Eastern Europe, differs from the Roman Church on both theological issues and aspects of ritual and worship. These churches respect the primacy of the patriarch of Constantinople and include reverence for the Holy Trinity as a central spiritual tenet of the faith. Veneration of holy icons is an important devotion leading ultimately to worship of God the Father, God the Son, and God the Holy Spirit. Currently the term *Eastern Orthodox Church* refers to four ancient patriarchates

(Constantinople, Alexandria, Antioch, and Jerusalem), as well as a number of other churches such as those of Russia and Romania, Cyprus, Greece, Egypt, and Syria (Farrugia, 1990, p. 306).

The term *Protestant* generally refers to the churches that originated during the 16th-century Reformation (Gros, 1990). Some characteristics of original Protestantism are "the acceptance of the Bible as the only source of revealed truth, the doctrine of justification by faith alone, and the universal priesthood of all believers" (Livingstone, 1990). Protestant Christians generally regard Baptism and Holy Communion as important sacraments, although denominations may differ on associated rituals. Some of the major Protestant denominations are Adventist, Baptist, Church of the Brethren, Church of the Nazarene, Episcopal (Anglican), Friends (Quakers), Lutheran, Mennonite, Methodist, and Presbyterian.

Christianity is based on the worship of God and promotion of the Kingdom of God through the living out of the Gospel message of Jesus of Nazareth. For the Christian patient, the nurse will need to be sensitive to a multiplicity of religious beliefs and rituals associated with such health-related events as birth, childbearing, organ donation, and death. For example, infant Baptism is required by Roman Catholics and Episcopalians, and Last Rights or the Sacrament of the Sick is optional for some Protestant groups, but traditional for Eastern Orthodox Christians (Krekeler & Yancey, 1993). In a study of Christian patients' attitudes toward spiritual care, Conco (1995) found that three key themes emerged from interview data. Christian patients described the spiritual care they received as "enabling transcendence for higher meaning and purpose," which helped the patients find meaning in their illness and suffering; "enabling hope," which included the belief that the patients could find a better future; and "establishing connectedness," a theme which spoke to the support provided by the caregiver in terms of such activities as touching, listening, and being present to the patient (pp. 271–272).

Other Western churches of which the practicing nurse should be aware include Christian Science, Church of Jesus Christ of Latter Day Saints (Mormons), Jehovah's Witnesses, and Unitarian Universalist Association of Churches (Taylor, Lillis, & LeMone, 1997, p. 886).

Islam is frequently viewed as having been founded by the prophet Muhammed in the seventh century, with the revelation of the Holy Qur'an. Muslims themselves, however, do not regard Islam as a new religion; "they believe that Allah is the same God who revealed His will to Abraham, Moses, Jesus and Muhammed" (Esposito, 1990). A key tenet of Islam is *Tauhid*, which means faith in the total Lordship of Allah as ruler of heaven and earth; allied with this concept is the understanding that one's life must be centered on this belief (Abdil-Haqq Muhammad, 1995). Important religious practices for Muslims include the ritual prayer, prayed five times each day (preceded by ritual washing) while facing Mecca (the east); honoring Ramadan, the month of fasting from sunup to sundown, which occurs in the ninth lunar month of the Islamic calendar; and the experience of a *hajj*, a pilgrimage to Mecca, once in one's lifetime, if possible. Spiritual care for a hospitalized Muslim patient should be focused on providing the time (about 15 minutes) and the setting (a quiet, private place) for the five-times-daily ritual prayer (Kemp, 1996, p. 88). Most hospitals have access to the services of a Muslim spiritual leader, an imam, if requested by the patient (Rassool, 2000).

A Muslim registered nurse, Selia, spoke about some of the needs of Muslim patients who have entered into the health care system:

> A Muslim patient, what they need during their sickness is similar to what a Christian patient needs: they need a faith in God; they need someone to listen to them; someone to talk about God with them; to know the support coming from God. We have some people in Islam, Muslim women, like who you might say is a "nun," and they are very prayerful and we might ask them to visit and to pray for someone who is sick. We also have in Islam, an imam, who is the spiritual leader of the mosque; he can be called to visit and pray with patients.

Selia also spoke of the importance of faith in helping her own sister accept a diagnosis of cancer. "The staff nurse helped her see that the cancer was not a punishment from God. The nurse sat with her and prayed with her in Arabic and after this she was able to accept her chemotherapy. The 'spiritual' was the most important thing in helping my sister accept her cancer and her treatment." Selia noted that if a patient was not physically able to pray facing Mecca during an illness or treatment, "They can pray while they are lying in bed; they can pray in their minds, even if they are not able to talk. Nurses should encourage Muslim patients to pray to accept their disease because it will help them to cope." She added, "One does not mourn if a family member dies from an illness; they accept this as the will of Allah and one does not contradict this."

Selia continued, "Although a Muslim patient who is very ill is not required to pray five times each day, Muslim hospitals usually prepare prayer rooms; one for women and one for men, who are able to move about. During Ramadan, a patient is not required to fast. The Qur'an says that the sick person, after he gets well, can fast then. She explained, however, that some patients "insist on fasting because they think it is like a prayer; it is something from God."

Finally, Selia spoke of the importance in Islam of visiting the ill:

> The Prophet Mohammed, in the Holy Qur'an, it is written in his own words, that each Muslim should visit patients who are sick and support them and pray with them. It is a must for each Muslim to pray; to ask Allah to help that patient and to help all patients all over the world, whatever their religion.

Eastern Religious Traditions

The major Eastern traditions—Buddhism, Hinduism, and Confucianism—incorporate beliefs about God that differ significantly from those of religions of the Western tradition.

Buddhism derives its beliefs and practices from the life and teachings of the Buddha, the "enlightened one," who lived in India some 2,500 years ago (Borelli, 1990). Myriad Buddhist traditions are associated with the cultures of particular geographical communities, such as Tibetan Buddhism or Chinese Buddhism. Wherever Buddhists are found, there are usually monasteries of monks, and sometimes nuns, who preserve the Buddhist teachings and liturgies. Buddhists believe that suffering can be ended by following the eightfold path: "right understanding, right intention, right speech, right action, right livelihood, right effort, right mindfulness and right contemplation" (Borelli, 1990, p. 146). Buddhists do not revere any particular sacraments.

Hinduism does not embrace one particular body of beliefs and practices; the name *Hindu* is derived from the geographical region of the Indus river valley and the subcontinent, Hindustan, where many of those who practice Hinduism reside (Cenkner, 1990). Key concepts in Hinduism relate to reincarnation or rebirth and the idea of *karma*, or "the law by which one's personal deeds determine one's present and future status in this life and in future lives" (Cenkner, 1990, p. 467). Hindus who have lived well do not fear death; it is seen as the preparation for reincarnation into another life.

Confucianism is an Eastern tradition derived primarily from the personal philosophy of the ancient Chinese scholar Confucius. Inherent in Confucian thought is belief in the importance of maintaining harmony and balance in the body. Two potentially conflicting forces are thought to occur in the world, the "yin" and the "yang"; it is critical that these dimensions of function be kept in balance in order to achieve and maintain a good and productive life.

NURSING THEORY AND SPIRITUAL CARE

In the ideal world of nursing, clinical practice would be based on and directed by well-validated nursing theory; this includes the practice of spiritual care. Nursing theory, however, is still relatively new, having been developed primarily over the past three decades. And in a number of the grand theories of nursing, the spiritual needs of the ill person are given only minimal attention. As more grand nursing theory, as well as theory of the middle range, is generated, scholars anticipate that spirituality will be an important concept of interest. One example is the work of Judith Allen Shelly and Arline Miller, *Called to Care: A Christian Theology of Nursing* (1999).

Speaking from the practitioner's perspective, hospital charge nurse Andrew Oldnall (1995) decried the fact that many nurse theorists have either omitted discussion of the concept of spirituality from their models or have "referred to it only implicitly" (p. 417). There has, however, been a recent reawakening to the importance of the spiritual nature of the human person among contemporary nurse theorists. Barbara Barnum (1995) posited three reasons for what she describes as a "spiritual resurgence" in nursing; these include "a major shift in the normative world view," "a spiritual focus in the growing self-help movement," and "a renewed drive on the part of traditional religious groups and individuals within nursing" (p. 24). Barnum's suggestion that the "self-help movement" has been a catalyst for nursing's current interest in spirituality may be related to the holistic health care concept, a central premise of the holistic approach being patient autonomy and participation in therapeutic planning.

In examining the writings of some of the key nurse theorists of past and present, one finds significant variability in terms of interest in spirituality or the spiritual needs of the ill person. One of the earliest theorists, Virginia Henderson, writing with Harmer in 1955, observed that "sickness may threaten the patient's faith in the ultimate 'goodness' of life. He cannot believe in a God that lets terrible things happen; or he may fear he has lost favor in the sight of God, considering illness a punishment for real or imagined sins" (p. 74). In her later work, Henderson (1966) identified as one of 14 "Components of Basic Nursing Care" provision for "Worship according to one's faith" (p. 17); she did not, however, explore this precept in any detail. Faye Abdellah (Abdellah & Levine, 1979), in "Criterion Measures of Patient Care," also included a patient care component related to personal faith "to facilitate progress toward achievement of personal spiritual goals"; Abdellah, like Henderson, viewed attention to the patient's spiritual needs as a key component of nursing care.

Joyce Travelbee, in her theory of illness as a "self-actualizing experience," was more explicit in her concern with both the patient's and the nurse's spirituality, observing, "It is believed the spiritual values a person holds will determine, to a great extent, his perception of illness. The spiritual values of the nurse or her philosophical beliefs about illness and suffering will determine the degree to which he or she will be able to help ill persons find meaning, or no meaning, in these situations" (1971, p. 16). Travelbee further asserted that a patient's religious beliefs will greatly influence the experience of, and the ability to cope with, suffering (p. 64). She admitted, however, that the degree to which a person actually practices his or her religion is a mediating factor in relation to coping with distress and suffering (p. 71).

Nurse theorist Betty Neuman's systems model is a conceptual framework that addresses the spiritual dimension and needs of the ill person. In Neuman's model, the patient system is assessed holistically from five perspectives: physiological, psychological, developmental, sociocultural, and spiritual (Sohier, 1997, p. 112). For Neuman, the spiritual dimension of a person supports and permeates all other systems (Fawcett, 1989, p. 172). In her earlier work, Betty Neuman placed less emphasis on the spiritual; the spiritual aspects of her theory were first significantly displayed in her 1989 understanding of the patient system (Mclcis, 1991, p. 294). In the third edition of the theorist's book *The Neuman Systems Model*, Neuman's "spiritual variable" is described as the pivot on which the framework centers and as having important implications for patients from a variety of world cultures (Curran, 1995, p. 581).

Callista Roy's adaptation model, which focuses on the adaptive needs of the ill person and family, includes a self-concept adaptive mode that emphasizes the psychological and spiritual characteristics of an individual. This mode addresses the "self-consistency, self-ideal and moral-ethical-spiritual self" of a patient (Phillips, 1997, p. 177). Religion or religious practice is considered one of the significant cultural influences on a patient's adaptation. Although Roy identified the concept of religion as primarily associated with the major organized traditions of Eastern and Western society, she noted that this cultural category may also include "spiritual beliefs, practices and philosophies that are not necessarily attached to institutional forms of religion" (Sato, 1984, p. 69). Callista Roy views religion as an important variable in the adaptive process, as she perceives religiosity or religious practice as potentially influencing all dimensions of a person's life view and functional capacity, especially in terms of attitudes and behaviors related to health and illness.

Two other nursing theories that indirectly address the concept of the patient's spiritual nature in terms of phenomenological and humanistic approaches are the models of Parse (1981) and Paterson and Zderad (1976). Parse accepted the transcendent nature of humanity. "Nursing is unfolding in simultaneous mutual interchange with the world transcending with greater diversity and complexity" (p. 172). Paterson and Zderad viewed the human person as "an incarnate being, always becoming, in relation with men and things in a world of time and space" (p. 19).

And finally, nurse theorist Jean Watson (1985), whose conceptualization of caring is discussed in chapter 1, explained the nature of personhood by placing significant emphasis on the existence of the "human soul [spirit or higher sense of self] that is greater than the physical, mental and emotional existence of a person at any given point in time" (p. 45). Sarter (1992) asserted that Jean Watson is the only nurse theorist who explicitly describes the concept of the soul (p. 152).

In examining the writings of the select group of nursing theorists mentioned, one finds key words related to patients' spiritual needs, including faith, worship, spiritual goals, spiritual values, transcendence, human soul, higher authority, and organized religion. Identifying the patient's understanding of these concepts is important for a nurse undertaking the practice of spiritual care.

NURSING INTERVENTION: THE PRACTICE OF SPIRITUAL CARE

Admittedly, a nurse may not know precisely which nursing therapeutics to employ when faced with a patient experiencing spiritual need. Simple guidelines presented in an earlier publication may provide some basic ground rules for spiritual care:

> The nurse must attempt to respect and understand a patient's religious beliefs and practices, even if very different from his or her own. The nurse must take time to allow the patient to express religious, ethical, or philosophical views, as well as any fears and anxieties related to the patient's spiritual belief system. The nurse must be spiritually supportive, assisting the patient whenever it is within the realm of his or her understanding or expertise, and recognize the need to seek outside spiritual or ministerial counseling, either personally or for the patient, when the situation warrants (O'Brien, 1982, p. 108).

Nurses should keep two important principles of spiritual intervention in mind when ministering to those who are ill. First, because each person has a unique spirituality, the provision of spiritual care cannot be derived from a procedure book of orders; and second, to intervene in the spiritual needs of others, the nurse must first understand his or her own spirituality or relationship to God (Fish & Shelly, 1979, p. 68).

In his best-selling book, *Care of the Soul*, Thomas Moore (1992) observed that spiritual caring forces one to transcend the self and to "recover a sense of the sacredness of each individual life" (p. 19). Moore asserted that spiritual care of the soul incorporates the mystery of suffering and does not deny life's problems (pp. 19–20). Ultimately, Moore contended that spiritual care "requires craft (*techne*), skill, attention and art" (p. 285).

NURSING INTERVENTION IN SPIRITUAL DISTRESS

A patient's experience of spiritual suffering, or spiritual distress, may pose unique challenges for nursing intervention (Kahn & Steeves, 1994). Spiritual distress may be experienced by any ill person questioning the reason for his or her suffering (Harrison, 1993). Defining characteristics of spiritual distress include questioning one's relationship with God, attempting to identify religious idols, guilt feelings, and a variety of somatic symptoms (Heliker, 1992, p. 16); questioning the meaning and purpose of life; expressing anger toward God; refusing to participate in usual religious practices; regarding illness as God's punishment; and seeking spiritual assistance, other than usual spiritual or religious support (Tucker, Canobbio, Paquette, & Wells, 1996, p. 52).

The nurse does not need religious training to meet the needs of a patient in spiritual distress (DiMeo, 1991, p. 22); nurses continually engage in the process of assessing, planning, intervening, and evaluating (the nursing process) related to physical and emotional nursing diagnoses. In assessing spiritual need, the nurse must determine whether he or she may provide the spiritual care, such as listening and counseling, or whether referral should be made to a chaplain or formally trained minister of the patient's denomination (Duff, 1994).

Counseling a person in spiritual distress can constitute a growth experience for the nurse while also providing support for the patient (Burnard, 1988). This was validated in the observations of Gail, a 16-year veteran of nursing interviewed by the author:

> Spiritual care, listening, advising is so important, because people
> are hurting so much. They suffer a lot and the main thing is to listen

and let them tell you their pain. I can't tell them there's a cure and they know that; they lean on God, because there is no other answer. Sometimes chaplains come up and do a "quickie": "I'll keep you in my prayers." But sometimes the patient just needs somebody to sit and listen to her, and be with her. . . . I have seen and listened to much more spiritual distress in patients than I would ever have imagined, and I think it has made me grow spiritually. It's helped me to think about Christ's forsakenness. Suffering in itself can be a prayer.

Spiritual care interventions were identified in response to a nursing diagnosis of spiritual distress in a 41-year-old AIDS patient who demonstrated symptoms of fear of death and questioning belief in God. These nursing therapeutics included assisting the client to explore the spiritual meaning of coping with the HIV experience, providing support for the expression of feelings, and allowing the patient to proceed through the grief process related to physical and psychosocial losses (O'Brien & Pheifer, 1993, p. 314).

The Problem of Suffering

Perhaps the most difficult challenge a practicing nurse may face in attempting to carry out the theological mandate of caring is addressing a patient's suffering. In some cases, the nurse's therapeutic toolbox will contain instruments to alleviate the suffering, at least for a time. In other situations, the pain, whether physical, emotional, or spiritual, seems to take on a life of its own; no techniques or supplies in the nurse's armamentarium prove effective. At such an impasse the nurse, like the chaplain, must wrestle with the imponderable "why." And for the caregiver with a strong religious foundation, be it of the Judeo-Christian tradition or some other belief system, the "why" of suffering may take on a powerful spiritual élan. Why does an all-powerful God allow an infant to be born with multiple congenital anomalies? Why does a loving and compassionate God not intervene to alleviate a teenage cancer patient's intractable pain? Why does a merciful God not use his strength to heal a terminally ill mother whose death will leave orphaned children?

The nurse may also be called on to respond to patients' and family members' inability to understand or accept the reason for an injury or illness. Joyce Travelbee (1971) focused specifically on this point when she defined the purpose of nursing as being "to assist an individual, family or community to prevent or cope with the experiences of illness and suffering, and, if necessary, to find meaning in their experiences" (p. 16). Often, however, it is difficult to articulate a profound existential meaning in an illness experience; thus, the nurse must indeed draw on Moore's thesis of accepting suffering as mystery and of not attempting to offer a patient or family false hope or an unreal prognosis.

Several years ago, the author spent a summer as a chaplain intern at a research medical center whose treatment was directed primarily to those with life-threatening illness. Most of the patients were coping with the potential for a relatively imminent death or at least a shortened life; many were burdened with pain and suffering, both physical and spiritual. For the patients, the families, the staff, and the chaplains, the "why" question always seemed to be lurking in the background. Sometimes it was spoken aloud; at other times it could be read in the eyes of the patients and those who loved and cared for them. The following excerpt from the author's chaplaincy journal describes a mother's distress over the suffering of her son:

> This morning Catherine, the mother of a teenage son, Michael, who was facing mutilating surgery in hope of slowing the progress of advanced rhabdomyosarcoma, came to me in great spiritual pain; she said: "I need you to answer a question: Why? Why my beautiful, generous, loving son? Why not me; I've lived a full life? Why is the God I pray to letting this happen to him? I don't understand." I tried to respond to Catherine's question with some thoughts about the mystery of God's ways; mostly I just listened. Catherine spoke for over an hour, pouring out all of the pain in her heart, all of the love for her son, stopping only once to remind me gently, "You still haven't answered my question: Why?"
>
> At the end of our meeting Catherine said, "Thank you for spending this time with me; it's helped more than I can ever tell you." She did not raise the "why" question again; I breathed a sigh of relief.

When this experience was shared with other medical center chaplains, one observed, "I'm sure that mother knew in her heart there was no answer to the question, 'why?'; she just needed someone to be with her while she asked it."

Most patients and families who suffer, especially those with spiritual foundations, understand that in the realm of the Holy Mystery, the why question has no answers that we, as humans, can comprehend. Rather, what they ask of us as caregivers is, like Catherine, that we be there with them while they ask the questions, that we accept with them the mystery of human suffering, and that we offer no false illusions. This is the essence, the heart of spiritual caregiving.

Suffering as a concept has been defined as "any experience that impinges on an individual's or a community's sense of well being" (Sparks, 1993, p. 950). Sparks added that suffering may be "physical, psychological, interpersonal or spiritual," though he commented that generally it is a combination of all four (p. 950). Suffering is usually understood as a state rather than an incident. It is described not "by sharp pains and moments of terror but by an almost unbearable duration and inescapability" (Maes, 1990, p. 29). Suffering defines an ongoing and consistent state of distress, not merely a brief encounter with painful stimuli. Many of those who are chronically ill well understand the notion of an ongoing state of distress; they may experience, at any one time, a combination of physical, emotional, and spiritual suffering related to an illness condition.

A dimension of suffering frequently encountered in the health care setting and explored in the theological literature relates to the question of "why"; what or who is responsible for the suffering? Suffering, religious faith, and illness have long been associated concepts (Hufford, 1987). The "why" query is highlighted in the classic biblical story of Job. "They [Job's friends] sat down upon the ground with him seven days and seven nights, but none of them spoke a word to him, for they saw how great was his suffering" (Job, 2:13). Job was, seemingly, a good man, and yet he suffered great physical trials, which both he and his friends questioned. In his anger and frustration Job cried out to God, "Why?" According to the Scripture, God never answered Job's question but simply asked him to have faith, which ultimately Job accepted. Theologians agree that the story of Job, often quoted in relation to suffering, leaves the "why" question unanswered and supports the need for absolute faith in God (Baird, 1994; Bergant, 1990; Kidner, 1983).

Robert, a young man who had been living with cancer for more than five years, described a kind of "Job-like" anger at God. Like Job, Robert ultimately was able to trust in his long-standing faith relationship with his creator:

> When I found out I had cancer I was depressed and really mad at God. But then, because I was so scared, I started to pray. And, you know, I learned about praying and about how you really can talk to God. God has always been with me and he'll be with this too. I just have to trust his love.

Robert's conclusion is supported by theologian Kathleen O'Conner's commentary on the "Job Story." O'Conner (1990) observed that the book of

Job is not really about suffering but about one's relationship to God while experiencing suffering (p. 104). She asserted, like Robert, that the lesson to be learned is to pray, to ask God for answers, and then to accept and trust.

In discussing religious interpretations of sickness-related suffering, Emeth and Greenhut (1991) decried explanations claiming that illness is a form of God's punishment or that God gives illness and suffering to those He loves (p. 63). While obviously God allows suffering and may use a suffering experience to draw an ill person to Him, most contemporary theologians would argue that a loving God could not purposely choose to hurt or cause pain. This thinking was reflected by Eriksson (1994) who warned against attempting to find "premature" or "quick-fix" explanations for suffering, asserting that to do so might block an individual from discovering his or her own phenomenological understanding of the meaning of a suffering experience (p. 7). As Eriksson observed, "Suffering in itself has no meaning, but people could, having lived through it, realize that it was in fact meaningful to do so" (p. 7).

In a pastor's response to the suffering experience, especially as related to illness, Rabbi Harold Kushner, author of the best-selling book *When Bad Things Happen to Good People*, asserted, "The God I believe in does not send us the problem; He gives us the strength to cope with the problem" (1981, p. 127). Rabbi Kushner's position is reflected in the comments of Paul, a middle-aged cancer patient:

> God doesn't design diseases; He is a God of love. Why does God allow His people to suffer from sickness? I don't know! But I do know He holds us up. We are His. We belong to Him and He will sustain us. We may walk the way of suffering but we will not be alone.

For the individual who denies or is uncertain about the existence of God, the condition of human suffering is more difficult to manage. Nurses need to be aware of the secular humanist philosophy of such a person. In the case of a patient who professes to be either an atheist or an agnostic, the listening, loving presence of a caring nurse may provide spiritual support and comfort in an experience of suffering.

The most difficult suffering for a nurse to work with is that which is unrelieved. Hospice physician Ira Byock (1994), in discussing persistent suffering, admitted that he sometimes asks himself the question, "how complete is my commitment?" (p. 8). Sister Rosemary Donley (1991) believes that part of the nurse's mission is to "be with people who suffer, to give meaning to the reality of suffering"; it is in these activities, Donley asserted, that the "spiritual dimension" of nursing lies (p. 180).

SPIRITUAL AND RELIGIOUS RESOURCES

In order to provide spiritual care to patients from a variety of religious traditions, the nurse must have some familiarity with the available resources, particularly pastoral care, prayer, Scripture, religious rituals, devotional articles, and sacred music.

Pastoral Care

Pastoral care describes the interventions carried out by religious ministers in response to the spiritual or religious needs of others. The activities of the pastoral caregiver, "including sacramental and social ministries, can be as informal as conversational encounters and as formal as highly structured ritual events" (Studzinski, 1993, p. 722). Howard Clinebell (1991), identified five specific pastoral care functions: "healing, sustaining, guiding, reconciling, and nurturing" (p. 43). Such spiritual care interventions may promote significant healing on the part of ill persons.

Shelly and Fish (1988) noted the importance of the clergy as a resource in spiritual care of the ill; they asserted that spiritual care given by clergy and nurses should be complementary (p. 138). For such complementarity to exist, three conditions are suggested: mutuality of goals in the caregiving, a delineation of role responsibilities, and communication (p. 138). The activities of the minister or pastoral caregiver offer an important religious comfort dimension by providing the patient with familiar symbols and experiences (Atkinson & Fortunato, 1996, p. 99). A pastoral advisor understands the patient's religious belief system and can plan care to be congruent with the individual's religious heritage (Krekeler & Yancey, 1993, p. 1010).

In making a pastoral care referral, the nurse may contact a priest, minister, rabbi, imam, or other spiritual advisor of the patient's acquaintance and tradition, or refer the patient to a health care facility's department of pastoral care. To facilitate a pastoral care visit, the nurse may prepare a place close to the patient for the spiritual minister to sit, provide privacy to the degree possible in the setting, and cover the bedside table with a white cover if a sacrament such as Anointing of the Sick is to be administered (Taylor, Lillis, & LeMone, 1997, p. 896).

A renal failure patient, Catherine, spoke about the importance of pastoral ministry in helping her cope with the acute onset of her disease:

> When I first went on dialysis and was in the hospital, I was sick as a
> dog. I had pneumonia plus the kidney failure and I thought I might
> die. But the response that I got from my minister and the church

was just fantastic. The minister prayed for me, and I had everybody wanting to know how's my dialysis going, and I got a list of 35 people from the church, especially the deacons, who were willing to drive me anyplace I need to go.

Prayer

The word *prayer* is generally understood as a request or a petition to obtain some good outcome. A number of other kinds of prayer, such as prayers of thanksgiving, as well as specific methods of prayer, including vocal prayer, contemplation, and centering prayer, are described in chapter 5.

Spiritual writer Carlo Carretto (1978) observed that "we can never define what prayer is . . . prayer is communicating with the mystery" (p. 75). Prayer is envisioned as the spiritual action one takes to bring an individual "into connection with God" (Johnson, 1992, p. 148). Prayer, whether formal or informal, may be central to healing the sick (Normille, 1992, p. 74). Healing prayer has been described as bringing oneself and a situation of disease before God, "with at least one other person to listen, discern, speak and respond, so that healing in relation to or with God can take place" (Bacon, 1995, p. 15).

Although prayer may be engaged in individually by a patient, and often is, it is important to remember that illness, especially acute illness, may create a "barrier to personal prayer" (Shelly & Fish, 1995, pp. 9–10). In such instances a nurse's prayer for and with the patient can be an important spiritual care intervention. Shelly and Fish remind the nurse that his or her prayer should reflect what the patient would pray for if capable of doing so; they advised, "The most helpful prayer is usually a short, simple statement to God of the patient's hopes, fears and needs, and a recognition of God's ability to meet the patient in his [or her] situation" (p. 11). Prayer as a nursing intervention was described by a practicing nurse as "possible in any setting, as long as we ask people's permission" (Mason, 1995, p. 7). Mason believes that prayer can be an important source of peace and comfort for an ill person (p. 7).

In a 1995 editorial in the *Journal of Christian Nursing*, editor Judith Shelly posed the rhetorical question, "Is prayer unprofessional?" In answering, decidedly in the negative, Shelly cited an address by Florence Nightingale to students at the Nightingale School of Nursing. Nightingale commented, in part, "Did you ever think how Christ was a nurse; and stood by the bedside, and with His own hands, nursed and did for the suffering?" (p. 3). In supporting prayer as an appropriate dimension of holistic nursing, Lewis (1996) also drew on the wisdom of Florence Nightingale as mentor and guide. "Nightingale recognized that the use of prayer attuned the inward man to the universal laws of God . . . and . . . contended that prayer could be applied to daily life for health, wholeness and healing" (p. 309).

Two chronically ill persons experiencing bouts of acute exacerbation of their conditions described the comfort personal prayer afforded them. Agnes, a maintenance hemodialysis patient who was hospitalized at the time, reported, "I believe in a hereafter, and in a God someplace, and that makes you feel like, OK, I can go on. If I feel bad, I can lay in bed and talk to Him, when I don't want to talk to anybody else about my feelings. That's it. That's what religion is all about." Nicholas, an AIDS patient suffering from acute symptoms of cytomegalovirus, admitted, "Sometimes when I'm having a bad day, you know, Why is this happening to me? I say to God, 'could you give me a little hand here?' And usually what happens is I get overwhelmed with gratitude, and I get a sense that God's saying, 'You can handle it, Nicholas; I'm right here.' Sometimes His words actually come to me. I mean, I don't hear a booming voice, but I hear real words in my heart."

A family member of an AIDS patient who had recently died in the ICU after a bout with *pneumocystis carinii* pneumonia, described the importance of a nurse's prayer in the unit:

> I was particularly touched when [she] prayed for Jonathan in the hospital. I didn't say it at the time but when she prayed aloud it was like I was burning inside. And I prayed too. She really had a way with words and I hoped to emulate that.

As advised by Shelly and Fish, the nurse praying aloud for a patient should try to pray as the patient would. An example is a prayer said by the author while in chaplaincy training. Michael, a 36-year-old hospitalized patient suffering from an anaplastic astrocytoma, had described himself as a born-again Christian. Michael loved to talk to and about Jesus in a very direct and simple manner; however, it was difficult for him to articulate a prayer, so he asked that it be done for him. The prayer, recorded in a clinical pastoral education report, is as follows:

> Lord Jesus, put your arms around Michael as he prepares for his chemo treatment. Let him know that he is not walking on this path alone, that you are right there by his side; you are holding him up and supporting him with your strength. Let him know that you are holding his hand. Remind Michael that his name is written on the palm

of your hand. [Michael frequently responded, "Amen" or "Thank you, Jesus."] Michael knows you, Jesus, and knows that you are His Lord. Help him to feel your love and care during this illness. Bless the doctors and the nurses who are giving Michael his treatments, that their hands may be Your Hands as they care for him on this journey. God, our Father, you know what Michael needs in these days, and you know the prayers that are in his heart. Bless his prayer, protect him, guide him and comfort him, we ask this in the name of your son, our Lord Jesus. Amen.

Michael responded to the prayer by saying, "Thank you, your coming here and ministering means a lot to me."

Scripture

Scripture, or the "word of God," is written material that represents venerated and guiding principles for many religious traditions. For the Jewish community, the Hebrew Scripture as contained in the Torah represents God's word and laws for his people. For a Christian, both Old (or "First") and New Testaments contained in the Bible are revered. The Old Testament, shared with the Jewish religion, contains "the story of God's work in the world from creation to the period of the second temple (built in 515 B.C.E.)"; the second, or "New Testament . . . begins with the story of Jesus, and contains documents and letters and visions of the early Christian community in the 1st century CE" (Nowell, 1993, p. 857). *Merriam-Webster's New Collegiate Dictionary* (1976) defines the term *scripture*, not only as "the books of the Old and New Testaments," but also, broadly, as "the sacred writings of a religion" (p. 775). Thus, other scriptural materials, comforting for patients of the appropriate denominations, might include the Holy Qur'an (for Muslims) or the Book of Mormon (for members of the Church of Jesus Christ of Latter Day Saints).

Shelly and Fish (1988) cautioned that a "principle of appropriate timing" should govern the nurse's use of Scripture (p. 121). If a patient is angry or depressed, or experiencing severe discomfort, such as that accompanying acute pain, the seemingly glib quoting, even of an apparently comforting Scripture passage, may seem like "rubbing salt into the wounds" of the sufferer. If, however, it seems that a patient might benefit from a Scripture passage, the nurse can always ask permission in a noncontrolling manner, leaving the patient free to refuse without discomfort. Related to nurses' sensitivity to timing in the use of Scripture, a study of the spiritual caring behaviors of 303 nurses (Hall & Lanig, 1993) revealed that of three types of interventions (conversing, praying, and reading Scripture), nurses were least likely to read Scripture to their patients (p. 736). Ultimately, Piles (1990) suggested that prior to a nurse initiating the sharing of Scripture with patients, he or she should have acquired some sense of when the use of Scripture is an "appropriate intervention" (p. 39).

When a nurse feels comfortable sharing a passage of Scripture with a patient or family member, the reading can represent an important and valid dimension of spiritual care. Following are some suggested Scripture passages and their underlying messages:

For comfort in times of fear and anxiety—Psalm 23; Philippians 4:4–7; 1 Peter 5:7; Romans 8:38–39.

For fear of approaching death—Psalm 23; John 14:17.

For one in need of healing—Isaiah 53:4–6.

For one seeking God's care and protection—Isaiah 43:2; Isaiah 40:28–31; Psalm 25; Psalm 121; Psalm 139:11–19; Deuteronomy 8:2–3; Jeremiah 29:11; Matthew 10:26–33; Luke 12:22–31.

For one seeking God's mercy and forgiveness—Isaiah 1:18; Isaiah 53:5–6; Hebrews 4:14–16; 1 John 1:9.

For one who is fatigued by illness or life stress—Isaiah 40:31.

Religious Rituals

One must observe the proper rites. . . . What is a rite? asked the little prince.
These are actions too often neglected said the fox.

SAINT-EXUPERY, *The Little Prince*

The concept of rite or ritual may be understood theologically as "a social, symbolic process which has the potential for communicating, creating, criticizing and even transforming meaning" (Kelleher, 1990, p. 906). Religious rituals are sets of behaviors that reflect and honor spiritual or religious beliefs on the part of the participant. There can be a profoundly healing value in participation in religious ritual, especially for the acutely ill person (Texter & Mariscotti, 1994). Thus, the use of or support for religious rituals meaningful to a patient should be an integral part of spiritual care intervention provided by a nurse.

A number of religious rituals may be appropriate for an ill person, whether at home or in the hospital setting. For the Muslim patient whose theology is anchored in the five pillars of Islam, formal prayer (*salat*) is prayed five times daily, facing the east (Mecca). To support the Muslim's daily prayer requirement, a nurse may provide a prayer rug facing the east, situated in a place of privacy, as well as facilities for the ritual washing of hands and face. Advice from an imam may have to be sought regarding fasting if a Muslim falls ill during the holy period of Ramadan. Some other important Muslim rituals are those associated with birth and death. At the birth of an infant the husband stands near his wife's head; when the infant is born, the new father whispers a prayer from the Qur'an in the child's ear. Usually a dying Muslim chooses to lie facing Mecca (the east); he or she may also wish to confess prior sins and to recite the words, "There is no God but Allah, and Muhammed is His prophet."

The Orthodox Jewish patient is required to pray three times each day. A male patient, if able, may wish to wear a yarmulke (skull cap) and prayer shawl, as well as phylacteries (symbols of the Ten Commandments) when praying (Charnes & Moore, 1992, p. 66). On the eighth day after birth, a Jewish male child must be circumcised. Circumcision may be done in the hospital, if necessary, or in the home by a *mohel* or Jewish rabbi trained in the procedure. When a Jewish patient is dying, family and friends consider it a religious duty to visit and pray with the dying person and his or her family. In the case of an Orthodox Jew, the nursing personnel may not need to perform postmortem care, as a group from the patient's synagogue, the "burial society," will come to care for the body.

For the Christian person who is ill, the sacraments, as mentioned earlier, as well as prayers particular to each denomination, may be an important part of the healing process. Some years ago, a Roman Catholic could only receive Anointing, then called Extreme Unction, when death was perceived to be imminent. Current Church teaching allows the Catholic patient to request the anointing in the revised ritual of the Sacrament of the Sick at any point during an illness experience. Receiving Holy Communion at that time, or at any time during one's illness, is an important religious ritual for the Catholic and also for many Protestant patients.

Infant Baptism is also an important Roman Catholic ritual. Ordinarily it is carried out in the parish church several weeks after mother and baby have left the hospital. If, however, an infant is in danger of death, any nurse may perform an emergency Baptism by pouring a small amount of water on the child's head and reciting simultaneously, "I baptize you in the name of the Father and of the Son and of the Holy Spirit." Many other Christians practice infant Baptism; some of these church groups include the Episcopal, Lutheran, Methodist, and Presbyterian denominations. Baptismal rites may vary slightly. For example, in the Methodist tradition, "the one baptizing should put his or her hands in the water and then place the wet hand on the baby's head and repeat the baptismal words. In the Lutheran rite, the water is poured on the head three times, while saying the baptismal words" (Reeb & McFarland, 1995, p. 27).

Rosemarie, an operating room nurse for more than 20 years, described a situation in which she felt that she was providing spiritual care by supporting a patient's religious ritual belief, even though she was of a different faith.

> In this situation I was a fairly new nurse, and the patient came in [to the OR suite], and I just had a sense that this patient was going to die. The patient was very ill; he was elderly and had a bowel obstruction. He had come in the middle of the night for emergency surgery. The man was Catholic, and I thought, "well if this man is this bad, then he needs to see a priest." I felt strongly about supporting that and the surgeon got angry with me for not taking the patient in. I literally stepped in front of the gurney, and didn't let the patient get rolled into the OR until the priest came and he was able to give his last confession. That patient died on the table! . . . It was scary for me. I don't know why I felt so strongly; normally I wouldn't go up against an authoritative role like the surgeon. I don't know what drove me to do it but it was based on my own religious beliefs. . . . The wife of the patient was so grateful that I insisted on waiting for the priest; the family never got to see him alive again.

Devotional Articles

Frequently the first clue to an ill patient's religious beliefs and practices is the presence or use of religious or devotional articles. A Jewish person, especially one of the Orthodox tradition, may use a prayer shawl and phylacteries during times of prayer. A Muslim may choose to read passages from the Holy Qur'an, or to pray with prayer beads, which identify the 99 names of Allah. A Christian patient, as well as reading sacred books such as the Bible or the Book of Mormon, will often display devotional items such as relics, medals, crosses, statues, and holy pictures with symbolic meaning for the person. For example, an ill Mexican American of the Christian tradition will frequently carry a medal or picture of Santo Niño de Atocha, a religious personage believed to be instrumental in healing the sick. Other religious symbols an ill person might display include sacred threads tied around the neck of a Hindu, Native American medicine bags, or mustard seeds used by Mediterranean groups to ward off the "evil eye" (Morris & Primomo, 1995, p. 111).

A medical–surgical nurse caring for acutely ill patients validated the notion that the visible presence of patients' devotional articles signaled religious belief and practice. "Usually we get a cue; if you see a Bible or a prayer book, or if they have a cross or a rosary, you think the patient probably has an interest in spiritual matters."

Sacred Music

Music, especially music reflecting an interest in the transcendent, expresses the depth of feeling of one's spirit. Music is a part of all cultures and religious traditions, especially as a central dimension of religious worship (Hurd, 1993, p. 75). Music is frequently used by individuals to relieve stress, and music therapy may be used as an adjunct to healing (Keegan, 1994, p. 169). In a nursing study exploring the use of music in the postoperative recovery period, researchers learned that experimental group patients reported that the music served to relax them, as well as serving as a distracter from pain and discomfort (Heiser, Chiles, Fudge, & Gray, 1997).

Karen Sutherland observed that "the first recorded use of music as an instrument of healing is in the Bible" and cited the story of the young shepherd David who was "summoned to play his music to heal King Saul's emotional and spiritual distress" (2005, p. 29). "The therapy was so successful," Sutherland adds, "Saul requested that David remain in his service (1 Samuel 16:14–23)" (p. 29). The story of a contemporary David is reported in *The nurse with an alabaster jar: A biblical approach to nursing.* The author was told an anecdote about a hospitalized elderly end-stage emphysema patient who was experiencing severely compromised breathing. While she received prescribed nebulizer treatments periodically throughout the day, her breathing and her anxiety became more and more pronounced toward the end of each afternoon. Thus, "a young respiratory therapist, who had been working with the patient, asked the head nurse if he could try an intervention with music; he was a folk guitarist. The head nurse, desperate for any kind of relief for her patient, agreed. The respiratory therapist brought his guitar to the unit and began to play gently for the patient during the periods when her breathing became extremely labored. Everyone, including the head nurse, was amazed at how this gentle 'folk guitar therapy' eased the rapid, labored breathing of the anxious patient" (O'Brien, 2006, p. 104).

Religious music ranges from religious rock, folk, or country-western music, which may appeal to younger patients, to the traditional religious hymns and classical religious pieces such as Handel's *Messiah,* often preferred by the older generation. Playing a recording of religious music, or even softly singing a hymn with a patient, may be incorporated into spiritual care (Folta, 1993, p. 29), if nurse and patient find it meaningful.

Anna, a 13-year-old Ewing's sarcoma patient from a Christian missionary family, loved the traditional hymns of her church. Anna was very ill and experiencing severe pain from her disease; she also required periodic painful bone marrow exams to determine the side effects of her chemotherapy. Anna's mother and the nursing staff decided that singing hymns would be a good way to distract her during the procedure. It was deeply moving to hear the gentle singing of "Abide with me, fast falls the eventide" coming from the pediatric clinic treatment room during Anna's "bone marrows."

If a nurse believes that a patient of any religious tradition might find comfort and support in sacred music, yet the ill person has little experience with religious music, one suggestion might be the beautiful ecumenical chants of Taize, known throughout the world. The community of Taize, founded by Lutheran Brother Roger Shutz, has become a center of ecumenical prayer and reconciliation for people from all countries and of all religious traditions. The simple and beautiful chants were created so that Taize visitors of all cultures and religious persuasions might be able to sing together as one choir. Recordings of the Taize chants, which include a short scripture verse or brief prayer, with refrains such as "Alleluia," "Bless the Lord," and "Stay with us O Lord," are available at most religious bookstores.

This chapter describes the importance of the nurse's role in spiritual care. Many contemporary nurses find assessment, and in some cases intervention, relative to patients' spiritual needs to be a treasured part of their clinical practice. It is nevertheless important to reiterate that not all nurses will feel competent or comfortable undertaking nursing therapeutics in the area of spiritual care. These nurses should, however, be sensitive to the importance of nursing assessment of patients' spiritual needs; referral to a pastoral caregiver for support or intervention is always an acceptable option.

REFERENCES

Abdellah, F. G., & Levine, E. (1979). *Better patient care through nursing research.* New York: Macmillan.

Abdil-Haqq Muhammad, K. (1995, June). What Muslims believe and why. *Muslim Community News,* 1–2.

Atkinson, L. J., & Fortunato, N. M. (1996). *Berry & Kohn's operating room technique*. St. Louis, MO: C. V. Mosby-Yearbook.

Bacon, J. (1995). Healing prayer: The risks and the rewards. *Journal of Christian Nursing, 12*(1), 14–17.

Baird, R. H. (1994). On bad luck: Job and Jesus. *Journal of Religion and Health, 33*(4), 305–312.

Barnum, B. S. (1995, Spring). Spirituality in nursing. *Nursing Leadership Forum, 1*(1), 24–30.

Beck, S. E., & Goldberg, E. K. (1996). Jewish beliefs, values and practices: Implications for culturally sensitive nursing care. *Advanced Practice Nursing Quarterly, 2*(2), 15–22.

Bergant, D. (1990). The book of Job (introduction). In D. Senior, M. Getty, C. Stuhlmueller, & J. Collins (Eds.), *The Catholic study Bible* (pp. 611–612). New York: Oxford University Press.

Black, J. M., & Matassarin-Jacobs, E. (1997). *Medical–surgical nursing: Clinical management for continuity of care* (5th ed.). Philadelphia: W. B. Saunders.

Borelli, J. (1990). Buddhism. In J. A. Komonchak, M. Collins, & D. A. Lane (Eds.), *The new dictionary of theology* (pp. 144–147). Collegeville, MN: The Liturgical Press.

Brennan, M. R. (1997). Value-belief patterns. In G. McFarland & E. McFarlane (Eds.), *Nursing diagnosis and intervention: Planning for patient care* (pp. 852–862). St. Louis, MO: C. V. Mosby.

Broten, P. (1997). Spiritual care documentation: Where is it? *Journal of Christian Nursing, 14*(2), 29–31.

Bruner, L. (1985). The spiritual dimension of holistic care. *Imprint, 31*(4), 44–45.

Burnard, P. (1988). Spiritual distress and the nursing response: Theoretical considerations and counseling skills. *Journal of Advanced Nursing, 12*(3), 377 382.

Byock, I. R. (1994). When suffering persists. *Journal of Palliative Care, 10*(2), 8–13.

Carretto, C. (1978). *Summoned by love*. Maryknoll, NY: Orbis Books.

Carroll, B. (2001). A phenomenological exploration of the nature of spirituality and spiritual care. *Mortality, 6*(1), 81–98.

Cenkner, W. (1990). Hinduism. In J. A. Komonchak, M. Collins, & D. A. Lane (Eds.), *The new dictionary of theology* (pp. 466–469). Collegeville, MN: The Liturgical Press.

Ceronsky, C. (1993). Creative models of spiritual care. *Health Progress, 74*(4), 58–61.

Charnes, L., & Moore, P. (1992). Meeting patients' spiritual needs: The Jewish perspective. *Holistic Nurse Practitioner, 6*(3), 64–72.

Clark, C. F., Cross, J. R., Dean, D. M., & Lowry, L. W. (1991). Spirituality: Integral to quality care. *Holistic Nursing Practice, 5*(3), 67–76.

Clinebell, H. (1991). *Basic types of pastoral care and counseling.* Nashville, TN: Abington Press.

Conco, D. (1995). Christian patients' views of spiritual care. *Western Journal of Nursing Research, 17*(3), 266–276.

Curran, G. (1995). The spiritual variable, a world view. In B. Newman (Ed.), *The Neuman systems model* (3rd ed., pp. 581–589). Stamford, CT: Appleton & Lange.

Dennis, P. (1991). Components of spiritual nursing care from the nurse's perspective. *Journal of Holistic Nursing, 9*(1), 27–42.

DiMeo, E. (1991). Patient's advocate: Rx for spiritual distress. *RN, 54*(3), 22–24.

Donley, R. (1991). Spiritual dimensions of health care. *Nursing and Health Care, 12*(4), 178–183.

Duff, V. (1994). Spiritual distress: Deciding to care. *Journal of Christian Nursing, 11*(1), 29–31.

Edmision, K. W. (1997). Psychosocial dimensions of medical–surgical nursing. In J. M. Black & E. Matassarin-Jacobs (Eds.), *Medical–surgical nursing: Clinical management for continuity of care* (5th ed., pp. 50–74). Philadelphia: W. B. Saunders.

Emblen, J., & Halstead, L. (1993). Spiritual needs and interventions: Comparing the views of patients, nurses and chaplains. *Clinical Nurse Specialist, 7*(4), 175–182.

Emeth, E. V., & Greenhut, J. H. (1991). *The wholeness handbook.* New York: Continuum.

Eriksson, K. (1994). Theories of caring as health. In D. A. Gaut & A. Boykin (Eds.), *Caring as healing: Renewal through hope* (pp. 3–20). New York: National League for Nursing Process.

Esposito, J. L. (1990). Islam. In J. A. Komonchak, M. Collins, & D. A. Lane (Eds.), *The new dictionary of theology* (pp. 527–529). Collegeville, MN: The Liturgical Press.

Farrugia, E. G. (1990). Oriental orthodoxy. In J. A. Komonchak, M. Collins, & D. A. Lane (Eds.), *The new dictionary of theology* (pp. 306–310). Collegeville, MN: The Liturgical Press.

Fawcett, J. (1989). *Analysis and evaluation of conceptual models of nursing* (2nd ed.). Philadelphia: F. A. Davis.

Fine, J. (1995). Long-term care in the Jewish tradition. *The Nursing Spectrum, 5*(22), 2.

Fish, S., & Shelly, J. A. (1979). *Spiritual care: The nurses role.* Downer's Grove, IL: InterVarsity Press.

Folta, R. H. (1993). Music: Arousing the human spirit. *Journal of Christian Nursing, 10*(2), 27–28.

Greenstreet, W. M. (1999). Teaching spirituality in nursing: A literature review. *Nurse Education Today, 19*(8), 649–658.

Gros, J. (1990). Protestantism. In J. A. Komonchak, M. Collins, & D. A. Lane (Eds.), *The new dictionary of theology* (pp. 811–815). Collegeville, MN: The Liturgical Press.

Hall, C., & Lanig, H. (1993). Spiritual caring behaviors as reported by Christian nurses. *Western Journal of Nursing Research, 15*(6), 730–741.

Harmer, B., & Henderson, V. (1955). *Textbook of the principles and practice of nursing* (5th ed.). New York: Macmillan.

Harrison, J. (1993). Spirituality and nursing practice. *Journal of Clinical Nursing, 2*(3), 211–217.

Heiser, R., Chiles, K., Fudge, M., & Gray, S. (1997). The use of music during the immediate postoperative recovery period. *Association of Operating Room Nurses Journal, 65*(4), 777–785.

Heliker, D. (1992). Re-evaluation of a nursing diagnosis: Spiritual distress. *Nursing Forum, 27*(4), 15–20.

Henderson, V. (1966). *The nature of nursing: A definition and its implications for practice, research and education.* New York: Macmillan.

Hufford, D. J. (1987). The love of God's mysterious will: Suffering and the popular theology of healing. *Listening, 22*(2), 115–126.

Hurd, B. (1993). Music. In M. Downey (Ed.), *The new dictionary of Catholic spirituality* (pp. 674–677). Collegeville, MN: The Liturgical Press.

Ignatavicius, D. D., Workman, M. L., & Mishler, M. A. (1995). *Medical–surgical nursing: A nursing process approach.* Philadelphia: W. B. Saunders.

Johnson, R. P. (1992). *Body, mind, spirit: Tapping the healing power within you.* Liguori, MO: Liguori Publications.

Kahn, D. L., & Steeves, R. H. (1994). Witnesses to suffering: Nursing knowledge, voice and vision. *Nursing Outlook, 42*(6), 260–264.

Karns, P. S. (1991). Building a foundation for spiritual care. *Journal of Christian Nursing, 8*(3), 11–13.

Keegan, L. (1994). *The nurse as healer.* Albany, NY: Delmar.

Kelleher, M. M. (1990). Ritual. In J. A. Komonchak, M. Collins, & D. A. Lane (Eds.), *The new dictionary of theology* (pp. 906–907). Collegeville, MN: The Liturgical Press.

Kemp, C. (1996). Islamic cultures: Health-care beliefs and practices. *American Journal of Health Behavior, 20*(3), 83–89.

Kidner, D. (1983). Poetry and wisdom literature. In D. Alexander & P. Alexander (Eds.), *Eerdmans' handbook to the Bible* (pp. 316–369). Grand Rapids, MI: W. B. Eerdmans.

Kozier, B., Erb, G., Blais, K., & Wilkinson, J. (1995). *Fundamentals of nursing: Concepts, process and practice* (5th ed.). Menlo Park, CA: Addison-Wesley.

Krekeler, K., & Yancey, V. (1993). Spiritual health. In P. A. Potter & A. G. Perry (Eds.), *Fundamentals of nursing: Concepts, process and practice* (3rd ed., pp. 1000–1013). St. Louis, MO: C. V. Mosby.

Kumar, K. (2004). Spiritual care: What's worldview got to do with it? *Journal of Christian Nursing, 21*(1), 24–27.

Kushner, H. (1981). *When bad things happen to good people.* New York: Avon.

Labun, E. (1988). Spiritual care: An element in nurse care planning. *Journal of Advanced Nursing, 13*(3), 314–320.

Lane, J. A. (1987). The care of the human spirit. *Journal of Professional Nursing, 3*(6), 332–337.

Lewis, P. J. (1996). A review of prayer within the role of the holistic nurse. *Journal of Holistic Nursing, 14*(4), 308–315.

Livingstone, E. A. (1990). *The concise Oxford dictionary of the Christian church.* New York: Oxford University Press.

Maes, J. (1990). *Suffering: A caregiver's guide.* Nashville, TN: Abington.

Mason, C. H. (1995). Prayer as a nursing intervention. *Journal of Christian Nursing, 12*(1), 4–8.

Meleis, A. I. (1991). *Theoretical nursing, development and progress* (2nd ed.). Philadelphia: J. B. Lippincott.

Merriam-Webster's new collegiate dictionary (7th ed.). (1976). Springfield, MA: Merriam-Webster.

Moore, T. (1992). *Care of the soul.* New York: HarperCollins.

Morris, D. L., & Primomo, J. (1995). Nursing practice with young and middle-aged adults. In W. J. Phipps, V. L. Cassmeyer, J. K. Sands, & M. K. Lehman, (Eds.), *Medical–surgical nursing: Concepts and clinical practice* (5th ed., pp. 45–64). St. Louis, MO: C. V. Mosby.

Narayanasamy, A. & Owens, J. (2001). A critical incident study of nurses' responses to the spiritual needs of their patients. *Journal of Advanced Nursing, 33*(4), 446–455.

Nelson, B. (1984). Who should give spiritual care? *Journal of Christian Nursing, 1*(2), 20–26.

Nightingale, F. (1859). *Notes on nursing: What it is and what it is not.* London: Hamson, Bookseller to the Queen.

Nolan, P. (2000). Learning from the past, not living in it. *Nursing Review, 17*(4), 92–95.

Normille, P. (1992). *Visiting the sick: A guide for parish ministers.* Cincinnati, OH: St. Anthony Messenger Press.

Nowell, I. (1993). Scripture. In M. Downey (Ed.), *The new dictionary of Catholic spirituality* (pp. 854–863). Collegeville, MN: The Liturgical Press.

Nutkiewicz, M. (1993). Jewish spirituality. In M. Downey (Ed.), *The new dictionary of Catholic spirituality* (pp. 561–565). Collegeville, MN: The Liturgical Press.

O'Brien, M. E. (1982). The need for spiritual integrity. In H. Yura & M. Walsh (Eds.), *Human needs and the nursing process* (Vol. 2, pp. 85–115). Norwalk, CT: Appleton Century Crofts.

O'Brien, M. E., & Pheifer, W. G. (1993). Physical and psychosocial nursing care for patients with HIV infection. *Nursing Clinics of North America, 28*(2), 303–315.

O'Brien, M. E. (2006). *The nurse with an alabaster jar: A biblical approach to nursing.* Madison, WI: NCF Press.

O'Conner, K. M. (1990). *The wisdom literature.* Collegeville, MN: The Liturgical Press.

Oldnall, A. S. (1995). On the absence of spirituality in nursing theories and models. *Journal of Advanced Nursing, 21*(3), 417–418.

Parse, R. R. (1981). *Man, living, health: A theory for nursing.* New York: Wiley.

Paterson, J. G., & Zderad, L. T. (1976). *Humanistic nursing.* New York: Wiley.

Pawlikowski, J. (1990). Judaism. In J. Komonchak, M. Collins, & D. A. Lane (Eds.), *The new dictionary of theology* (pp. 543–548). Collegeville, MN: The Liturgical Press.

Phillips, K. D. (1997). Roy's adaptation model in nursing practice. In M. R. Alligood & A. Marriner-Tomey (Eds.), *Nursing theory: Utilization and application* (pp. 175–198). St. Louis, MO: Mosby-Yearbook.

Phipps, W. J., Cassmeyer, V. L., Sands, J. K., & Lehman, M. K. (1995). *Medical–surgical nursing: Concepts and clinical practice* (5th ed.). St. Louis, MO: C. V. Mosby.

Piles, C. L. (1990). Providing spiritual care. *Nurse Educator, 15*(1), 36–41.

Potter, P. A., & Perry, A. G. (1997). *Fundamentals of nursing: Concepts, process and practice* (4th ed.). St. Louis, MO: C. V. Mosby.

Praill, D. (1995). Approaches to spiritual care. *Nursing Times, 91*(34), 55–57.

Rassool, G. H. (2000). The crescent and Islam: healing, nursing and the spiritual dimension. *Journal of Advanced Nursing, 32*(6), 1476–1484.

Reeb, R. H., & McFarland, S. T. (1995). Emergency baptism. *Journal of Christian Nursing, 12*(2), 26–27.

Sarter, B. (1992). Philosophical sources of nursing theory. In L. H. Nicoll (Ed.), *Perspectives on nursing theory* (2nd ed., pp. 147–156). Philadelphia: J. B. Lippincott.

Sato, M. K. (1984). Major factors influencing adaptation. In C. Roy (Ed.), *Introduction to nursing: An adaptation model* (2nd ed., pp. 64–87). Englewood Cliffs, NJ: Prentice-Hall.

Sellers, S. C. (2001). The spiritual care meanings of adults residing in the Midwest. *Nursing Science Quarterly, 14*(3), 239–248.

Shelly, J. A. (1995). Is prayer unprofessional? (Editorial). *Journal of Christian Nursing, 12*(1), 3.

Shelly, J. A., & Fish, S. (1988). *Spiritual care: The nurse's role* (3rd ed.). Downer's Grove, IL: InterVarsity Press.

Shelly, J. A., & Fish, S. (1995). Praying with patients. *Journal of Christian Nursing, 12*(1), 9–13.

Shelly, J. A., & Miller, A. (1999). *Called to care: A Christian theology of nursing.* Downer's Grove, IL: InterVarsity Press.

Sims, C. (1987). Spiritual care as a part of holistic nursing. *Imprint, 34*(4), 63–65.

Simsen, B. (1988). Nursing the spirit. *Nursing Times, 84*(37), 32–33.

Smeltzer, S. C., & Bare, B. G. (1996). *Brunner and Suddarth's textbook of medical–surgical nursing* (8th ed.). Philadelphia: J. B. Lippincott.

Sohier, R. (1997). Neuman's systems model in nursing. In M. R. Alligood & A. Marriner-Tomey (Eds.), *Nursing theory: Utilization and application* (pp. 109–127). St. Louis, MO: Mosby-Yearbook.

Sparks, R. (1993). Suffering. In M. Downey (Ed.), *The new dictionary of Catholic spirituality* (pp. 950–953). Collegeville, MN: The Liturgical Press.

Stephenson, C., & Wilson, K. (2004). Does spiritual care really help? A study of patient perceptions. *Journal of Christian Nursing, 21*(2), 26–29.

Studzinski, R. (1993). Pastoral care and counseling. In M. Downey (Ed.), *The new dictionary of Catholic spirituality* (pp. 722–723). Collegeville, MN: The Liturgical Press.

Sutherland, K. (2005). Can music help heal us? The first recorded use of music as an instrument of healing is in the Bible. *Journal of Christian Nursing, 22*(3), 29–31.

Taylor, C., Lillis, C., & LeMone, P. (1997). *Fundamentals of nursing: The art and science of nursing care* (3rd ed.). Philadelphia: J. B. Lippincott.

Texter, L. A., & Mariscotti, J. M. (1994). From chaos to new life: Ritual enactment in the passage from illness to health. *Journal of Religion and Health, 33*(4), 325–332.

Travelbee, J. (1971). *Interpersonal aspects of nursing* (2nd ed.). Philadelphia: F. A. Davis.

Treloar, L. L. (2001). Spiritual care: Safe, appropriate, ethical. *Journal of Christian Nursing, 18*(2), 16–20.

Tucker, S., Canobbio, M., Paquette, E., & Wells, M. (1996). *Patient care standards: Collaborative planning guides.* St. Louis, MO: C. V. Mosby.

van Leeuwen, R., & Cusveller, B. (2004). Nursing competencies for spiritual care. *Journal of Advanced Nursing, 48*(3), 234–246.

Watson, J. (1985). *Nursing: Human science and human care.* Norwalk, CT: Appleton Century Crofts.

7 ✸ Spiritual Needs of the Patient with an Acute Illness

Waiting for tomorrow ... asks for ... a deep faith in the value and mean-
ing of life, and a strong hope which breaks through the boundaries of death.

HENRI NOUWEN
The Wounded Healer (1979)

The spiritual needs of the adult patient suffering from an acute illness vary greatly depending on such factors as age, religious tradition, and the seriousness of the condition. These and other variables are explored in this chapter, which describes the spiritual needs of patients experiencing conditions including congestive heart failure, septicemia, pneumonia, myasthenia gravis (myasthenic crisis), toxoplasmosis, acute renal failure, and acute pain. Data documenting the importance of personal spirituality and religious support were obtained through the author's interviews of and interaction with patients, family members, and nurse caregivers of patients with acute illness.

THE CASE OF ACUTE ILLNESS

Current nursing texts distinguish between acute and chronic illnesses, differentiating the two phenomena as distinct entities. Taylor, Lillis, and LeMone (1997) described acute illness as "a rapidly occurring illness that runs its course, allowing the person to return to his or her previous level of functioning" (p. 1451), whereas Potter and Perry (1997) defined it as "characterized by symptoms that are of relatively short duration, are usually severe, and affect the functioning of the client in all dimensions" (p. 1475). These conceptualizations are appropriate to describe a multiplicity of illness conditions such as pneumonia, influenza, bronchitis, gastritis, herpes zoster ("shingles"), and a host of other self-limiting disease processes. With an uncomplicated acute illness, an individual may pass rapidly through the stages of initial symptom development, treatment and "sick role" behavior, and recovery.

However, a number of "chronic" disease conditions may begin or end with an acute illness phase or manifest acute symptoms during periods of exacerbation over the course of the illness trajectory. One example is that of chronic renal failure (CRF), which may, if undiagnosed, initially manifest in a state of acute renal failure, necessitating emergency dialytic therapy and, in some cases, critical care nursing. Human immunodeficiency virus (HIV) infection, another condition currently being categorized as chronic, may be initially diagnosed by the acute onset of an opportunistic infection such as *pneumocystis carinii* pneumonia (PCP) or cytomegalovirus. Patients suffering from various types of carcinoma may experience acute illness symptoms related to a therapeutic regimen incorporating radical surgery and/or chemotherapy.

During periods of acute illness, whether self-limiting or associated with a chronic disease, the patient may experience significant physical discomfort and anxiety, especially if symptoms are severe or life threatening. Patients with self-limiting illness may need comfort and support in coping with the sequelae of an infectious process, such as the acute pain accompanying a bout with herpes zoster ("shingles"). Individuals experiencing acute exacerbations of a potentially life-threatening chronic illness may need help in coping with the prognosis as well as the diagnosis of their condition. For the acute renal failure patient faced with the possibility of a future of dependency on medical technology, quality of life may become questionable; in a few cases, patients have elected to die rather than continue living supported by continuous dialytic therapy (O'Brien, 1982b). Thus the need for spiritual care and assessment of spiritual concerns are important aspects of holistic nursing care during periods of acute illness.

SPIRITUAL NEEDS IN ACUTE ILLNESS

Spiritual beliefs and, for some, religious practices, may become more important during illness than at any other time in a person's life (Kozier, Erb, Blais, & Wilkinson, 1995, p. 314). While an individual is enjoying good mental and physical health, spiritual or religious practices may be relegated, in terms of both time and energy, to a small portion of one's life activities. With the onset of acute illness, however, especially if associated with the exacerbation of a chronic condition, some significant life changes may occur both physically and emotionally. First, the ill person is usually forced to dramatically curtail physical activities, especially those associated with formal work or professional involvement. This may leave the individual with a great deal of uncommitted time to ponder the meaning of life and the illness experience. Such a time of forced physical "retreat" may effect considerable emotional change in one's assessment of past and future attitudes and behaviors.

The remarks of a 32-year-old male patient reflected such an experience during an episode of acute renal failure. "It enlightened me as to just how fast I was really going. It made me reevaluate my life. Now I can place my needs before my wants. It hasn't been so difficult in looking at the good advantages. This thing has made me think a lot about the way I used to live, and put different values on things" (O'Brien, 1983, p. 146). A 47-year-old male renal failure patient who had also suffered a serious bout of acute illness at the time of disease onset, commented in a similar vein. "This illness definitely made me think; get my mind together. I know all things happen for the good. It turned me around spiritually and mentally. Now I listen better. I try to be more patient, and I have more to learn from others" (O'Brien, 1983, p. 146).

Of the 126 renal failure patients studied, 93 individuals (approximately 74 percent of the total group) reported that religious or spiritual beliefs were, to some degree, responsible for their ability to accept their disease and its prognosis.

Despite a possible positive effect, however, the onset of a sudden and unanticipated acute illness may pose serious emotional and spiritual problems related to fear of possible death or disability. Psychological depression may occur as a result of severe physical symptoms such as acute pain and fatigue. Some patients question God's will and even express anger toward God for allowing the illness to occur. At this point, especially, the nurse must be alert and astute in assessing the spiritual concerns and needs of an acutely ill patient. Although a diagnosis of spiritual distress may be masked by the physical and emotional symptoms of an illness, the patient's remarks can provide a hint as to the presence of spiritual symptoms in need of attention. For example, comments such as "God help me," or "I wonder where God is in all of this?" can give the nurse an opening for informal spiritual assessment.

In essence, meeting the spiritual needs of the acutely ill may encompass basic concepts of spiritual care such as listening, being present, praying or reading Scripture (if acceptable to the patient and comfortable for the nurse), and/or making a referral to a chaplain or other pastoral caregiver. These activities, however, must be handled sensitively, related to the severity of patient symptoms such as pain, nausea, or fatigue. Appropriate spiritual care behaviors for the acutely ill person might include sitting quietly at the patient's bedside for a brief period, saying a short prayer aloud or offering a silent prayer, or sharing a comforting Scripture passage that may help to focus the patient away from the present suffering.

SPIRITUAL HEALTH IN ACUTE ILLNESS

Even though an acutely ill person may be facing a potentially life-threatening situation, the concept of spiritual health is not only possible, but may be the key factor in his or her coping successfully with the physiological deficit. In discussing the spiritual health of the acutely ill patient, Peterson and Potter (1997) suggested that "the strength of a client's spirituality influences how he or she copes with sudden illness, and how quickly he or she can move to recovery" (p. 443).

Spiritual health can be defined as "a state of well-being and equilibrium in that part of a person's essence and existence which transcends the realm of the natural and relates to the ultimate good. Spiritual health is recognized by the presence of an interior state of peace and joy; freedom from abnormal anxiety, guilt or a feeling of sinfulness; and a sense of security and direction in the pursuit of one's life goals and activities" (O'Brien, 1982a, p. 98). Spiritual health is also understood as relating to the ability to identify and describe one's purpose in life (Chapman, 1986; Levin & Schiller, 1987). Health care researchers found a significant correlation between spiritual health and an individual's subjective evaluation of overall physical health (Michello, 1988), and that spiritual health can be predictive of how a person confronts his or her personal mortality (Hart, 1994). In emphasizing the value of the concept, Seidl (1993) argued that, as spiritual health organizes the values, meaning, and purpose in one's life, it also motivates an individual to "optimize" personal health so that he or she can serve God and community (p. 48). This places the notion of spiritual health in a religious context, which indeed is appropriate for many persons. An individual who professes no particular religious beliefs, however, may also be in a state of spiritual health. The terms *spiritual* and *religious* are not synonymous. Spirituality may, however, undergird religious practice, and thus, both concepts become relevant to a discussion of spiritual health (Fahlberg & Fahlberg, 1991).

An acutely ill person who is spiritually healthy can find comfort and strength in his or her spiritual or religious philosophy of life. This is reflected in the comments of Evan, HIV-positive for three years, who had recently experienced an acute episode of an opportunistic infection, *pneumocystis carinii* pneumonia. "It's the spiritual dimension of religion that I want to practice. I meditate a lot. I sing the refrain from 'Day by Day.' Remember that? That's what I want to do; love Him more dearly. That's the most important thing in my life right now, with this disease" (O'Brien, 1992, pp. 47–48).

For the atheist or the agnostic who may be struggling to find a state of spiritual health, coping with the acute symptoms of an illness may be expressed very differently and, for some, may be much more difficult. Atheism, denial of the existence of God, or agnosticism, uncertainty about the existence of God, may leave a person diagnosed with serious illness struggling to find meaning and purpose in the experience. Burnard (1988) pointed out that patients with such beliefs also have spiritual needs, however, and nurses must be creative and compassionate in carrying out assessment and interventions.

Kent, an HIV-positive patient with cytomegalovirus, described his belief system as basically universal. "I believe in a superior force or being. It's an energy that I tap into. It's everywhere and it speaks to everything. I call on it when I need some reinforcement and encouragement in dealing with the stress of this illness" (O'Brien, 1992, p. 48).

Gerry, still in the process of recovering from a bout with toxoplasmosis, poignantly expressed the distress of his personal struggle to find spiritual health. "I don't think I believe in God. But it is hard not to believe in God because I am so afraid of death. If there is no God, then death is really going to be the 'death' that I am afraid of, which is nothingness" (O'Brien, 1992, p. 48).

For an acutely ill patient such as Evan, the nurse might anticipate spiritual needs related to traditional religious belief and practice as reflected in his comment about wanting to love God more dearly. For patients such as Kent and Gerry, however, whose belief systems are either humanistic or currently in a state of crisis, spiritual care must be creative and tailored to assist the patient in relation to his or her faith or lack of faith.

The comments of those living with acute sequelae of HIV and AIDS demonstrate that spiritual health correlates importantly with one's ability to cope with an illness experience. The patients themselves recognized that their spiritual or religious beliefs or lack thereof were significantly related to their adaptation to living with their illness conditions.

As well as being associated with the acute illness conditions and the acute phases of chronic illness, serious physiological and psychological challenges requiring spiritual support are also present in such experiences as the perioperative journey, the critical care experience, the emergency room experience, and the experience of pain; these are reflected in the following sections.

SPIRITUAL NEEDS OF THE PERIOPERATIVE PATIENT

The term *perioperative* refers to the period encompassing the preoperative, intraoperative, and postoperative experiences for a surgical patient. Specifically, the preoperative phase begins with the plan to carry out surgery and ends with the actual transfer of the patient to the operating room (OR);

the intraoperative phase covers the period of the actual surgical procedure; and the postoperative phase begins with the transfer of the patient out of the OR to recovery, and continues through the healing process to the time of discharge from the physician's care. The perioperative client may be found in a hospital, a community-based surgery center, or, for minor procedures, a physician's office.

The perioperative patient and family may pose significant challenges to the nursing staff related to the anxiety experienced prior to, during, and immediately after the surgery; yet, the perioperative nurse often has little time to develop a relationship with the patient due to the fast-paced nature of the nursing (Dearing, 1997). Some of the most frequently identified causes for fear in the preoperative period are "fear of the unknown," "fear of pain or death," and "fear of changes in body image and self concept" (Taylor, Lillis, & LeMone, 1997, pp. 676–677); fear of the unknown may encompass the other fears. Fear of the unknown may also include fear of the postoperative diagnosis, especially if the surgical procedure is focused on an exploration to determine the possible presence of a malignancy. Fear of surgical death or of a painful postoperative death lurks in the minds of most patients and families during the intraoperative period. Even if the surgery has been described as a "simple procedure," preoperative patients often express fear of "going under the knife" or going under anesthesia, especially if general anesthesia is used.

A dimension of the perioperative nurse's role is to provide comfort and support to patients and families, especially during the pre- and postoperative periods (Fairchild, 1996). Meeker and Rothrock (1995) described the perioperative nurse's role as including a "continuous awareness of the dignity of persons and their physical, emotional, cultural, ethnic, and spiritual needs." In a 1994 statement, the Association of Operating Room Nurses asserted that "the perioperative nurse designs, coordinates, and delivers care to meet the identified physiologic, psychologic, sociocultural and spiritual needs of patients whose protective reflexes or self-care abilities are potentially compromised because they are having invasive procedures. The nursing activities address the needs and responses of patients and their families or significant others" (cited in Atkinson & Fortunato, 1996, p. 22).

The perioperative nurse can identify a patient's spiritual beliefs through use of the nursing history and thus can provide spiritual care through "acceptance, participation in prayer, or referral to clergy or chaplain" (Taylor, Lillis, & LeMone, 1997, p. 678). Although some nurses may feel that raising spiritual issues may be threatening to the patient, Burns asserted that regardless of religious tradition, discussing spiritual concerns is therapeutic during the perioperative period (1996, p. 361). Burns believes that simply asking if a perioperative patient's pastor is aware of impending surgery is a supportive approach (p. 361).

The model of perioperative nursing developed by Phippen, Wells, and Martinelli (1994) contains the earlier identified assumption of the appropriateness of holistic health care, including attention to the patient's spiritual nature (p. 3). The individual's spiritual component is viewed as the "animating" principle of life, and this spiritual dimension of the patient is influenced by underlying "religious and philosophical beliefs" (p. 4). If the nurse diagnoses "spiritual distress" manifested by symptoms of fear of death, anger at God, or disruption of spiritual practices on the part of a perioperative patient, appropriate spiritual care interventions may be carried out. The strategy suggested by Phippen et al. involves an exploration of the type of spiritual or religious practices to which the patient relates (e.g., spiritual reading or a visit with a chaplain); the nurse may then intervene by providing materials or making an appropriate referral (p. 66).

In a study of perioperative nurses' perceptions of caring practices, McNamara (1995) found that spiritual care was viewed as primarily including those activities and behaviors that "comforted patients or increased their feelings of security" (p. 385). The perioperative nurses interviewed in McNamara's study asserted the importance of avoiding judgmental attitudes about patients' religious beliefs and practices. Listening and being aware of the patient's religious tradition was considered essential to spiritual care. Several nurses reported praying with patients; others made referral to a pastor of the patient's choice (p. 385). In a discussion of the meaning of spirituality to perioperative nurses and their patients, Rothrock (1994) advocated supporting hope as a "healing force." Heiser, Chiles, Fudge, and Gray (1997) advocated that perioperative nurses use music therapy in the immediate postoperative recovery period as a contemporary spiritual intervention strategy.

Carol, a nurse anesthetist with 18 years of experience in perioperative nursing, explained the importance of spiritual care in the immediate preoperative period:

> I try to talk to patients when they arrive in the OR suite. They are just scared to death. I might be the last person to talk to them before they go to sleep. I talk to them outside the OR while the surgeons are changing clothes. We usually have a few minutes of privacy. I listen to their concerns. I listen to hear if they say anything like, "I'm in God's hands," and then I just take it from there. I say it's OK to put all

your trust in God; He'll be with you in there [the OR]. Especially if a person is in for cancer surgery, I reassure them of God's love and care during the surgery. This is when people are at their most vulnerable; they feel like they are losing all control of their lives. They don't know what the surgery will bring and their future is in the balance. This is the most logical time to think of God, to think, "Am I ready to die?" This is the time they really need some spiritual care. . . . I pray silently while the patient is under anesthesia; if they're having a hard time, I ask God to give them strength.

Diane, a master's-prepared operating room nurse with 19 years of experience, spoke of spiritual care as "being with" the patient during the intraoperative phase; she also incorporates touch in her caring. "I think there isn't a patient that has gone to sleep here that I haven't held their hand while they're being put to sleep. That is spiritual care as far as I'm concerned. You stand beside them and hold their hand and talk to them. I consider all that part of spiritual care." Diane also admitted that she prayed for patients during surgery, while performing her duties as a scrub nurse or circulating nurse. "I especially pray for the 'open hearts.' When they go on and off that pump, believe me, I'm praying like crazy. When open heart surgery patients are in the OR and on the pump, and we are literally touching their hearts; that's the time when I especially pray for that patient." Diane added, "I serve God through being present for my patients."

Opportunities for spiritual care of the perioperative patient in the postoperative period may vary significantly depending on the nature of the surgical procedure. Many patients currently experiencing less complex surgeries, classified as "same day surgery," are in and out of the hospital very quickly. Nevertheless, a gentle touch or a word of comfort or support may still be possible during the recovery room stay. This is also a time when anxious family members or friends greatly welcome a kind word of encouragement from the nursing staff. For the patient immediately postoperative from a complex surgical procedure, such as a coronary artery bypass graft (CABG) who may emerge from the OR on mechanical ventilation, the intensive care unit (ICU) will be the setting where spiritual intervention is needed and much appreciated by both patients and families.

SPIRITUAL NEEDS OF THE ICU PATIENT

In the contemporary critical care unit, with its ever more complex therapeutic technology, the persona of the patient may seem lost in the myriad tubes, wires, and sophisticated monitoring devices. Obviously, a central responsibility of the critical care nurse is to skillfully employ the technology at hand in the service of intensive patient care. If the nurse is to provide truly holistic care to the critically ill patient, however, attention to the needs of the mind and the spirit must accompany the delivery of high-quality physical care. Dossey, Guzzetta, and Kenner, in the introduction to their text *Critical Care Nursing: Body, Mind, Spirit* (1992), admitted that their subtitle may seem inappropriate to some readers who might regard the emphasis on mind and spirit as irrelevant to contemporary science. The authors argued, however, that sensitivity to the patient's emotional and spiritual needs is an essential dimension of the subfield of critical care nursing. They suggested that during a period of critical illness "patients frequently search for how to create new perceptions for their life as well as to find wholeness and spirituality" and that they "need guidance in their transformation" (p. 11). Dossey et al. explained that the critical care nurse, therefore, needs to be sensitive to a variety of factors in order to help patients deal with spiritual issues, including the pluralism of spiritual beliefs and religious practices that patients may adhere to, the difference between spiritual and religious concepts, and the nurse's own possible personal confusion in regard to spiritual or religious values (p. 12).

Critical care units (CCUs) or intensive care units (ICUs), first created in the early 1960s, were developed to sustain individuals who might not otherwise survive a serious physiological deficit or complex surgical procedure, such as acute myocardial infarction or a coronary artery bypass graft. The critical care patient in the ICU is considered physiologically unstable and at great risk for developing life-threatening complications (Kidd, 1997). Like acutely ill patients in general, ICU patients may include persons experiencing bouts of severe symptomatology related to a chronic illness, such as myasthenic crisis in a myasthenia gravis patient, or a sudden onset acute illness or trauma, as in the case of patients diagnosed with meningococcal meningitis or multiple fractures sustained in an accident.

Among the current variety of specialized critical care units are neonatal ICUs (NICUs), pediatric ICUs (PICUs), surgical ICUs (SICUs), medical ICUs (MICUs), neurological and neurosurgical ICUs, and coronary care units (CCUs). These contemporary critical care units, as centers for advanced health care technology, are host to many medical "machines" such as cardiac, hemodynamic, and intracranial pressure monitors, ventilators, and defibrillators, the sight of which may be anxiety provoking to patients and their families. Another particularly frightening aspect of the ICU environment is the potential for observing crisis intervention in another patient

(Hopkins, 1993, p. 1564); a patient or family member might unexpectedly be witness to an emergency intubation or a "code blue" occurring close to their own assigned space in the unit.

Virtually all cognitively aware adult patients report significant stress associated with the ICU experience. As well as those discussed already, other identified stressors include "social isolation, enforced immobility, pain from procedures, poor communication with staff, excessive noise and lack of sleep" (Dracup, 1995, pp. 12–13). Lack of personal autonomy (Walleck, 1989) and a feeling of utter helplessness (Niklas & Stefanics, 1975, p. 75) are perhaps the most devastating emotions that the ICU patient experiences. This may result in an overwhelming sense of depersonalization as a result of such factors as "powerlessness, emotional/touch deprivation, loss of privacy, invasion of personal space, and transfer anxiety" (Clochesy, 1988, p. 193). Thus, concepts such as prayer and spirituality are becoming more and more sought after as dimensions of care by critically ill patients and their families (Holt-Ashley, 2000).

Related to the stress of critical illness, with its painful sequelae, as well as the sometimes persistent fear of death and the added stressor of hospitalization in a critical care unit, Busch (1994) recognized that the experience may either enhance or challenge a patient's spiritual or religious beliefs (p. 16). A first step in providing spiritual care for the critically ill patient, then, is to carry out an assessment of the person's spiritual and/or religious beliefs, practices, and current needs. Some pertinent information about spiritual or religious history may be obtained from the patient's chart and from the family; hopefully, information about current spiritual needs will emerge through personal interaction between patient and nurse.

Because of the patient's possible isolation from usual religious practices, such as attending worship services or reading Scripture or other spiritual books, and because of the fear and anxiety about his or her illness condition, the nurse may diagnose spiritual distress in the ICU patient. Twibell, Wieseke, Marine, and Schoger (1996) identified some defining characteristics of a spiritual distress diagnosis for a critically ill patient, including a request of spiritual guidance or support, the verbalization of distress over not being able to carry out usual religious practices, expression of "spiritual emptiness," questioning the credibility of one's belief system, and expressing anger or frustration over the meaning of the present illness experience (p. 249). Following such a diagnosis, the nurse may intervene or may elect to contact a chaplain or other pastoral care provider. Bell (1993) advised that if the nurse chooses to pray with the critically ill patient, using "the patient's own words" in relation to illness-related needs may be comforting (p. 27).

Gillman, Gable-Rodriguez, Sutherland, and Whitacre (1996) identified some basic postures in providing spiritual care in a critical care setting: "inclusion," meaning that the nurse should try to imagine what the ICU experience must actually be like for the patient; "confirmation," that the nurse should support the patient's personal spiritual goals; and "mutuality," a spirit of cooperation between nurse and patient in seeking healing (p. 13). Stromberg (1992) described the role of the spiritual care provider in a coronary care unit as encompassing three tasks: listening empathetically, confronting reality, and being a "fellow pilgrim" on the patient's current spiritual journey (p. 127). Listening and "being there" are central to spiritual care in the ICU. The concept of presence, "enhanced by empathetic listening," reflects the nurse's sense of "genuineness, trust and positive regard," which will allow the patient freedom to express his or her spiritual needs or concerns (Shaffer, 1991, p. 45). Beverly Hall (1997), in discussing the nurse's role as spiritual caregiver in life-threatening illness, observed that "what patients need from us is not psychology or theology but caring and presence while they seek answers" (p. 93). As well as providing a listening presence for the critically ill patient in the ICU, and praying with him or her if acceptable to the patient, nurses should refer patients to clergy when appropriate (Bardanouve, 1994; Bucher, Wimbush, Hardie, & Hayes, 1997; Reed, 1991; Shelly & Fish, 1995).

A sometimes neglected yet no less important dimension of spiritual care for the ICU patient that should be included in the nurse's role is that of providing care and support to the patient's family (Chesla & Stannard, 1997). The ICU hospitalization of one of its members may create great anxiety on the part of the rest of the family (Rukholm, Bailey, & Coutu-Wakulczyk, 1991); thus, spending even a brief period of time with family visitors is an important dimension of spiritual care (DiSarcina, 1991, p. 23).

ICU nurse Joyce Hahn related a poignant anecdote about taking the times allocated for her mealtime and break in order to sit with a dying patient's husband. After his beloved wife's death, the husband returned with a lovely poem he had written for their nurse. The meditation included the thought that he had experienced an "angel clothed in white" and ended with the words, "It was one of God's children, a nurse from the ICU" (Hahn, 2001, p. 32).

For the majority of critical care patients, regardless of professional credentials or life history, the ICU experience is new and exceedingly traumatic. This concept was clearly exemplified in the case of an ordained minister who was hospitalized in the same ICU where he himself ministered to others. Pastor Norton, who was a longtime myasthenia gravis patient, was brought to the unit late one evening in myasthenic crisis; he was immediately intubated and placed on mechanical ventilation. He remained on ventilatory support for approximately two weeks. Shortly after his critical care experience, Pastor Norton admitted that although the physical and technical care had been excellent, he had in fact felt isolated during the intubation period and longed for more caring "touch." There were times, the minister admitted, when he would have liked a nurse simply to come and sit by the bed, take his hand, and be with him. As he reflected on the experience, Pastor Norton's conclusion about the lack of "spiritual care" related to his personal identity as a minister; he speculated that the staff probably felt shy about attempting to comfort or support him spiritually, thinking that he already possessed a vast store of resources to draw on. With honesty and humility, Pastor Norton confessed that despite his own strong faith, he had experienced significant feelings of anxiety, loneliness, and helplessness during his stay in the intensive care unit.

An older female patient, Mrs. McCarthy, who was experiencing an exacerbation of a chronic endocrine disorder, and who had also been intubated for several weeks, admitted to feelings of devastating helplessness while on mechanical ventilation, as had Pastor Norton. Mrs. McCarthy, who reported after extubation that her nursing care had been fine, confessed that while on the ventilator she had fantasized that because of the physical deterioration of her body, an ICU staff member, questioning the quality of her life, might "pull the plug" while she was sleeping. This was very threatening to her as she was looking forward to the high school graduations of two of her grandchildren. Obviously, the ICU nursing staff expressed shock when told of this fear. Mrs. McCarthy's frightening fantasy, however, was a reminder of the fragility of the ICU patient's emotional state, and of the constant need for reassurance and support.

In the case of a confused or comatose patient, caregivers should provide spiritual care and support directly toward the family of the person receiving intensive care. One such case was that of a 67-year-old patient, Mr. Lundquist, who was critically ill as the result of a rampant septicemia following bowel surgery; he was mechanically ventilated and his physiological functioning was being maintained by the continual use of pharmacologic agents (the use of multiple "pressors"). As his illness progressed, Mr. Lundquist was only minimally responsive to verbal or tactile stimuli. Mr. Lundquist's family, including his wife and several adult children, spent many hours in the critical care waiting room, as well as at the bedside. Their pastor visited frequently and helped them begin the process, on the physician's advice, of facing the patient's imminent death. The adult children's concern, which was verbalized on several occasions to the nursing staff, especially as new therapeutic procedures were initiated, was, "how long would Dad want to live like this?" They were very concerned about their father's suffering. Mr. Lundquist's wife and children reported that he had never discussed his wishes in regard to the use of "extraordinary measures" to prolong life. A nurse researcher working with patients and families in the ICU was able to spend time at Mr. Lundquist's bedside and also be with the family in order to provide a caring presence when such issues as the "DNR" (Do Not Resuscitate) option were discussed. The family expressed gratitude for this supportive nursing presence in a note sent after Mr. Lundquist's death.

The critical care nurses involved in the study described in chapter 5 frequently commented on the need for the nursing practice of spiritual care in the ICU. Margaret, a relatively new ICU staff nurse, observed:

> My patients are all very sick, and communication is a key issue. When I talk to them about religious things, they often exhibit strengths related to how they are handling their illness. For some of these patients it's really tough, like with young bone marrow transplants in the MICU flunking the second transplant, and they're not going to live and they know it and the family knows it. They really need spiritual support. The physicians get to leave the room but it's the nurses who have to stay and be with the patients while they suffer. . . . I'm trying to work on the nonpharmacologic approach to decreasing anxiety. Patients may be anxious because of unmet spiritual needs, so we're trying to use music, listening, visitors, communication . . . just being open to whatever the patients' spiritual needs are, whether they're religious like associated with a church or just their own spirituality.

Coleen, a 22-year veteran of ICU nursing, spoke about critically ill patients' fear of death:

> I've worked in critical care for many, many years and I can't even count the number of patients who have said to me, "Am I going to die?" This is the biggest opening for spiritual care that anybody could present. Usually what I say back is, "Do you mean if or when?" Then we can get down to what's really bothering them. The only answer you can give is "I don't know"; it also depends on where the nurse is spiritually herself. If you're Christian and the patient is, you can give them a parable like the man who built his house on rock and it will

not be blown away, or if the patient is Jewish, something "Old Testament." You can pray out loud with the patient or silently, and just help them be at peace. . . . Most people will let you know if they have a religious background and want you to pray or read the Scripture with them. Sometimes you just have to go with the Holy Spirit, and hope you say what the Holy Spirit wants you to say.

Coleen related a personal prayer experience in the ICU:

I've been reading about some scientific research where nurses were praying for cardiac surgical patients; an experimental group who got prayers and a control group that didn't, and the experimental group didn't have any complications and did a lot better than the control group. I had a hint of that last year when one of the unit nurses I was working with said, "Watch my patient; I'll be right back." There wasn't anything to do so I just started to pray for the patient. When his nurse came back she said, "Coleen, what did you do? His O_2 sat [oxygen saturation] has never been this good!"

Coleen concluded with advice about spiritual intervention in the ICU:

You want to be careful to respect the religious practice of the patient. You don't want to shock anybody by a religious practice that might seem strange or different, or inappropriate in their eyes. When we are going to do spiritual care for patients I think that it is better to be on the conservative side until they give us clues as to what they want or need, if it's prayer or whatever. If you have the love of God in you, they are going to respond to that regardless of what their religious affiliation is.

Judith, a master's-prepared nurse with 24 years of experience in critical care nursing, shared her perception of the change in attitude toward the provision of spiritual care by the ICU nurse:

When I first went into critical care I did it because of the focus on the technical aspect, but shortly into my career I really kept looking for the person; that you are not just taking care of the equipment, but that there is a person there in the bed. I believe there's been a change, especially in the last five to eight years. Patients are not afraid to share how they feel spiritually. It used to be, years ago, I remember, that the nurse never talked about God or church or praying with a patient. The minister came and prayed with the patient and everybody else left the room. What I've seen over these last few years is nurses being less anxious and more comfortable in their own spirituality; then they can comfort others. . . . Sometimes you are really busy in ICU and you don't have much time to talk to the patient about spirituality but you can find out where they are with it and maybe call the chaplain. You can get the ball rolling for the chaplain to come in. We are the ones right there at the bedside, especially in critical care. You can sense what the patient needs and pick up on it. . . .

I'm not Catholic, but this past week I had a Catholic patient who was really anxious, and one of the other nurses was Catholic so she went and they had a talk. She gave the patient a little "Lady of Perpetual Help" charm [medal], pinned it on her, blessed her with some holy oil, and shared prayer with her. . . . I think that is a prime example of a nurse attending to a patient's spiritual needs. We shouldn't ever foster one religion over another, and sometimes we don't know what a person believes really, but just to be there with them. Death is really hard in the ICU so just sitting with a family, I am sometimes at a loss for words but just to be there, I think is part of caring.

An excerpt from the author's research journal, maintained during the course of a five-year study of the nursing needs of persons living with HIV and AIDS, presents a final example of spiritual care that a practicing nurse might carry out in the ICU setting.

It was a clear, crisp Friday morning in autumn, my favorite season, as I headed off to a local medical center, but my heart was heavy. I had just received a phone call from Luke, the friend of Jonathan, an AIDS patient with whom I had been working. Luke apologized for calling early but, he said, "Jonathan asked that I get in touch with you. He was admitted to ICU during the night and they're putting him on the ventilator; it doesn't look good."

As I drove to the hospital I tried to imagine, or perhaps to not imagine, what condition I would find Jonathan in. I couldn't help but reminisce about when we had first met some two years previously; it was shortly after he had been diagnosed with HIV infection. I was searching for persons living with HIV to participate in a five-year NIH-supported study of coping strategies, and Jonathan had agreed to speak with me. His enthusiasm for the study matched his enthusiasm for life: it was infectious. During the past months we had laughed and worried and cried over the strange twists and turns which the human immunodeficiency virus had introduced into his life, but always, underneath it all, Jonathan maintained a serenity and a joy that were exquisite to behold.

When I arrived in the intensive care unit, Jonathan had already been placed on the ventilator and was barely conscious; Luke was standing at his bedside. After filling me in on the events of the past few hours, Luke looked across the bed and said, "Mary Elizabeth, would you do something for Jonathan?" I immediately responded, "Of course," wondering, considering the setting, what it could be. I assumed Luke's request was for some nursing task, a comfort measure perhaps, yet Jonathan appeared to be resting peacefully, at least as peacefully as one can when attached to a ventilator, IVs, and the multiple system monitoring devices usual to the ICU environment. Luke, who was an aeronautical engineer, explained, "Religion is not something that is very big with me; as a scientist I have difficulty with the mystery, but for Jonathan it's important. He didn't go to church a lot but faith in God was a real part of his life. Would you say a prayer for him?"

My first reaction was something akin to panic [this occurred prior to my chaplaincy training]; where is a chaplain? I thought. As a nurse I'm not "credentialed" in prayer. But I quickly realized that since it was I, the nurse, whom Luke had asked, surely God would compensate for my perceived weakness in the prayer department.

I cannot recall the exact prayer that I prayed that morning in the medical center intensive care unit. I remember that I reached out and took one of Jonathan's hands; I also grasped Luke's hand, so that we three could be connected, as a small worship community in our makeshift chapel. The words were simple, I think. I asked God to put His arms around Jonathan and hold him close, to give him strength and comfort, to let him know how deeply he was loved and cherished as one of God's own. The musical accompaniment was provided by the rhythmic hum of the ventilator as it coaxed and supported Jonathan's labored breathing; the choir, the hushed whispers of the nurses and technicians as they quietly worked in the background. Together, hand in hand, amidst the tubes and lines and wires apropos of contemporary intensive care, our small community celebrated a liturgy. When we had finished Luke's eyes filled with tears and he whispered, "Thank you"; my eyes also filled with tears and I silently prayed "Thank you" to the God of love who carries us in His arms when we feel most fragile.

The experience with Jonathan and Luke taught me that we, as nurses, are indeed called to a lived reality of God's love which may be manifested in terms of spiritual care, as well as physical and emotional support. I recognized the importance of allowing myself to be "used" as God's instrument in the midst of feelings of personal inadequacy. Although I did not feel competent to minister spiritually, through prayer, at the time, the Spirit provided the courage and the words. Luke told me several days later, after Jonathan's death, that he felt peace after we prayed together; that this was a turning point, and that he had now begun to think about his own spiritual life and how he might understand God. I believe that not only the praying together, but also our joining hands, as a worshipping community, was an important dimension of our ICU liturgy. Through the intimate touch of palm against palm, we became aware of our connectedness both as a human family and as the spiritual family of God. We were thus able to support and strengthen each other, even as we sought the support and strength of our Creator.

SPIRITUAL NEEDS OF THE EMERGENCY ROOM PATIENT

An emergency is defined as "any sudden illness or injury that is perceived to be a crisis threatening the physical or psychological well-being of a person or a group" (Lazure & DeMartinis, 1997, p. 2501). Although most large hospitals house emergency departments to care for those persons and groups, it is well known that a number of individuals seek care at an emergency room for non-life-threatening, and even routine, problems. This occurs most frequently in large urban inner-city areas, where indigent and homeless individuals have no other available and accessible source of medical care.

The goal of emergency departments is to provide care for "the acutely sick and injured" (Santacaterina & Stein-Spencer, 1990, p. 3). Most hospital ERs are also involved in prehospital care, provided prior to arrival at the health care facility; for example, care provided at an emergency scene by emergency medical technicians (EMTs) and carried on during ambulance transport. Sophisticated telemetry systems may connect the EMTs with the hospital emergency room staff physicians and nurses (Robinson, 1992).

The Emergency Nurses Association defines emergency nursing care as "assessment, diagnosis and treatment of perceived, actual or potential, sudden, or urgent physiological or psychosocial problems that are primarily episodic or acute. These may require medical care or life support measures, client and significant other education, appropriate referral, and knowledge of legal limitations" (Lazure & DeMartinis, 1997, p. 2503). A key role of the emergency department nurse is that of triage, or initial nursing assessment of the patient's condition in order to determine priority care needs (Blair & Hall, 1994, pp. 21–23). Following triage, the patient may be assigned to one of several types of ER space such as "major trauma or arrest room, minor suture room, gynecologic examination room, psychiatric room, family room, or general examination room" (MacPhail, 1992, p. 7).

The Emergency Nurses Association has articulated comparative standards for working with individual patients. Standard 1, Assessment, states, "The emergency nurse initiates accurate and ongoing assessment of physical, psychological and social problems of patients within the emergency care system" (Emergency Nurses Association, 1995, p. 16). The consideration of the ER patient's psychological and social problems, as well as physical assessment and triage, as part of the emergency nurse's role, is underscored in a list of ER nurse activities. This is identified in a contemporary fundamentals of nursing text, which includes caring for the patient with severe anxiety (Long, 1993, p. 1540). The current philosophy of emergency care has become so broad as to consider an emergency "whatever the patient or family considers it to be" (Miller, 1996, p. 2000).

Spiritual care and support may be an important need for both patient and family in an emergency situation, especially if the admitting diagnosis contains a life-threatening dimension. In 1993, Eileen Corcoran (1993), president of the Emergency Nurses Association, posed the question, "Is it reasonable to believe that the emergency room nurse's role includes addressing spiritual needs of patients and their families?" (p. 183). In posing her rhetorical question in the *Journal of Emergency Nursing*, Corcoran admitted that a significant amount of the ER nurse's time must be spent on meeting the patient's physical needs, but she argued that this does not relieve the ER nurse from attention to spiritual needs. Some suggestions Corcoran offered for spiritual care intervention by emergency nurses include establishing a trusting relationship with the patient; maintaining a supportive environment, including providing privacy for patient and family if necessary and identifying religious resources such as the availability of on-call clergy; and finally, recognizing the role of the nurse in "healing the whole person" (p. 184).

Anecdotal reports in the nursing literature document emergency room patients questioning God's will. See "Has God forsaken the emergency department?" (Schlintz, 1987) and "Would God listen to me now?" (Schlintz,

1988). Guthrie (1985), an ER nurse, also recorded the distress of ER patients. Three contemporary emergency department nurses spoke of the need for and experiences in spiritual care in their setting.

Pat, a 19-year ER nursing veteran, worried:

> In the ER you really see the need for spiritual care but sometimes you are moving and working; you feel you are not able to provide much. With death, you always ask, "Would you like us to call a chaplain?" But there are a lot of other needs to minister to, like thinking from a staff nurse's point, dealing with abuse cases, especially the kids.

Ann, with eight years of ER experience, expressed gratitude for her own spirituality:

> Having my own spiritual base really helped me because I've done so much work in the ER and trauma. You see so much death and dying. You only have a few minutes with the patient before you see them die, and you have to support them in that little bit of time. You also deal with supporting the families; they need a lot of spiritual care. It makes you look at life differently; it makes you a different person. . . . Sometimes the chaplains don't get there at the time of a crisis and you are the only one giving support. I can think of many times when I have been the only one there to talk with a family who had just lost a patient. . . .
>
> Nurses need to know how to do ministry especially in the crisis times. I see nursing as a ministry, no question about it. Taking care of these patients in the ER is a ministry in and of itself. There are individuals who incorporate that into their nursing. There are some nurses who may not consciously think about it all the time, but they allow themselves to be used by God. . . . I think that nurses have to work at being truly spiritual people. I think that my own spirituality leads me to being a more feeling individual, to see a client through their own eyes instead of mine.

Helen, head nurse of an emergency department for five years, spoke of spiritual care interventions she had carried out in the ER:

> My coping comes out of a belief that there is a God and that He is loving and generous and forgiving. I always believe that He allows things for a reason and that we can learn from it, the trials and tribulations.

For my patients it's the idea that I am given the gift of taking care of them in the ER, to get them through this crisis. I spend a lot of time talking and listening to them. I touch their hand. I believe there are energies from God that we are not necessarily aware of. I think nursing supports the person in giving this kind of spiritual care.

Finally, Helen spoke about her ER nursing staff:

I am very proud of the spiritual care they give; that is one of our strong points. Sometimes we need to get someone in on the patient, and we call pastoral care to come and sit with the family. It works well in our ER. You need a sense of your own spirituality to function well and take care of patients. I think ideally you address the patients' needs by knowing what you believe in yourself.

SPIRITUAL NEEDS OF THE PATIENT IN PAIN

Although no common definition of pain exists, many nurse clinicians still rely on the pragmatic description first articulated in 1968 by McCaffery. "Pain is whatever the experiencing person says it is, existing whenever the experiencing person says it does" (p. 95). A more contemporary, yet also practical, definition identifies pain as "the state in which an individual experiences and reports the presence of severe discomfort or an uncomfortable sensation" (Gunta, 1993, p. 1538). *Pain* is broadly understood as a word used to reflect a "subjective perception of distress"; the concept may be divided into three major categories: acute pain, chronic pain, and the pain of malignancy (Gildenberg & DeVaul, 1985, pp. 4–5). Acute pain is described as that which "follows acute injury, disease or surgical intervention, and has a rapid onset, varying in intensity [mild to severe], and lasting for a brief time (Potter, 1997, p. 1160). Chronic pain has been characterized as pain that "persists longer than three months," "cannot be eliminated," "often becomes diffuse," "may originally have been acute," and has an "insidious onset" (Watt-Watson & Long, 1993, p. 167). The chronic pain of malignancy is identified as pain that lasts for more than six months, "after tissue damage has healed or in the absence of evident tissue damage" (Gunta, 1993, p. 1541).

Pain, whether acute, chronic, or related to a malignancy, is influenced by a multiplicity of physiological, psychological, sociocultural, and spiritual factors. Therapeutic interventions for the relief of pain include pharmacological (e.g., analgesic drugs) and physiological (e.g., acupuncture, acupressure, cutaneous stimulation, surgery) measures, as well as nonpharmacological measures such as biofeedback, meditation, relaxation, and guided imagery.

Potter (1997) advised that in attempting to provide relief for those in pain, the nurse must remember that the patient interprets and experiences both pain and comfort in light of his or her own "physiological, social, spiritual, psychological, and cultural characteristics" (p. 1154). The National Institute of Nursing Research report, submitted by the priority expert panel on symptom management of acute pain, while including spiritual factors as influential in pain perception and response, also identified the religious ethic as a mediating variable (National Institute of Nursing Research, 1994, p. 30).

Any pain diagnosis may, as noted, be influenced by or contain within its boundaries a spiritual dimension; thus, a nursing diagnosis of spiritual distress may be identified in a patient experiencing chronic pain such as that of malignancy. In a study to explore the management of "spiritual distress in patients with advanced cancer pain," Georgensen and Dungan (1996) identified a list of questions to be used in the assessment of spiritual distress, including, "Has your illness affected your faith/belief system?" "Do you pray? What do you think the power of prayer means?" "Is God or other power important to you?" "How can I assist you in maintaining spiritual strength?" and "Are there religious rituals that are important to you now?" (p. 379). Some defining characteristics for the diagnosis of spiritual distress in patients with advanced cancer pain were anger at God, expressions of helplessness, questioning the meaning and purpose in life, grief, and concerns regarding religious beliefs (p. 381).

Religious beliefs can be particularly important to the pain experience as they may provide support and strength through such activities as prayer (Springhouse Corporation, 1985, p. 21). Religious or spiritual beliefs may also provide the person in pain with a vehicle for finding meaning in suffering, or for "offering" the pain experience to God, in expiation for one's failings or the failings of others. Some individuals, however, may also view pain or suffering as a punishment from God, for example, the concept of *castigo* (punishment) in the Mexican American culture. A nurse or pastor familiar with contemporary theology may be helpful in counseling a patient with this negative perception of God and of the pain experience (Kumasaka, 1996). (The concept of *spiritual pain*, as a distinct dimension of the pain experience, is discussed in chapter 3.)

As well as recommending or participating in prayer (if acceptable to the patient in pain) and seeking counsel of a chaplain, another therapeutic spiritual care activity that the nurse may recommend and teach is the use of spiritual imagery (Ferszt & Taylor, 1988). A suggestion that the patient imagine God as a loving parent holding him or her in His arms and gently loving and caring may do much to comfort the person in pain. Some other spiritual care strategies for alleviating patients' pain include listening with a caring manner to the individual's fears and anxieties related to the pain experience, and facilitating the participation of family members or other significant persons who may be a primary source of support (Turk & Feldman, 1992; Warner, 1992).

Ultimately, as described in spiritual care of acutely ill patients in general, sometimes simply the nurse's presence is an important spiritual intervention. Molly, an advanced cancer patient, although medicated with self-administered analgesics, was experiencing acute pain during her final hospitalization at a clinical research facility. Molly had consistently refused the ministrations of a pastoral caregiver with the excuse that she was too tired and in too much pain to be bothered. One day a chaplain desperate to provide some support for Molly asked gently if she might just sit by her bed and pray silently; the chaplain promised not to talk. Molly acquiesced. She seemed to drowse during most of the chaplain's visit, but opened her eyes periodically to see if the pastoral caregiver was still there. A few days later, as Molly was dying, she asked the staff to call the chaplain to be with her. Molly told the staff, "She's the only one who knows what to say!"

Spiritual care is an important dimension of holistic care for the person with an acute illness or an acute exacerbation of a chronic condition. Spiritual care is also essential for persons experiencing a serious physical or psychosocial challenge related to a perioperative experience, a critical care experience, an emergency room experience, or a pain experience. Often the nurse must employ creative strategies to intervene spiritually for persons who may be experiencing a crisis of faith as well as a serious illness. Ultimately, however, spiritual care is appropriate and acceptable for the nurse working with acutely ill patients.

REFERENCES

Atkinson, L. J., & Fortunato, N. M. (1996). *Berry & Kohn's operating room technique*. St. Louis, MO: Mosby-Yearbook.

Bardanouve, V. E. (1994). Spiritual ministry in the ICU. *Journal of Christian Nursing, 11*(4), 38–39.

Bell, N. (1993). Caring: The essence of critical care nursing. In N. M. Holloway (Ed.), *Nursing the critically ill adult* (4th ed., pp. 14–29). New York: Addison-Wesley.

Blair, F., & Hall, M. (1994). The Klein nursing process: Assessment and priority setting. In A. Klein, G. Lee, A. Manton, & P. Parker, (Eds.), *Emergency nursing core curriculum* (4th ed., pp. 3–23). Philadelphia: W. B. Saunders.

Bucher, L., Wimbush, F., Hardie, J., & Hayes, E. (1997). Near death experiences: Critical care nurses' attitudes and interventions. *Dimensions of Critical Care Nursing, 16*(4), 194–201.

Burnard, P. (1988). The spiritual needs of atheists and agnostics. *The Professional Nurse, 4*(3), 130–132.

Burns, L. (1996). Preoperative nursing management. In S. C. Smeltzer & B. G. Bare (Eds.), *Brunner and Sudarth's textbook of medical–surgical nursing* (8th ed., pp. 357–367). Philadelphia: J. B. Lippincott.

Busch, K. D. (1994). Psychosocial concepts and the patient's experience with critical illness. In C. M. Hudak, B. M. Gallo, & J. J. Benz (Eds.), *Critical care nursing: A holistic approach* (pp. 8–22). Philadelphia: J. B. Lippincott.

Chapman, L. S. (1986, Summer). Spiritual health: A component missing from health promotion. *American Journal of Health Promotion,* 38–41.

Chesla, C., & Stannard, D. (1997). Breakdown in the nursing care of families in the ICU. *American Journal of Critical Care, 6*(1), 64–71.

Clochesy, J. M. (1988). *Essentials of critical care nursing.* Rockville, MD: Aspen Systems.

Corcoran, E. (1993). Spirituality: An important aspect of emergency nursing. *Journal of Emergency Nursing, 19*(3), 183–184.

Dearing, L. (1997). Caring for the perioperative client. In P. A. Potter & A. G. Perry (Eds.), *Fundamentals of nursing: Concepts, process and practice* (pp. 1379–1427). St. Louis, MO: C. V. Mosby.

DiSarcina, A. (1991). Spiritual care at a code. *Journal of Christian Nursing, 8*(3), 20–23.

Dossey, B. M., Guzzetta, C. E., & Kenner, C. (1992). Body, mind, spirit. In B. M. Dossey, C. E. Guzzetta, & C. V. Kenner (Eds.), *Critical care nursing: Body, mind, spirit* (pp. 10–16). Philadelphia: J. B. Lippincott.

Dracup, K. (1995). Key aspects of caring for the acutely ill. In S. G. Funk, E. M. Tornquist, M. T. Champagne, & R. A. Wise (Eds.), *Key aspects of caring for the acutely ill* (pp. 8–22). New York: Springer.

Emergency Nurses Association. (1995). *Standards of emergency nursing practice* (3rd ed.). St. Louis, MO: Mosby-Yearbook.

Fahlberg, L. L., & Fahlberg, L. A. (1991). Exploring spirituality and consciousness with an expanded science. *American Journal of Health Promotion, 5*(4), 273–281.

Fairchild, S. S. (1996). *Perioperative nursing: Principles and practice* (2nd ed.). Boston: Little Brown and Company.

Ferszt, G. G., & Taylor, P. B. (1988). When your patient needs spiritual comfort. *Nursing '88, 18*(4), 48–49.

Georgensen, J., & Dungan, J. M. (1996). Managing spiritual distress in patients with advanced cancer pain. *Cancer Nursing, 19*(5), 376–383.

Gildenberg, P. L., & DeVaul, R. A. (1985). *The chronic pain patient: Evaluation and management.* New York: Karger.

Gillman, J., Gable-Rodriguez, J., Sutherland, M., & Whitacre, J. (1996). Pastoral care in a critical care setting. *Critical Care and Nursing Quarterly, 19*(1), 10–20.

Gunta, K. E. (1993). Chronic pain. In J. M. Thompson, G. K. McFarland, J. E. Hirsch, & S. N. Tucker (Eds.), *Mosby's clinical nursing* (3rd ed., pp. 1538–1543). St. Louis, MO: C. V. Mosby.

Guthrie, J. (1985). E.R.: One nurse's struggle with problem patients and self-righteousness. *Journal of Christian Nursing, 2*(4), 20–21.

Hahn, J. (2001). Ministry in ICU. *Journal of Christian Nursing, 18*(2), 31–32.

Hall, B. A. (1997). Spirituality in terminal illness. *Journal of Holistic Nursing, 15*(1), 82–96.

Hart, C. W. (1994). Spiritual health, illness, and death. *Journal of Religion and Health, 33*(1), 17–22.

Heiser, R., Chiles, K., Fudge, M., & Gray, S. (1997). The use of music during the immediate postoperative recovery period. *Association of Operating Room Nurses Journal, 65*(4), 777–785.

Holt-Ashley, M. (2000). Nurses pray: Use of prayer and spirituality as a complimentary therapy in the intensive care setting. *AACN Clinical Issues: Advanced Practice in Acute and Critical Care, 11*(1), 60–67.

Hopkins, M. (1993). Care of the patient in a critical care unit. In B. Long, W. J. Phipps, & V. L. Cassmeyer (Eds.), *Medical–surgical nursing: A nursing process approach* (3rd ed., pp. 1565–1585). St. Louis, MO: C. V. Mosby.

Kidd, P. S. (1997). Caring for the critically ill patient: Patient, family and nursing considerations. In P. S. Kidd & K. D. Wagner (Eds.), *High acuity nursing* (2nd ed., pp. 3–24). Stamford, CT: Appleton & Lange.

Kozier, B., Erb, G., Blais, K., & Wilkinson, J. (1995). *Fundamentals of nursing: Concepts, process and practice* (5th ed.). Menlo Park, CA: Addison-Wesley.

Kumasaka, L. (1996). My pain is God's will. *American Journal of Nursing, 96*(6), 45–47.

Lazure, L. A., & DeMartinis, J. E. (1997). Basic concepts of emergency care. In J. H. Black & E. Mahassarin-Jacobs (Eds.), *Medical–surgical nursing: Clinical management for continuity of care* (5th ed., pp. 2501–2516). Philadelphia: W. B. Saunders.

Levin, J. S., & Schiller, P. L. (1987). Is there a religious factor in health? *Journal of Religion and Health, 26*(1), 9–36.

Long, B. C. (1993). Problems encountered in emergencies and disasters. In B. Long, W. J. Phipps, & V. L. Cassmeyer (Eds.), *Medical–surgical nursing: A nursing process approach* (3rd ed., pp. 1537–1560). St. Louis, MO: C. V. Mosby.

MacPhail, E. (1992). Overview of emergency nursing and emergency care. In S. Sheehy (Ed.), *Emergency nursing principles and practice* (pp. 1–8). St. Louis, MO: Mosby-Yearbook.

McCaffery, M. (1968). *Nursing practice theories related to cognition, bodily pain, and man–environment interaction.* Los Angeles: University of California at Los Angeles.

McNamara, S. (1995). Perioperative nurses' perceptions of caring practices. *Association of Operating Room Nurses Journal, 61*(2), 377–388.

Meeker, M. H., & Rothrock, J. C. (1995). *Alexander's care of the patient in surgery* (10th ed.). St. Louis, MO: C. V. Mosby.

Michello, J. A. (1988). Spiritual and emotional determinants of health. *Journal of Religion and Health, 27*(1), 62–70.

Miller, K. (1996). Emergency nursing. In S. C. Smeltzer & B. B. Bare (Eds.), *Brunner and Suddarth's textbook of medical–surgical nursing* (8th ed., pp. 2000–2018). Philadelphia: J. B. Lippincott.

National Institute of Nursing Research. (1994). Symptom management: Acute pain, a report of the NINR priority expert panel. Bethesda, MD: Author.

Niklas, G. R., & Stefanics, C. (1975). *Ministry to the hospitalized.* New York: Paulist Press.

Nouwen, H. J. M. (1979). *The wounded healer.* Garden City, NJ: Image Books.

O'Brien, M. E. (1982a). The need for spiritual integrity. In H. Yura & M. B. Walsh (Eds.), *Human needs and the nursing process* (Vol. 2, pp. 85–115). Norwalk, CT: Appleton Century Crofts.

O'Brien, M. E. (1982b). Religious faith and adjustment to long-term hemodialysis. *Journal of Religion and Health, 21*(1), 68–80.

O'Brien, M. E. (1983). *The courage to survive: The life career of the chronic dialysis patient.* New York: Grune & Stratton.

O'Brien, M. E. (1992). *Living with HIV: Experiment in courage.* Westport, CT: Auburn House.

Peterson, V., & Potter, P. A. (1997). Spiritual health. In P. A. Potter & A. G. Perry (Eds.), *Fundamentals of nursing: Concepts, process and practice* (4th ed., pp. 441–456). St. Louis, MO: C. V. Mosby.

Phippen, M. L., Wells, M. P., & Martinelli, A. M. (1994). A conceptual model for perioperative nursing practice. In M. L. Phippen & M. D. Wells (Eds.), *Perioperative nursing practice* (pp. 3–67). Philadelphia: W. B. Saunders.

Potter, P. A. (1997). Comfort. In P. A. Potter & A. G. Perry (Eds.), *Fundamentals of nursing: Concepts, process and practice* (4th ed., pp. 1153–1190). St. Louis, MO: C. V. Mosby.

Potter, P. A., & Perry, A. G. (1997). *Fundamentals of nursing: Concepts, process and practice* (4th ed.). St. Louis, MO: C. V. Mosby.

Reed, P. (1991). Preferences for spiritually related nursing interventions among terminally ill and non-terminally ill hospitalized adults and well adults. *Applied Nursing Research, 4*(3), 122–128.

Robinson, K. (1992). Pre-hospital care. In S. Sheehy (Ed.), *Emergency nursing: Principles and practice* (3rd ed., pp. 9–18). St. Louis, MO: Mosby-Yearbook.

Rothrock, J. C. (1994). The meaning of spirituality to perioperative nurses and their patients. *Association of Operating Room Nurses Journal, 60*(6), 894–895.

Rukholm, E. E., Bailey, P. H., & Coutu-Wakulczyk, G. (1991). Family needs and anxiety in ICU: Cultural differences in Northeastern Ontario. *The Canadian Journal of Nursing Research, 23*(3), 67–81.

Santacaterina, S., & Stein-Spencer, L. (1990). Emergency medicine services. In S. Kidd & J. Kaiser (Eds.), *Emergency nursing: A physiologic and clinical perspective* (pp. 3–12). Philadelphia: W. B. Saunders.

Schlintz, V. (1987). Has God forsaken the emergency department? *Journal of Christian Nursing, 4*(1), 18–19.

Schlintz, V. (1988). Would God listen to me now? *Journal of Christian Nursing, 5*(2), 14–16.

Seidl, L. G. (1993, September). The value of spiritual health. *Health Progress,* 48–50.

Shaffer, J. (1991). Spiritual distress and critical illness. *Critical Care Nurse, 11*(10), 42–45.

Shelly, J. A., & Fish, S. (1995). Praying with patients. *Journal of Christian Nursing, 12*(1), 9–13.

Smeltzer, S. C., & Bare, B. G. (1996), *Brunner and Suddarth's textbook of medical–surgical nursing* (8th ed.). Philadelphia: J. B. Lippincott.

Springhouse Corporation. (1985). *Nursing now series: Pain.* Springhouse, PA: Author.

Stromberg, R. (1992). The voices on coronary care: A confrontation with vulnerability. In L. E. Holst (Ed.), *Hospital ministry: The role of the chaplain today* (pp. 127–138). New York: Crossroad.

Taylor, C., Lillis, C., & LeMone, P. (1997). *Fundamentals of nursing: The art and science of nursing care* (3rd ed.). Philadelphia: J. B. Lippincott.

Turk, D. C., & Feldman, C. S. (1992). Facilitating the use of noninvasive pain management strategies with the terminally ill. *The Hospice Journal, 8*(1), 193–214.

Twibell, R., Wieseke, A., Marine, M., & Schoger, J. (1996). Spiritual and coping needs of critically ill patients: Validation of nursing diagnosis. *Dimensions of Critical Care Nursing, 15*(5), 245–253.

Walleck, C. A. (1989). Spinal cord injury. In K. T. Von Rueden & C. Walleck (Eds.), *Advanced critical care nursing* (pp. 181–203). Rockville, MD: Aspen Systems.

Warner, J. E. (1992). Involvement of families in pain control of terminally ill patients. *The Hospice Journal, 8*(1), 155–170.

Watt-Watson, J. H., & Long, B. C. (1993). Pain. In B. Long, W. J. Phipps, & V. L. Cassmeyer (Eds.), *Medical–surgical nursing: A nursing process approach* (3rd ed., pp. 163–179). St. Louis, MO: C. V. Mosby.

8 ✦ Spiritual Needs of the Chronically Ill Person

Those who wait for the Lord shall renew their strength, they shall mount up
with wings as eagles, they shall run and not be weary, walk and not faint.

ISAIAH 40:31

For the chronically ill individual, personal spirituality and/or religious beliefs and practices often constitute an important, even critical, dimension of coping with the life changes necessitated by the illness experience. This was clearly recognized in the author's longitudinal research with persons facing long-term adaptation to such illnesses as chronic renal failure (CRF) and HIV infection. The corporate élan of both groups was reflected in the titles of books reporting their coping strategies: *The Courage to Survive: The Life Career of the Chronic Dialysis Patient* (O'Brien, 1983) and *Living with HIV: Experiment in Courage* (O'Brien, 1992). For the CRF and HIV-positive study participants, as for many persons living with serious, life-threatening chronic illnesses, it is exquisitely courageous to go on about the business of living, knowing that each new day may possess myriad physical or emotional threats to one's quality of life. For many persons living with chronic illness, transcendent belief and experience provide the impetus to live and to love in the midst of significant pain and suffering. As one eight-year survivor of an HIV-positive diagnosis put it:

> God is the one reliable constant in my life. When I'm feeling unsure
> about everything else, I know that God is with me. I feel it. It's not a
> "head thing." It's in my heart. I almost think I'm being arrogant but
> it really is indescribable, the feeling of the presence of God; it's like
> the hymn puts it: "Standing on Solid Rock." (O'Brien, 1995, p. 129)

This chapter documents spiritual needs in chronic illness as identified in interviews with persons living with such conditions as cancer (including

189

Burkitt's lymphoma), chronic renal failure, depression, and multiple chronic sequelae of HIV infection and AIDS. The patients' spiritual needs are further explained through analysis of interview data elicited from families and professional nurse caregivers. In addition, practicing nurses report and describe specific instances of spiritual care in a variety of settings.

THE CASE OF CHRONIC ILLNESS

Any experience of illness may bring about a degree of disruption in a person's life. Usual patterns of life activity are temporarily, or in some cases permanently, changed or modified to cope with the situation. The need for a major life change occurs more frequently in patients facing chronic illness. Corbin (1996) defined chronic illness as "a medical condition or health problem with associated symptoms or disabilities that require long-term management" (p. 318). Taylor, Lillis, and LeMone (1997) described chronic illness as having the following characteristics: results in "permanent change," "causes or is caused by irreversible alterations in normal anatomy and physiology," "requires special client education for rehabilitation," and "requires a long period of care or support" (p. 61). Currently, chronic illness is considered the "primary health problem in the United States," with some 50% of the population experiencing one or more conditions (Ignatavicius, Workman, & Mishler, 1995, p. 213).

Chronic illness symptoms may range from mild to severe, and often fluctuate between periods of exacerbation and remission (LeMone & Burke, 1996, p. 44). Medical sociologists point out that in cases of chronic illness, frequently the fulfillment of previous roles and responsibilities becomes impossible, and significant reorganization of an individual's patterns of behavior is required. Major changes may occur in social relationships and future life plans, as well as in personal self-concept and self-esteem (Turk & Rudy, 1986, p. 309). The family, especially, may be significantly disrupted by the chronic illness of one of its members, especially when well family members are intimately involved with the care and support of the ill person. Both current and prior nursing research suggest that spiritual well-being is, for many chronically ill persons, a key factor in successful long-term adaptation to the illness condition (Landis, 1996).

SPIRITUAL CARE OF THE CHRONICALLY ILL PATIENT

If, as the literature suggests, an individual's spiritual well-being is central to coping with the physical and psychosocial sequelae of chronic illness, what interventions may a nurse initiate in the provision of spiritual care for a chronically ill patient? And, in what setting(s) will spiritual care for the chronically ill person need to be provided?

The chronically ill person, although most frequently living at home, may also be found in a hospital or clinic setting; the latter in times of illness exacerbation or during the carrying out of diagnostic or therapeutic procedures. The kind of spiritual care provided by the nurse will be influenced by the setting and also by the type and degree of the patient's disability. Physical disability, such as being unable to ambulate freely, may necessitate a creative strategy to facilitate participation in religious rituals, if desired by the client. Spiritual care may also be directed toward the emotional sequelae of chronic illness, which may affect overall spiritual well-being, such as "low self-esteem, feelings of isolation, powerlessness, hopelessness, and anger" (Soeken & Carson, 1987, p. 606). Spiritual interventions that a nurse can initiate in response are an affirmation of God's love and care for each person, encouragement to participate in rituals shared with others, and support for an individual's hope in God's protection (pp. 608–609).

In discussing a "spirituality for the long haul," Muldoon and King (1991) observed that the challenge for the chronically ill person is to integrate the illness experience into his or her self-concept (p. 102). Central to accomplishing this is the support of one's spiritual philosophy undergirding the ultimate meaning and purpose in life.

Spiritual care interventions for the chronically ill *are* similar to those proposed for the acutely ill patient. They include listening to and being with the patient, which may facilitate the integration of spirituality into coping behaviors; praying with a patient, if the patient so desires; reading Scripture, if appropriate; providing spiritual books or other devotional materials; and referring the patient to a clergy member. These spiritual interventions need to be adapted, however, to particular illness conditions and their sequelae, such as mental illness and physical disability, and to specific settings, such as those involving home health care and homelessness, which are discussed later in this chapter. Obviously, careful attention to the patient's religious tradition should precede any spiritual interventions as well as the assessment of spiritual needs.

SPIRITUAL NEEDS IN CHRONIC ILLNESS

All individuals have spiritual needs, regardless of religious belief or personal philosophy of life. The experience of illness, especially of a long-term chronic illness, may be a time when spiritual needs previously unnoticed or neglected become apparent (Baldacchino & Draper, 2001). Spiritual needs may manifest in a multiplicity of symptoms, depending on the person's particular theology, religious tradition, or philosophical understanding of the meaning and purpose of life. For the adherent of one of the monotheistic Western religious groups, Judaism, Christianity, or Islam, spiritual needs are generally associated with one's relationship to God. Shelly and Fish (1988) identified God in the believer's life to be the source of "meaning and purpose, love and relatedness and forgiveness" (p. 38); they asserted that an absence of belief in any one of these factors will result in spiritual need (p. 39). Spiritual needs may also include hope and creativity (Highfield & Cason, 1983, p. 188), as well as reassurance and self-esteem (Cassidy, 1992).

Although assessment of a patient's spiritual needs may be more readily carried out by a practicing nurse, it is often at the stage of intervention that difficulties arise. Although most nurses profess to practice holistic patient care, Forbis (1988) asserted that "they often avoid dealing pragmatically with the spiritual realm" (p. 158). In interviewing nurses prior to designing a course on spiritual care, Ellis (1986) found that many nurses were uncomfortable discussing spiritual issues with patients and were decidedly uneasy about praying with their patients (p. 76). Nurses need to develop an understanding of and comfort with their own spiritual beliefs in order to be at ease discussing spiritual matters with others (Burnard, 1988; McSherry, 1996).

In a study of nurses' perceptions of patients' spiritual needs, Boutell and Bozeht (1988) identified the concepts of faith (in religious beliefs), peace (inner strength), hope, and trust (in the importance of religious practices) (p. 174). Additional needs, those of courage and love, were reflected in nursing research data elicited from chronic renal failure and AIDS patients (O'Brien, 1983, 1992, 1995). The spiritual needs of hope, trust, courage, faith, peace, and love on the part of chronically ill persons are explored in the following pages; examples of these characteristics are drawn from the comments of individuals experiencing such illness conditions as cancer, HIV infection and AIDS, and chronic renal failure.

Hope

And now, O Lord, what do I wait for? My hope is in you.

PSALM 39:7

Hope, as a general term, relates to an anticipation that something desired will occur. Hope, or the act of hoping, defined theologically for a member of a monotheistic religious tradition, is the "focusing of attention, affectivity and commitment to action toward the future goal of fulfillment in God, the realization of the reign of God" (Hellwig, 1993, p. 506). Shelly and Fish (1988) pointed out that placing one's hope in God does not mean an immediate end to suffering or anxiety; rather, hoping relates to trust in God's support during a crisis (p. 44). Both clinical anecdotes and research have documented the fact that when a patient loses hope and the will to live, death may result (Ross, 1994, p. 440). Thus, supporting and nurturing hope is described as a "vital ingredient" in a nurse's plan of spiritual care (Gewe, 1994; Le Peau, 1996; Thompson, 1994).

Phillip, a young adult cancer patient who described himself as a born-again Christian, manifested a beautifully direct sense of hope as he faced his illness:

> I put all my hope in Jesus, in the Cross. I have my daily minute with Him. I mean, it's about an hour, but I call it my "minute." I try to always have the special "minutes." I pray to Jesus; He is with me. Jesus is my hope.

Because of his disease, an anaplastic astrocytoma, Phillip's speech patterns were sometimes difficult to follow; by listening carefully, however, one could understand his meaning; his eyes were very expressive as he spoke about his relationship with Jesus. On a page in his Bible, Phillip had written "Born again in Jesus"; he explained, "That's when I accepted Him, and now He's always with me."

Trust

I trust in you, O Lord, I say, "You are my God."

PSALM 31:14

The concept of trust indicates having confidence in something or someone. Theologically, the term is considered to be a relational one, "describing the quality of a relationship among two or more persons" (Schreiter, 1993, p. 982). The Hebrew word for trust, which occurs frequently in the Old Testament, "refers most often to trust in God" (p. 982). Possessing the ability to trust in others is considered "essential to spiritual health" (Simsen, 1988, p. 33).

In discussing adaptation to chronic illness, nursing scholar Ruth Stoll (1989) noted that "a dynamic spiritual belief system enables us to trust that somehow tomorrow will not be beyond our capacities" (p. 195). Trusting, for the ill person who is a believer, will give a sense of security that God's healing power will be operative in his or her life (Johnson, 1992, p. 92). It is important to recognize, however, that the "healing" that occurs may be of a spiritual or emotional nature, rather than a physical healing.

A recently married and newly diagnosed Burkitt's lymphoma patient, David, spoke eloquently to the concept of trust:

> Well, this is not what I had expected at this time in my life but this is the Cross, the folly of the Cross they say, so I put it in the hands of the "man upstairs." I mean I'm really with Him and He's with me, you know. . . . I have to tell you, though, even with my faith, we're all human, and I was really scared in the beginning. When they first brought me in to the hospital, they rolled me into that ICU, through the doors, and I saw all that equipment and those monitors, I thought: "Whoa! Is this the Cross?" But you know that God is going to be walking beside you.

David's life had, he admitted, been "turned upside down" by his diagnosis and hospitalization, and yet he described a sense of comfort in knowing that this, for him, was God's will. He laughingly commented that this kind of attitude would, he knew, be considered "folly" by some; for David it was, quite simply, a matter of trust.

Courage

> *I took courage for the hand of the Lord, my God, was upon me.*
>
> EZRA 7:28

Courage, or emotional strength, is described not as the absence of fear, but rather as "the ability to transcend one's fears, to choose to actively face what needs to be" (Stoll, 1989, p. 196).

Martha, an adult woman in midlife diagnosed with chronic renal failure and experiencing maintenance hemodialysis, spoke openly about the need for courage to face a life dependent on technology:

> You have to get yourself together and face the thing; be courageous about it because nobody is going to do it for you. I think adjusting to kidney failure and dialysis is very difficult because I can't answer why. Why did this happen to me? But my faith says that all things

have a reason, and God won't put anything on us that we can't bear. . . . But it's still difficult because chronic illnesses may be with you a long time before they lead to dying; you have to have some courage about it.

We, as nurses, long to do something for those with whom we work: to heal, to cure, to alleviate the suffering of our courageous patients and their families. Yet frequently we must accept that such accomplishments are beyond our power; we must learn to accept that our desire to comfort and our empathy are, of themselves, an important dimension of nursing care.

Faith

Daughter, your faith has made you well.

LUKE 8:48

Faith means belief or trust in someone or something. From a theological perspective, faith is the basis of our personal relationship with God "on whose strength and absolute sureness we can literally stake our lives" (Fatula, 1993, p. 379). Faith is identified as "a prerequisite for spiritual growth" (Carson, 1989, p. 28), and faith in God is often a critical element in surviving a loss (Sandin, 1996) or coping with an illness experience (Ross, 1994). A holistic nursing philosophy suggests that religious faith may give one the strength to "combat disease and facilitate healing" (Kennison, 1987, p. 29).

An example of the support provided by personal faith in coping with an advanced cancer diagnosis was reflected in Matthew's perception of his condition:

I can't question how I got this disease or what God's plan is for me. But I know my faith will get me through. At a time like this, faith is the key. My faith makes me strong. Chemo is tough but God's in that too. I don't know; I just know my faith will get me to the place I need to be.

Peace

May the Lord give strength to His people, may the Lord bless His people with peace.

PSALM 29:11

Peace is a sense of being undisturbed, a feeling of freedom from anxiety and fear. Theologically, peace is described as being derived from "a right relationship with God, which entails forgiveness, reconciliation and union" (Dwyer, 1990, p. 749). In a study of spiritual well-being (SWB), researcher David Moberg found that, according to most respondents' perceptions, two significant indicators of SWB were "peace with God" and "inner peace" (1979, p. 9).

Two chronic renal failure patients on maintenance hemodialysis described the peace their religious faith afforded them in relation to their disease and treatment regimens. Carolyn, who had been on dialysis for over three years, asserted:

> Well, I think if I didn't believe in God and have the religious beliefs I have, I don't think I'd be able to survive this. I don't think I'd have any peace. I think I probably would have attempted suicide at one time or another. But my faith helps me be optimistic about it; it really helps.

And Elizabeth, a two-year veteran of dialytic therapy, reported that the illness experience had a positive effect on her personal spirituality:

> My faith has really strengthened. I'm still a good old "knee-slapping" Baptist. I still love my pastor and I enjoy going to church on Sunday. I pray a lot, but I don't want to ask too much. I'm at peace. If healing is for me, then it will come to me. I just take the attitude that I don't worry about it. God will provide.

Love

How precious is your steadfast love, O God.

PSALM 36:7

To love means to care for or to treasure someone or something. Love, from a religious perspective, relates to "God's benevolent love"; thus, "by association, God's love encompasses human love for God, human love for neighbor, human love for creation, and self-love" (Dreyer, 1993, p. 613). Shelly and Fish (1988) asserted that God's love will be with one, unconditionally, during a crisis such as illness (pp. 46–47), and that His supportive love is best reflected in the Old Testament Scripture, Isaiah 43:2–3:

When you pass through raging waters, I will be with you;
in the river you shall not drown.
When you walk through fire, you shall not be burned;
the flames shall not consume you.
For I am the Lord, your God, the Holy One of Israel,
your savior.

Mary Grace, a cancer patient, described the importance of God's love as manifested by her church:

Well the one thing that helps you deal with this is that you know that your church is behind you. The pastor, he remembers to call you and the church members come to visit and the deacons bring me my Communion to the house. All those things make me feel good; they make me feel loved.

Tom, a 37-year-old lymphoma patient and a practicing attorney who described his personal spirituality as "secular humanism," also admitted the need for love in coping with his diagnosis:

I'm not sure about the "God thing"—I mean whether God exists or not. But I believe in human goodness and the responsibility we have to each other and to the universe. I don't lean on any religion to help me live with this disease, but I do rely on my family and friends who love me. That's what gets me through the day, knowing I'm loved.

Cancer, HIV/AIDS, and CRF are three chronic illness syndromes from which many individuals currently suffer. Examples of data-based spiritual needs of the oncology patient, the HIV-positive patient, and the CRF patient can serve to guide spiritual care therapeutics for persons suffering from other chronic illnesses that a nurse may encounter.

SPIRITUAL NEEDS OF THE CANCER PATIENT

The term *cancer* is a broad label that covers a family of diseases characterized by uncontrollable growth of mutated cells that may disseminate to various parts of the body. Cancerous growths originate in various tissues or organs, differ in size and appearance, develop in a variety of ways, and respond differently to therapeutic interventions (Petty, 1997, p. 533). Roughly 20 percent of all deaths in the United States are attributable to some form of the approximately 12 major and 50 minor types of cancer (LeMone & Burke,

1996, p. 306). Because of the serious, life-threatening nature of most cancer diagnoses, the spiritual needs of the patient may be significant. A study of 45 adult cancer patients (with diagnoses such as breast cancer, lung cancer, and leukemia) revealed that religious belief was a source of strength and comfort in coping with the illness (Moschella, Pressman, Pressman, & Weissman, 1997). Moschella et al. found that patients diagnosed with cancer reported an increase in faith, more time spent in prayer, and greater frequency of church attendance, despite the fact that their religious belief systems provided no theological explanation for suffering (1997, p. 17). Findings from research with 114 adult cancer patients indicated a positive association between high levels of spiritual well-being and lower levels of anxiety (Kaczorowski, 1989). Spiritual well-being, as evaluated in a study of 175 breast cancer patients, was demonstrated to be highest in those women who were classified as intrinsically religious, that is, those who internalized their religious belief as a core motivator in life (Mickley, Soeken, & Belcher, 1992). Highfield (1992) found the spiritual health of 23 primary lung cancer patients to be high when normed according to the current literature on spirituality and cancer. Highfield posited some reasons: the study participants' reliance on spiritual resources, and a greater degree of spiritual development, related either to age or the terminal diagnosis (p. 7).

Research on the attitudes and beliefs about spiritual care among Oncology Nursing Society members revealed that the community held the nurse's role of providing spiritual care in high regard (Taylor, Highfield, & Amenta, 1994). The study of 181 members of the Oncology Nursing Society reported spiritual care behaviors such as talking with patients about spiritual or religious matters; referring patients to other spiritual caregivers such as chaplains or clergy; praying with or for a patient; supporting a patient's family; facilitating the use of religious or devotional resources; and being with and touching the patient, with a supportive and nonjudgmental attitude (Taylor, Amenta, & Highfield, 1995, p. 36). Recent nursing research has also demonstrated the increasing role of spiritual caring among oncology nurses (Thomas & Retsas, 1999); the importance of the nurse's sensitivity to diverse cultural and religious traditions (Lackey, Gates, & Brown, 2001); and nurses' recognition of the uniqueness of individualized spiritual experience for oncology patients (Halstead & Hull, 2001; MacDonald, 2001).

Some additional research on the spiritual needs of cancer patients includes the work of McClain, Rosenfeld, and Breitbart in "Effect of Spiritual Well-Being on End-of-Life Despair in Terminally Ill Cancer Patients" (2003) and in "Spiritual Care Nursing: What Cancer Patients and Family Caregivers Want" (Taylor & Mamier, 2005).

Spiritual care for Mrs. Anna Smithfield, an advanced ovarian cancer patient participating in an experimental chemotherapy protocol, consisted primarily of listening and supporting the patient's existing spiritual and religious beliefs and traditions. Mrs. Smithfield's religious tradition was Methodist; her nurse, Beth, was Roman Catholic. At their first meeting, Beth and Mrs. Smithfield discussed their denominational differences; they agreed, however, that as Christians they really had more similarities in belief than differences. Mrs. Smithfield was receiving spiritual support from her pastor and church members. What she needed to talk to Beth about was her fear of leaving her husband of 26 years alone. She was also saddened over the fact that her young grandchildren would never get to know her as "grandmother." For Beth, the primary spiritual care intervention was to sit with Mrs. Smithfield, to listen, and to talk with her about her family; they also prayed together. Beth made a point to drop in when Mr. Smithfield visited, because the patient had expressed the wish that he meet her nurse; this provided Beth the opportunity to be available for Mr. Smithfield who also needed spiritual support in his anxiety over his wife's prognosis.

SPIRITUAL NEEDS OF THE HIV-INFECTED PERSON

Human immunodeficiency virus (HIV) infection, identified in 1983 under the acronym LAV (lymphadenopathy associated virus), and in 1984 as HTLV III (human t-cell lymphotropic virus) has progressed through many phases and mutations over the last 15 years; numerous therapeutic protocols have been tested on both the virus and related opportunistic infections with varying degrees of efficacy. Although HIV infection in the United States was originally a disease of white gay men, currently the condition is more prevalent in the black and Hispanic communities (Ungvarski & Matassarin-Jacobs, 1997). The clinical course of HIV infection is directed by the immune system response, with the development of opportunistic infection symptoms such as fever, malaise, sweating, headache, weight loss, sore throat, and rashes, among others (Lisanti & Zwolski, 1997). HIV infection may progress to a stage officially categorized as AIDS (acquired immunodeficiency syndrome) related to a variety of immune system parameters and symptomatology.

Countless psychosocial concerns related to both the seriousness and stigma of HIV infection have been identified in the nursing research literature; spiritual and religious needs are central among these (Belcher, Dettmore, & Holzemer, 1989; Carson, Soeken, Shanty, & Terry, 1990; Mellors, Riley, & Erlen, 1997; O'Brien, 1992; O'Brien, 1995; O'Brien & Pheifer, 1993;

Warner-Robbins & Christiana, 1989). There has also been a plethora of books published during the past decade on the topics of spirituality, religion, and pastoral care for people living with HIV and AIDS. Some examples that may prove useful resources for the nurse in providing spiritual care are *The Gospel Imperative in the Midst of AIDS* (Iles, 1989); *The Church with AIDS* (Russell, 1990); *Ministry to Persons with AIDS* (Perelli, 1991); *Embracing the Mystery: A Prayerful Response to AIDS* (Sandys, 1993); *AIDS, Ethics and Religion: Embracing a World of Suffering* (Overberg, 1994). Nevertheless, contemporary nursing literature suggests that spirituality remains a neglected area of concern in the assessment of HIV patients' needs (Newshan, 1998; Sherman, 2001). Nurses' current study and understanding of spirituality will help them identify spiritual needs and concerns among persons with HIV and AIDS (O'Neill & Kenny, 1998).

Spiritual care of the person living with HIV or AIDS may take many forms depending on the stage and current symptomatology of the illness. It is important to keep in mind that some HIV-positive persons who have become alienated from their churches may not be receiving formal religious ministry because of the stigma of the disease (Perelli, 1991). That, however, is a situation that can be remedied, if the patient and church desire. Some suggestions for spiritual care for the HIV-positive person that may be carried out by a nurse include listening to the patient's "stories" surrounding the illness (Crowther, 1991); offering small gestures of friendship, which may be missing in the alienated patient's life (AIDS Ministry Program, 1991); providing empathy and emotional support (Sunderland & Shelp, 1987); allowing the patient to take the lead in the offering of prayer (Christensen, 1991); and presenting the patient with a nonjudgmental attitude (Smith, 1988). For the HIV-positive individual who is physically and cognitively well enough to participate, activities such as creating and appreciating religious art or poetry may provide healing for the heart (Roche, 1992).

John Michael, who had lost many friends to AIDS and who had been living with an HIV diagnosis for over six years, began to write poetry as a way of coping with his illness. A nurse researcher provided spiritual support by listening to and appreciating John Michael's poetry. Reading the poetry often provided an opening to discuss spiritual issues related to both living and dying with the human immunodeficiency virus. One poem, entitled "The Touch of the Maestro," reveals the impact of the HIV experience on John Michael's personal spirituality. In the piece, the poet muses on how HIV disease has alerted him to the fragility of the human condition and has brought into focus the importance of transcendent issues; this is reflected in the final stanza:

*Never again, will I find satisfaction from a mundane
    ordinary success.
There is only one reward that needs to be filled,
That is the plucking of the instrument that is my heart, which now
    only sings at the touch of the Maestro.*

(O'Brien, 1995, p. 126,
reprinted with permission of the poem's author)

SPIRITUAL NEEDS OF THE CHRONIC RENAL FAILURE PATIENT

Matassarin-Jacobs (1997) defined chronic renal failure (CRF) as irreversible and "progressive reduction of functioning renal tissue such that the remaining kidney mass can no longer maintain the body's internal environment" (p. 1641). CRF may result from any one of a variety of diseases such as polycystic kidney disease, glomerulonephritis, and pyelonephritis; CRF may also accompany other illness conditions such as diabetes mellitus or hypertension. CRF, if undetected and untreated, generally progresses unilaterally through three stages: diminished renal function, renal insufficiency, and uremia. As a patient progresses toward the critical uremic stage, with symptoms of greatly decreased urine output, fatigue, nausea, and general malaise, dialytic therapy is usually considered. The four major modes of dialysis currently in use are hemodialysis, peritoneal dialysis, continuous ambulatory peritoneal dialysis (CAPD), and continuous cyclic peritoneal dialysis (CCPD). Hemodialysis employs a machine with a "semipermeable filtering membrane [artificial kidney] that removes accumulated waste products from the blood" (Kilpatrick, 1997, p. 1298). The peritoneal dialysis methods cleanse the blood by filling the abdominal cavity with dialysate (electrolyte solution) and using the peritoneum as a filter for waste not excreted by the kidneys. Any method of dialytic therapy, combined with the diagnosis of renal failure, may prove extremely stressful for the CRF patient and family (Flaherty & O'Brien, 1992; Korniewicz & O'Brien, 1994; O'Brien, 1990; O'Brien, Donley, Flaherty, & Johnstone, 1986).

Among the psychosocial sequelae of CRF and its treatment modality, perhaps the least studied yet possibly most important factor relates to the patient's spiritual or religious needs. In a recent nursing study of hemodialysis patients' needs, according to family perception, one of those most frequently identified was the patients' desire to feel "cared for" by their nurses (Wagner, 1996). For CRF patients "who live totally dependent upon [technology] for their continued existence, the need for truly caring nursing staff is key. For these patients, also, the quality of life may become questionable"; thus, a multiplicity of spiritual or ethical concerns can result for patients and families (O'Brien, 1983, p. 35).

The study of religious faith and long-term adaptation to CRF described in chapter 3 revealed that 78 percent of the 126 maintenance hemodialysis patients studied believed that religious beliefs were to some degree associated with their ability to cope with CRF and the related treatment regimen (O'Brien, 1983). Open-ended questioning of the same group of study respondents produced comments such as, "I knew everything would be alright [after cardiac arrest] because I asked God to carry me through. I know that He's got His arms around me." Another patient, after reporting that faith had been very important in coping with the illness, asserted, "A lot of people couldn't have gone through what I went through without faith in God" (O'Brien, 1982, p. 76).

For the CRF patient, often it is the therapeutic regimen, especially if consisting of maintenance hemodialysis carried out in a dialysis center, that is the most trying. One new hemodialysis patient admitted that the treatment regimen was the most difficult part of the CRF experience. "I pray to God all the time to help me stay on my treatment and to do what I have to do." The remarks of several other hemodialysis patients reflected a similar theme. "Without my religious faith, I couldn't make it"; "Religious faith really helps you go on"; "Without faith I don't know what I'd do"; and "If it hadn't been for my religion, I wouldn't even be here now" (O'Brien, 1983, p. 37).

Spiritual nursing care for the CRF maintenance dialysis patient should incorporate some element of spiritual or religious support that facilitates coping with the altered quality of life imposed by the disease and its treatment regimen. Virtually all dialysis patients report moderate to severe symptoms of fatigue and general malaise that periodically interfere with social and professional or work activities. As Joseph, a young businessman, described:

> You have to pull yourself up and do for yourself. You can't keep waiting for everybody else. Sometimes when I get up in the morning I feel bad, but I just get up and go to my business and make myself keep busy. You have to accept the fact that your kidneys are gone but you can still do things. A lot of it's in your own head, how you feel about it, how you accept it. (O'Brien, 1983, p. 40)

For a CRF patient who adheres to the theology of Reform Judaism, such as Joseph, a dimension of spiritual care might consist in exploring how his religious tradition views God's role in trials such as chronic illness. Joseph stated that "how you feel about" the illness influences "how you accept it." A comforting Scripture for Joseph might be Isaiah 43:2 ("When you pass through raging waters") or Jeremiah 29:11–12 ("For I know well the plans I have in mind for you, says the Lord, plans for your welfare, not for woe. Plans to give you a future full of hope."). Such a reading might provide the opportunity to discuss the need for hope in light of the CRF diagnosis and therapeutic regimen.

SPIRITUAL NEEDS OF THE MENTALLY CHALLENGED

The Person with Mental Illness

Mental health and *mental illness* are relative terms, existing along a continuum of attitude and behavior; the label *mental illness* covers a vast array of diagnostic categories, ranging from mild conditions, such as situational anxiety and depression, to the frank psychosis of schizophrenic disorders. The concepts are culturally determined also. What may be considered pathological in one society, such as the trancelike states entered into during some West Indian religious rituals, is normal according to the perception of that particular community. In order to determine functional mental status, some factors to be evaluated include "level of consciousness, orientation, memory, mood and affect, intellectual performance, judgement and insight and language and communication" (Bruegge, 1997, p. 715). Problems in any of these areas may reflect a deficit in one's mental health, whether of a temporary or a more lasting nature.

Mental health viewed from a Christian perspective is defined as "a state of dynamic equilibrium characterized by hope, joy and peace, in which positive self-regard is developed through love, relationship, forgiveness and meaning and purpose resulting from a vital relationship with God, and a responsible interdependence with others" (Shelly & John, 1983, p. 27). In exploring mental health for the person who does not embrace a monotheistic spirituality, this definition may be modified in terms of relationship with a deity.

The current standards of psychiatric mental health nursing identify spiritual variables as important to the nurse, who is advised to be attentive to the "interpersonal, systemic, sociocultural, spiritual or environmental circumstances or events which affect the mental and emotional well-being of an individual, family or community" (American Nurses Association, 1994, as cited in Carson, 1997, p. 144). Nurses who work with those categorized as mentally ill admit that assessing spiritual needs for the psychiatric patient is a difficult task. Frequently, the patient's manifestation of spiritual concerns is considered to be "part of the client's pathology" (Mickley, Carson, & Soeken, 1995; Peterson & Nelson, 1987, p. 34). Assessing the psychiatric patient's spiritual needs may be confounded by the individual's altered thought processes (Varcarolis, 1994; Walgrove, 1996), including religious delusions and hallucinations (Fontaine, 1995c, p. 305). Judith Shelly (1983) pointed out, however, that it is precisely the fact that so many psychiatric clients do manifest religiously oriented delusions or distortions in thinking that highlights the presence of spiritual need (p. 55). Shelly observed, "Clients tend to distort only those things that are intensely meaningful to them" (p. 56). It is important, in providing spiritual care to the mentally disturbed, that a nurse understand how a patient's religious or spiritual beliefs may interact with illness symptoms. For example, in the case of an individual who perceives suffering as a penance for past sins, prayer may be "as much a part" of the healing as therapy (Shoemaker, 1996, p. 298). Another facet of mental illness, which may be supported by prayer, is that of loss of faith in God or a distancing from God, which is "a common occurrence during depressive episodes" (Fontaine, 1995b, p. 243). Suggesting the use of prayer to a client needs to be done judiciously, related to the individual's personal spiritual and religious tradition; for the client with a theistic world view, however, prayer is identified as "one of the main spiritual tools for seeking God's help" (Walsh & Carson, 1996, p. 498). The lack of attention to spiritual care in some instances of mental health nursing has been associated with reliance on a medical model of care (Greasley, Chiu, & Gartland, 2001). It is suggested, nevertheless, that spiritual needs must be included in effective mental health nursing practice (Fry, 1998; Weaver et al., 1998).

To assist the nurse in distinguishing a psychiatric client's spiritual needs from those directly related to his or her mental health condition, John (1983) suggested a series of questions relating to such issues as whether a person's religious belief or behavior seems to contribute to the illness, whether religious concerns reflect a pathological inner conflict, whether religious beliefs and behavior bring comfort or distress, and whether religion is used merely as a context for psychotic delusions (pp. 81–83). In the case of a religiously oriented delusion, the role of the person providing spiritual care is to "support the person but not the delusion" (Wagner, 1992, p. 156). A case example offered by Wagner is that of a psychiatric patient who asserted that because he has not done God's will, God has "taken away his brain"; the patient questioned whether God will give it back. In this situation, Wagner contended, the spiritual caregiver should focus not on the delusion or any interpretations, but rather "support the reality of God's continued love and care" for the patient (p. 156). As noted throughout this discussion, a different strategy of spiritual support will need to be provided for the psychiatric client who is not from a monotheistic religious tradition.

An example of a nursing diagnosis associated with a moderately serious condition such as mood disorder is "Spiritual distress related to no purpose or joy in life; lack of connectedness to others; misperceived guilt" (Fontaine, 1995b, p. 253). Assessment of decreased spiritual well-being, associated with depression in older women, is also a diagnosis amenable to nursing intervention (Morris, 1996).

Angela McBride (1996) emphasized caring as a key dimension of the psychiatric–mental health nurse's role (p. 7); caring includes sensitivity to the values, beliefs, and practices of an individual, which is identified as the "first step" toward nursing competence in the provision of spiritual care for the patient with a mental health deficit (Campinha-Bacote, 1995, p. 24). In a study of 50 psychiatric–mental health nurses, the nurses' personal spiritual perspectives were found to be notably high (Pullen, Tuck, & Mix, 1996, p. 85). Spiritual interventions reported by the mental health nurses included "being with," or spending time with, the client; "doing for," or employing personal and environmental resources to care for the client; "encouraging the client to look inward for strength"; and "encouraging the client to look outward for people and objects that could be resources" (Tuck, Pullen, & Lynn, 1997, p. 351).

Finally, an article published by the American Psychiatric Association entitled "Psychiatrists Urge More Direct Focus on Patients' Spirituality" noted, "Many patients have spiritual needs that when addressed in psychiatric treatment help unearth important existential issues and strengthen the therapeutic relationship" (Bender, 2004).

Specific spiritual care interventions for the psychiatric client will vary greatly, depending not only on the patient's identified needs, but also on personal spiritual and religious history. For this patient population, especially, the nurse will need to employ the art, as well as the science, of nursing.

Mathias Johnson was a 66-year-old patient suffering from moderate depression associated with a multiplicity of physical ailments, as well as financial and situational stressors. Mr. Johnson's chart identified him as Baptist, although he admitted that he was not a frequent church attender. After spending about 15 minutes visiting with Mr. Johnson, during which time he spoke briefly about faith, his nurse Beth asked if he would like her to say a prayer before leaving. Mr. Johnson nodded in the affirmative. Beth took Mr. Johnson's hand and offered a brief prayer, asking God to give Mr. Johnson strength and comfort during his illness; she also prayed that God would let the patient feel his love and care. As Beth was concluding the prayer, she noticed that tears were streaming down Mr. Johnson's face; she handed him a tissue without comment. After taking a few deep breaths, Mr. Johnson looked up and said with a smile, "Thank you, I really needed that!"

Attempting to analyze and understand the spiritual needs of a mentally ill patient, especially a depressed individual, is extremely challenging to the nurse. Much time may be spent in simply encouraging the patient to verbalize his or her concerns. During the interaction, however, the nurse can communicate a sense of care and empathy, sometimes opening the door to the possibility of therapeutic intervention in the area of spiritual need.

The Cognitively Impaired Client

Cognitive functioning affects both physical and psychosocial dimensions of an individual's life. Although cognition is "primarily an intellectual and perceptual process, [it is] closely integrated with . . . emotional and spiritual values" (Arnold, 1996, p. 977). The cognitively disabled person may have been diagnosed from infancy with some degree or type of mental retardation; cognitive processes may have been injured during childhood or early to middle adulthood as a result of illness or traumatic injury; or a cognitive disability may have its onset only in the elder years, in cases such as senile dementia (the spiritual care of the senile dementia or Alzheimer's patient is discussed in chapter 9).

In the past, the religious community has raised some concern as to the role of the cognitively disabled individual in the church or worship setting. Some have questioned whether a person who is not cognitively functional can have a relationship with God, much less understand the meaning of religious practices. Reverend John Swinton (1997), a minister and former psychiatric–mental health nurse, admitted that theological confusion still exists about the spiritual and religious capabilities of persons with profound cognitive disabilities, and that some believe that to allow "sacramental participation without intellectual comprehension is dishonoring to God" (p. 21). Swinton argued, however, that "faith is not an intellectual exercise but relational reality," and that relationship to God is for any of us a mystery beyond intellectual understanding (pp. 21–22). True affective understanding of God, Swinton concluded, occurs at a much more interior level than that of intellectual comprehension (p. 23). Swinton's position is supported by ethicist Stanley Hauerwas (1995), who pointed out that, although including cognitively handicapped persons in worship services may not be easy, the extent to which they may bring about the unexpected is a reminder that "the God we worship is not easily domesticated" (p. 60). Hauerwas contended that "in worship the church is made vulnerable to a God who would rule this world not by coercion but by the unpredictability of love" (p. 60).

In a video entitled *We Are One Flock*, produced by the National Catholic Office for Persons with Disabilities (1990), a young woman with Down syndrome is shown assisting with the distribution of the Holy Eucharist during Mass. Her comments after the service reflect the validity of her active participation in the Eucharistic liturgy. "My idea about God is you feel it in your heart. When you really love God and you know He's around you, you feel it in your heart. And I feel it when I'm singing and when I'm ministering, and that brings me close to God, really close when I'm ministering."

A magnificent example of spiritual care for the profoundly cognitively impaired is that carried out in L'Arche (the Ark) communities founded by French Canadian philosopher Jean Vanier. Vanier (1975) began his work during a visit to the small town of Trosly, France, when he moved into a house with two mentally handicapped men. Gradually, other mentally challenged persons began to come, together with volunteers to live with and care for them. New L'Arche communities started to flourish under Vanier's spiritual philosophy of responsibility to care for one's brothers and sisters; this caring was to be done as in a family, where all are accepted and equal as God's children. Henri Nouwen, who spent his later years living in a L'Arche community in Canada, wrote, "Today, L'Arche is a word that inspires thousands of people all over the world . . . its vision is a source of hope" (1988, p. 13).

Evelyn, a veteran of 30 years in nursing, reported that she had worked for the past 13 years in an intermediate care facility (ICF), for the profoundly mentally retarded. Evelyn described her first encounter with the ICF patients:

> The youngest was about 12 and that's around the age my children were. They looked strange, and they acted strange. I didn't have any experience in this field of nursing. And I said, "I will never be able to do this!" I questioned God. I said, "Why? I just can't see the value of their lives. This is just too sad." . . . Every day I would walk home from work and every day I would cry, because I felt like I wouldn't ever be able to help them. I wouldn't ever have any impact on their lives. But then one day something just started to happen, and I started to realize how they were God's children and they began to have an impact on my life. And then, I began to see that each one has their own personality. They became special to me. And I started to think that even if they live on earth for only 20 or 30 years, they are going to live in heaven forever. . . .

Now they serve such purpose in my life, I couldn't imagine living my life without them. They have become so unique. Now I try to give them spiritual care. I try to anticipate their needs; I try to communicate with them and they do communicate, even if it is nonverbal. . . .

I don't get to do as much "hands on" as I would like to but when I do it's such a gift. I'm so grateful. There is something so holy. You say, "this person is completely dependent upon my hands and my compassion to be cared for." They depend solely upon you. If you let yourself be used by God, this is what spiritual care means to me.

Another ICF nurse, Sarah, commented that her Jewish faith supported her spiritual care of cognitively impaired patients. "I don't believe that God is sitting up somewhere looking down on us, but I believe He is all around us. I believe that the Spirit of goodness and giving all around us is God; that's how I live spirituality." Sarah spoke about her interaction with the ICF patients. "I talk to them as people, even the very lowest cognitively functioning person is still a person, so I try to explain things to them. I also try to see that they get the best possible care that we can give. I think there is a 'spirituality of touch' in the holding and the caring. I know we can't change their abilities, but we can make sure the quality of their lives is as good as possible." Sarah concluded, "I think that the patients understand a lot more than we think sometimes. I think we can bring our spirituality and our God to them, even though we think it is beyond their intellectual functioning ability. I think my caring brings them spirituality."

Marti, another nurse who had worked with cognitively impaired young adults for many years, added, "I feel very humble in working with the MRDD [mentally retarded, developmentally disabled] population. I know their intelligence and cognitive functioning isn't where ours is, but they have a perception of reality that is childlike and Godlike all at the same time. I think touching them and loving them is spiritual care."

SPIRITUAL NEEDS IN PHYSICAL DISABILITY AND REHABILITATION

Who are those persons on whom our society imposes the label "disabled"? Theologian Michael Downey (1993) believes that, excluding those who may temporarily require special attention such as infants and young children, the very elderly, and persons incapacitated for a time due to illness or accident, the term *disabled* generally describes individuals who are to some degree permanently impaired (p. 273). Downey defined the disabled as those

persons "whose capacities of mind or body are diminished in any way during the pre, peri or post natal period or at some later period in the course of
psychosomatic development, so as to necessitate particular attention or
special assistance in meeting basic human needs" (1993, p. 273).

Disability may affect all dimensions of an individual's life: physical,
social, emotional, and spiritual. The goal of rehabilitation is to return to the
disabled person as much preillness functioning in each of those life arenas
as possible. Ultimately the goal of the rehabilitation process is to help an
individual regain as much independence as possible. In analyzing the
"anatomy of illness," Schreiter (1988) posited that experiencing illness for a
disabled person is like taking a long journey to an unknown country: "disabled persons leave behind their accustomed ways of relating to their bodies, their friends, their workplaces, their families" (p. 7). McBride and
Armstrong (1995) suggested, additionally, that while no standardized tests
currently exist to measure "spiritual damage," "something does happen to
the spiritual development of a person who is traumatized" (p. 7). Theologian
Donald Senior (1995) pointed out that although an authentic response would
be to bear the illness in a "spirit of Faith," persons with disabilities need spiritual support in the process of achieving fullness of life (p. 17). Even though
Congress passed the Americans with Disabilities Act (ADA) in 1990, making
it illegal to discriminate against the handicapped, individuals who make up
our churches have not always internalized a supportive attitude for the disabled (Krafft, 1988).

In a book discussing the "psychospiritual aspects of rehabilitation,"
Carolyn Vash (1994) observed that "disability is a symbol we all fear"; this, she
asserted, is why religion has not well supported the disabled (p. 49). Vash
demonstrated through numerous examples from history that disabled individuals such as Helen Keller can use adversity to achieve significant life
goals. The rehabilitation nurse may refer to such role models in providing
spiritual care.

The concept of spiritual care is an appropriate dimension of rehabilitation nursing, which is concerned with the promotion of client wholeness
(Solimine & Hoeman, 1996, p. 628). Some suggested spiritual interventions
for a disabled patient experiencing rehabilitation are recommending a spiritual counselor; providing prayer materials, as denominationally appropriate; and introducing imagery, music, or meditative prayer to the client
(Solimine & Hoeman, 1996, p. 636). In regard to the latter activity, Solimine
and Hoeman suggested that through prayer, disabled individuals are able to
give over their situation to God and "trade their weakness for God's strength"
(p. 631). Accardi (1990) suggested three other pastoral care interventions for

the disabled: listening to the patient's "spiritually significant stories," that is, walking with the patient on his or her spiritual journey; "indwelling the stories," or expressing the empathy and compassion that results from entering into another's pain; and "linking the stories" with biblical references that may help the person find meaning in, or the ability to transcend, the disability (p. 91).

For the rehabilitation patient not associated with a religious tradition that employs devotional practices, Boucher suggested that spiritual care may draw on such basic needs as "the need to belong, to feel attachment to a person or group, to reach out beyond oneself, to have a meaningful life, and to be creative" (1989, p. 46). In general, spiritual care of the disabled person must focus on the acceptance of present life circumstances as a basis for future growth and accomplishment (Saylor, 1991). Some related activities include maximizing the client's wellness and assisting him or her to move out of the sick role, supporting the client's present talents and abilities, teaching the client to conserve energy and to avoid focusing on deficits, and promoting activities that enhance self-esteem (Davidhizar & Shearer, 1997, pp. 132–133).

The rehabilitation nurse may employ usual spiritual assessment skills to determine the religious beliefs and practices and spiritual support system of the patient prior to the occurrence of the disability (Davis, 1994, p. 298). The point, of course, is to help the disabled patient return to former spiritual and religious practices to the degree possible. Because the rehabilitation nurse may have more time to provide spiritual care than a nurse in an acute illness setting, Clifford and Gruca (1987) suggested setting aside time to discuss spiritual needs and concerns with the client, reading meditations or poetry to the client, or playing spiritual music (p. 332).

Two nurses who worked in a rehabilitation setting with partially disabled persons described their perceptions of spiritual care. One reported:

> For me, rehabilitation nursing of patients has to do with spiritual care, with establishing the quality of their lives. One patient considers himself rehabilitated because he can walk from his house to his car; now he can get out. To him that establishes his need to be connected to people.

A second nurse added:

> Spiritual care is about quality of life, and quality of life is whatever the patient wants to make it. I have a patient who is very disabled. He

can't walk, so they got him a wheelchair with a motor on it, so he can get around and do his church work . . . that's what makes his quality of life. (O'Brien, 1983, p. 41)

SPIRITUAL NEEDS OF THE CLIENT IN THE COMMUNITY

Nursing care of the client in the community is carried out in the overall context of community health nursing, which is identified as "a synthesis of nursing practice and public health practice applied to promoting and preserving the health of populations" (American Nurses Association, 1980, cited in Nies & Swanson, 1997, p. 10). The ANA definition goes on to explain that the primary responsibility of community health nursing is to the community as a whole or aggregate nursing (Nies & Swanson, 1997). In discussing the role of the community health nurse in providing spiritual care to clients, Burkhardt and Nagai-Jacobson (1985) advised that three questions may guide the initial assessment of need: Does the client's formal religious tradition or denomination provide a good structure for spiritual care?; Does the way in which the client speaks or does not speak of God reveal spiritual concerns or needs?; and Do the client's religious contacts seem to provide strength and comfort? (p. 194). The answers to such questions can then lead the nurse to a more detailed spiritual assessment and plans for intervention, if needed.

This section focuses on two specific dimensions of community health nursing: spiritual needs of the home health care client and spiritual needs of the homeless client.

The Home Health Care Client

McNamara (1982) defined home health care as "that component of comprehensive health care where services are provided to individuals and families in their places of residence for the purpose of promoting, maintaining or restoring health or minimizing the effects of illness and disability" (p. 61). Some examples of clients receiving home health care include acutely ill patients, especially those suffering from AIDS; terminally ill clients; the frail elderly; and at-risk women and children (Lyon, Bolla, & Nies, 1997, pp. 798–799). A primary component of home health care is nursing care, which is one of the largest contemporary nursing practice areas. Home health care nurses help clients manage their prescribed plans of care and also help them cope with the social and environmental factors that may influence the course of illness and treatment (Smith, 1997).

Dealing with illness in the home, the client or family has to coordinate the meeting of a multiplicity of needs that may require such items as medications, medical supplies, special diet, or physical therapy equipment; the nurse can serve as advisor in obtaining necessary therapeutic materials (Humphrey, 1994, p. 1). Some home health care clients are acutely ill, some have chronic debilitating health problems, and many are elderly. An individual must be seriously ill, homebound, and "in need of skilled nursing services" to receive home health care (Smeltzer & Bare, 1996, p. 18). A significant role identified for the home health nurse is that of client advocate (LeMone & Burke, 1996, p. 54); this title lends itself well to the inclusion of spiritual care as an appropriate activity in home health nursing.

Spiritual assessment and, if appropriate, the provision of spiritual care, are important activities for the home health nurse, as "hope and faith" have been identified as playing a major role in the home care client's adaptation to illness or disability (Rice, 1996, p. 47). Jaffe and Skidmore-Roth (1993) suggested several issues to be addressed in a spiritual assessment of the home health care patient: religious beliefs and practice, how one's belief (or lack of belief) in a supreme being relates to illness, specific people who provide spiritual support, religious symbols of importance (e.g., a Bible or Sabbath candles), religious restrictions (dietary, medical treatment), requirements for church attendance, and religious leaders (pp. 42–43). Bauer and Barron (1995) noted that spiritual nursing interventions are particularly important for the elderly client who lives alone in the community with no religiously based support system available; the community health nurse may be the only visitor who is able and willing to discuss spiritual issues with such a client. In their research with elderly community-based clients, Bauer and Barron found that older individuals especially wanted nurses to be respectful, caring, and sensitive to their religious beliefs and traditions.

Dorothy, a community health nurse for more than 17 years, described the caring relationship she developed in providing spiritual care to clients:

> In my clinical practice in community health, it's like the "I–thou" relationship, where you give of your own spiritual energy to the people you're working with. You have to respect their beliefs and where they are spiritually, and then go from there. Some people will ask you to pray with them, if they're having a hard time, or they'll say, "think of me," and I think they just want you to send them some energy. Sometimes a patient has something very deep, like being away from their church, and you need to call in a priest or a minister. But that's part of the nurse's job, especially the community health nurse.

Megan, another nurse, with an MSN in community health nursing and 23 years of experience, added:

> You have to be attuned to what the client is saying. Sometimes they don't say it in spiritual words or religious words, but really the thing they need is some spiritual care. You have to listen with your heart to what is behind the words they say.

The Homeless Client

Topics such as the "culture of poverty" and "care of the homeless client" are now being included in many fundamentals of nursing, community health nursing, and psychiatric–mental health nursing texts. The word *poverty* is a relative term; some defining characteristics may include homelessness, feelings of despair or hopelessness, unemployment, family instability, and lowered self-esteem and self-concept (Taylor, Lillis, & LeMone, 1997, p. 38). Although not all poor persons are homeless, most homeless people are poor, with the exclusion of those individuals who choose to be homeless as a result of a mental health deficit or because of religious or ascetic philosophies.

Homelessness has been defined by the federal government as "the absence of 'fixed, regular and adequate nighttime residence' "; this statement also encompasses the use of public or private shelters for sleeping (Virvan, 1996, p. 1025). Earlier in the century, the homeless were conceptualized primarily as derelicts of society; recently, a new homeless population consisting of women and children and families has emerged within urban communities (Vernon, 1997, p. 484). Fontaine (1995a) identified four subgroups of homeless people: the chronically mentally ill, individuals who abuse illegal drugs, teens living on the streets, and families with children (pp. 472–473). These homeless persons often lack not only shelter, but also adequate food, clothing, and health care.

Providing care for the homeless has been described as "problematic at best" for the community health nurse, with interventions representing mostly "downstream" or "band-aid" kinds of therapies (Hatton & Droes, 1997, p. 403). Such health care difficulties are well documented in David Hilfiker's poignant account of a doctor's journey with the poor, entitled *Not All of Us Are Saints* (1994). Community health nurses working with homeless people need to be sensitive to the many material and sociocultural needs of their clients, as well as being nonjudgmental in attitude (Smeltzer & Bare, 1996; Ugarriza & Fallon, 1994). The latter approach especially directs the nurse from a Judeo-Christian tradition, who is aware that both Old and New

Testament Scriptures identify the poor as those for whom one has a responsibility, as demonstrated in Exodus 22:21 ("You shall not wrong any widow or orphan") and Luke 10:30–34, the parable of the Good Samaritan.

What constitutes spiritual care of the homeless client who is poor? Murray (1993) described the spiritual care of homeless men as moving beyond the basic needs of food and shelter and involving such activities as providing the men with unconditional acceptance and speaking with them in a caring manner; providing small devotional materials supportive of spiritual practices that can be carried out privately; planning religious services that are supportive rather than condemning; and praying with a person if acceptable (p. 34). In a study of homeless women, Shuler, Gelberg, and Brown (1994) found that the use of prayer among clients was significantly associated with decreased alcohol and drug abuse, fewer worries, and less depression (p. 106). The authors also suggested the use of spiritual reading materials, such as religious books or the Bible, and clergy counseling, which together with the use of prayer can decrease the effects of stressful stimuli and increase coping strategies (p. 112).

Allie, a community health nurse who had worked for more than 16 years with the homeless in a large urban inner city, described her understanding of spiritual care:

> You really can just be with that person who is having a hard time and their life becomes more whole because you are there with them; nursing has to function in a much broader way now, as cocommunity. The homeless person is suffering so intensely from oppression: physical, spiritual, psychological. I need to try to help get things in balance, to get the person at peace, in their immediate life, in the life of the neighborhood, and the whole community. . . . We really do need to talk to homeless people about their spiritual needs, but not to proselytize, which is hard for some people to get the difference between. I mean listening and picking up on a patient's spirituality instead of preaching. One technique is to see if they ever carry a little Bible or prayer book, or to ask if they have a favorite psalm. You can always use "The Lord is my Shepherd" if somebody's in trouble, or you can ask if there's any church or synagogue you can call.
>
> My religious experiences with patients haven't been the "away on a mountain top" kind. But like with this one man I'm seeing now, Johnny; he's an addict. Some guys came to me on the street and said one of the fellows was hurt, and I followed this guy into the street and I found Johnny just about dead. His head was a mess; he looked

awful. I looked at him and I just had this shock, this shock image of the suffering Christ. . . . This is really where I meet Christ, in the street.

Personal spirituality and/or religious beliefs and practices may constitute an important mediating variable for the individual coping with a chronic illness. For the chronically ill patient, such concepts as hope, trust, courage, and love may take on new and deeper meaning following the illness onset. Nurses may support and facilitate the presence of positive attitudes and attributes in a patient's life through a variety of spiritual care interventions. As well as providing spiritual care for the hospitalized patient, contemporary nurses need to be sensitive to the spiritual needs and concerns of persons with a variety of other chronic conditions and in a variety of settings.

REFERENCES

Accardi, R. F. (1990). Rehabilitation: Dreams lost, dreams found. In H. Hayes & C. J. van der Poel (Eds.), *Health care ministry: A handbook for chaplains* (pp. 88–92). New York: Paulist Press.

AIDS Ministry Program, the Archdiocese of St. Paul and Minneapolis. (1991). *For those we love: A spiritual perspective on AIDS*. Cleveland, OH: The Pilgrim Press.

American Nurses Association. (1980). *A conceptual model of community health nursing* (ANA publication #CHI0). Kansas City, MO: American Nurses Association.

American Nurses Association. (1994). *A statement on psychiatric–mental health clinical nursing practice and standards of psychiatric–mental health clinical nursing practice.* Washington, DC: American Nurses Publishing.

Arnold, E. N. (1996). The journey clouded by cognitive disorders. In V. B. Carson & E. N. Arnold (Eds.), *Mental health nursing: The nurse–patient journey* (pp. 977–1019). Philadelphia: W. B. Saunders.

Baldacchino, D., & Draper, P. (2001). Spiritual coping strategies: A review of the nursing research literature. *Journal of Advanced Nursing, 34*(6), 833–841.

Bauer, T., & Barron, C. R. (1995). Nursing interventions for spiritual care. *Journal of Holistic Nursing, 13*(3), 268–279.

Belcher, A. E., Dettmore, D., & Holzemer, S. P. (1989). Spirituality and sense of well-being in persons with AIDS. *Holistic Nurse Practice, 3*(4), 16–25.

Bender, E. (2004). Psychiatrists urge more direct focus on patients' spirituality. *Psychiatric News, 39*(12), 30.

Boucher, R. J. (1989). Nursing process. In S. S. Dittmar (Ed.), *Rehabilitation nursing: Process and application* (pp. 45–62). St. Louis, MO: C. V. Mosby.

Boutell, K. A., & Bozeht, F. W. (1988). Nurses' assessment of patients' spirituality: Continuing education implications. *Journal of Continuing Education in Nursing, 21*(4), 172–176.

Bruegge, M. V. (1997). Assessment of clients with neurologic disorders. In J. M. Black & E. Matassmarin-Jacobs (Eds.), *Medical–surgical nursing: Clinical management for continuity of care* (5th ed., pp. 709–742). Philadelphia: W. B. Saunders.

Burkhardt, M. A., & Nagai-Jacobson, M. G. (1985). Dealing with spiritual concerns of clients in the community. *Journal of Community Health Nursing, 2*(4), 191–198.

Burnard, P. (1988, December). Discussing spiritual issues with clients. *Health Visitor, 61,* 371–372.

Campinha-Bacote, J. (1995). Spiritual competence: A model of psychiatric care. *Journal of Christian Nursing, 12*(3), 22–44.

Carson, V. B. (1989). Spiritual development across the lifespan. In V. B. Carson (Ed.), *Spiritual dimensions of nursing practice* (pp. 24–51). Philadelphia: W. B. Saunders.

Carson, V. B. (1997). Spirituality and patient care. In A. W. Burgess (Ed.), *Psychiatric nursing: Promoting mental health* (pp. 143–149). Stamford, CT: Appleton & Lange.

Carson, V. B., Soeken, K. L., Shanty, J., & Terry, L. (1990). Hope and spiritual well-being: Essentials for living with AIDS. *Perspective in Psychiatric Care, 26*(2), 28–34.

Cassidy, J. (1992, April). What keeps people well? A new paradigm for pastoral care. *Health Progress,* 34–36.

Christensen, M. J. (1991). *The Samaritans imperative: Compassionate ministry to people living with AIDS.* Nashville, TN: Abington Press.

Clifford, M., & Gruca, J. (1987). Facilitating spiritual care in the rehabilitation setting. *Rehabilitation Nursing, 12*(6), 331–333.

Corbin, J. (1996). Chronic illness. In S. C. Smeltzer & B. G. Bare (Eds.), *Brunner and Suddarth's textbook of medical–surgical nursing* (8th ed., pp. 317–324). Philadelphia: J. B. Lippincott.

Crowther, C. E. (1991). *AIDS: A Christian handbook.* London: Epworth Press.

Davidhizar, R., & Shearer, R. (1997). Helping the client with chronic disability achieve high level wellness. *Rehabilitation Nursing, 22*(3), 131–134.

Davis, M. C. (1994). The rehabilitation nurse's role in spiritual care. *Rehabilitation Nursing, 19*(5), 298–301.

Downey, M. (1993). Disability: The disabled. In M. Downey (Ed.), *The new dictionary of Catholic spirituality* (pp. 273–274). Collegeville, MN: The Liturgical Press.

Dreyer, E. (1993). Love. In M. Downey (Ed.), *The new dictionary of Catholic spirituality* (pp. 612–622). Collegeville, MN: The Liturgical Press.

Dwyer, J. A. (1990). Peace. In J. A. Komonchak, M. Collins, & D. A. Lane (Eds.), *The new dictionary of theology* (pp. 748–753). Collegeville, MN: The Liturgical Press.

Ellis, C. (1986, April). Course prepares nurses to meet patients' spiritual needs. *Health Progress*, 76–77.

Fatula, M. A. (1993). Faith. In M. Downey (Ed.), *The new dictionary of Catholic spirituality* (pp. 379–390). Collegeville, MN: The Liturgical Press.

Flaherty, M. J., & O'Brien, M. E. (1992). Family styles of coping in end-stage renal disease. *ANNA Journal, 19*(4), 345–350.

Fontaine, K. L. (1995a). Contemporary issues: AIDS and homelessness. In K. L. Fontaine & J. S. Fletcher (Eds.), *Essentials of mental health nursing* (3rd ed., pp. 467–477). New York: Addison-Wesley.

Fontaine, K. L. (1995b). Mood disorders. In K. L. Fontaine & J. S. Fletcher (Eds.), *Essentials of mental health nursing* (3rd ed., pp. 236–258). New York: Addison-Wesley.

Fontaine, K. L. (1995c). Schizophrenic disorders. In K. L. Fontaine & J. S. Fletcher (Eds.), *Essentials of mental health nursing* (3rd ed., pp. 300–321). New York: Addison-Wesley.

Forbis, P. A. (1988). Meeting patients' spiritual needs. *Geriatric Nursing, 9*(3), 158–159.

Fry, A. (1998). Spirituality communication and mental health nursing: The tacit interdiction. *Australian New Zealand Journal of Mental Health Nursing, 7*(1), 25–32.

Gewe, A. (1994). Hope: Moving from theory to practice. *Journal of Christian Nursing, 11*(4), 18–21.

Greasley, P., Chiu, L. F., & Gartland, M. (2001). The concept of spiritual care in mental health nursing. *Journal of Advanced Nursing, 33*(5), 629–637.

Halstead, M. T., & Hull, M. (2001). Struggling with paradoxes: The process of spiritual development in women with cancer. *Oncology Nursing Forum, 28*(10), 1534–1544.

Hatton, D. C., & Droes, N. S. (1997). The homeless. In J. M. Swanson & M. A. Nies (Eds.), *Community health nursing: Promoting the health of aggregates* (pp. 387–406). Philadelphia: W. B. Saunders.

Hauerwas, S. (1995). The church and mentally handicapped persons: A continuing challenge to the imagination. In M. Bishop (Ed.), *Religion as a disability: Essays in scripture, theology and ethics* (pp. 46–64). Kansas City, MO: Shead & Ward.

Hellwig, M. K. (1993). Hope. In M. Downey (Ed.), *The new dictionary of Catholic spirituality* (pp. 506–515). Collegeville, MN: The Liturgical Press.

Highfield, M. F. (1992). Spiritual health of oncology patients. *Cancer Nursing, 15*(1), 1–8.

Highfield, M. F., & Cason, C. (1983). Spiritual needs of patients: Are they recognized? *Cancer Nursing, 6*(6), 187–192.

Hilfiker, D. (1994). *Not all of us are saints: A doctor's journey with the poor.* New York: Hill and Wang.

Humphrey, C. J. (1994). *Home care nursing handbook.* Gaithersburg, MD: Aspen.

Ignatavicius, D. D., Workman, M. L., & Mishler, M. A. (1995). *Medical–surgical nursing: A nursing process approach.* Philadelphia: W. B. Saunders.

Iles, R. (Ed.). (1989). *The gospel imperative in the midst of AIDS.* Wilton, CT: Morehouse.

Jaffe, M. S., & Skidmore-Roth, L. (1993). *Home health nursing care plans.* St. Louis, MO: C. V. Mosby.

John, S. D. (1983). Assessing spiritual needs. In J. A. Shelly & S. D. John (Eds.), *Spiritual dimensions of mental health* (pp. 73–84). Downers Grove, IL: InterVarsity Press.

Johnson, R. P. (1992). *Body, mind, spirit: Tapping the healing power within you.* Liguori, MO: Liguori Publications.

Kaczorowski, J. M. (1989). Spiritual well-being and anxiety in adults diagnosed with cancer. *The Hospice Journal, 5*(3), 105–116.

Kennison, M. M. (1987). Faith: An untapped health resource. *Journal of Psychosocial Nursing, 25*(10), 28–30.

Kilpatrick, J. A. (1997). Urinary elimination. In P. A. Potter & A. G. Perry (Eds.), *Fundamentals of nursing: Concepts, process and practice* (4th ed., pp. 1293–1334). St. Louis, MO: C. V. Mosby.

Korniewicz, D., & O'Brien, M. E. (1994). Evaluation of a hemodialysis patient education and support program. *ANNA Journal, 21*(1), 33–38.

Krafft, J. (1988). *The ministry to persons with disabilities.* Collegeville, MN: The Liturgical Press.

Lackey, N. R., Gates, M. F., & Brown, G. (2001). African American women's experiences with the initial discovery, diagnosis and treatment of breast cancer. *Oncology Nursing Forum, 28*(3), 519–527.

Landis, B. J. (1996). Uncertainty, spiritual well-being and psychosocial adjustment to chronic illness. *Issues in Mental Health Nursing, 17*(1), 217–231.

LeMone, P., & Burke, K. M. (1996). *Medical–surgical nursing: Critical thinking in client care.* New York: Addison-Wesley.

Le Peau, P. J. (1996). Finding hope when everything's up for grabs. *Journal of Christian Nursing, 13*(1), 16–19.

Lisanti, P., & Zwolski, K. (1997). Understanding the devastation of AIDS. *American Journal of Nursing, 97*(7), 26–34.

Lyon, J. C., Bolla, C. D., & Nies, M. A. (1997). The home visit and home health care. In J. M. Swanson & M. A. Nies (Eds.), *Community health nursing: Promoting the health of aggregates* (pp. 798–821). Philadelphia: W. B. Saunders.

MacDonald, B. H. (2001). Quality of life in cancer care: Patients' experiences and nurses' contributions. *European Journal of Oncology Nursing, 5*(1), 32–41.

Matassarin-Jacobs, E. (1997). Nursing care of clients with renal disorders. In J. M. Black & E. Matassarin-Jacobs (Eds.), *Medical–surgical nursing: Clinical management for continuity of care* (5th ed., pp. 1625–1681). Philadelphia: W. B. Saunders.

McBride, A. B. (1996). Psychiatric–mental health nursing in the twenty-first century. In A. B. McBride & J. K. Austin (Eds.), *Psychiatric–mental health nursing* (pp. 1–10). Philadelphia: W. B. Saunders.

McBride, J. L., & Armstrong, G. (1995). The spiritual dynamics of chronic post traumatic stress disorder. *Journal of Religion and Health, 34*(1), 5–16.

McClain, C., Rosenfeld, B., & Breitbart, W. (2003). Effect of spiritual well-being on end-of-life despair in terminally ill cancer patients. *The Lancet, 361*(9369), 1603.

McNamara, E. (1982). Hospitals discover comprehensive home care. *Hospital, 56*(1), 60–66.

McSherry, W. (1996). Raising the spirits. *Nursing Times, 92*(3), 49–50.

Mellors, M. P., Riley, T. A., & Erlen, J. A. (1997). HIV, self-transcendence, and quality of life. *Journal of the Association of Nurses in AIDS Care, 8*(2), 59–69.

Mickley, J. R., Carson, V. B., & Soeken, K. L. (1995). Religion and adult mental health: State of the science in nursing. *Issues in Mental Health Nursing, 16*(1), 345–360.

Mickley, J. R., Soeken, K., & Belcher, A. (1992). Spiritual well-being, religiousness and hope among women with breast cancer. *Image Journal of Nursing Scholarship, 24*(4), 267–272.

Moberg, D. O. (1979). The development of social indicators of spiritual well-being for quality of life research. In D. O. Moberg (Ed.), *Spiritual well-being: Sociological perspectives* (pp. 1–13). Washington, DC: University Press of America.

Morris, L. E. (1996). A spiritual well-being model: Use with older women who experience depression. *Issues in Mental Health Nursing, 17*(1), 439–455.

Moschella, V. D., Pressman, K. R., Pressman, P., & Weissman, D. E. (1997). The problem of theodicy and religious response to cancer. *Journal of Religion and Health, 36*(1), 17–20.

Muldoon, M. H., & King, J. N. (1991). A spirituality for the long haul: Response to chronic illness. *Journal of Religion and Health, 30*(2), 99–108.

Murray, R. (1993). Spiritual care of homeless men: What helps and what hinders? *Journal of Christian Nursing, 10*(2), 30–34.

National Catholic Office for Persons with Disabilities. (1990). *We are one flock.* Washington, DC: Author.

Newshan, G. (1998). Transcending the physical: Spiritual aspects of pain in patients with HIV and/or cancer. *Journal of Advanced Nursing, 28*(6), 1236–1241.

Nies, M. A., & Swanson, J. M. (1997). Health: A community view. In J. M. Swanson & M. A. Nies (Eds.), *Community health nursing: Promoting the health of aggregates* (pp. 4–15). Philadelphia: W. B. Saunders.

Nouwen, H. (1988). *The road to daybreak: A spiritual journey.* New York: Doubleday.

O'Brien, M. E. (1982). Religious faith and adjustment to long-term hemodialysis. *Journal of Religion and Health, 21*(1), 68–80.

O'Brien, M. E. (1983). *The courage to survive: The life career of the chronic dialysis patient.* New York: Grune & Stratton.

O'Brien, M. E. (1990). Compliance behavior and long-term maintenance dialysis. *American Journal of Kidney Disease, 15*(3), 209–214.

O'Brien, M.E. (1992). *Living with HIV: Experiment in courage.* Westport, CT: Auburn House.

O'Brien, M. E. (1995). *The AIDS challenge: Breaking through the boundaries.* Westport, CT: Auburn House.

O'Brien, M. E., Donley, R., Flaherty, M., & Johnstone, B. (1986). Therapeutic options in end-stage renal disease: A preliminary report. *ANNA Journal, 13*(6), 313–318.

O'Brien, M. E., & Pheifer, W. G. (1993). Physical and psychosocial nursing care for patients with HIV infection. *Nursing Clinics of North America, 28*(2), 303–315.

O'Neill, D. P., & Kenny, E. K. (1998). State of the science: Spirituality and chronic illness. *Image, the Journal of Nursing Scholarship, 30*(3), 275–280.

Overberg, K. R. (Ed.). (1994). *AIDS, ethics and religion: Embracing a world of suffering.* Maryknoll, NY: Orbis Books.

Perelli, R. J. (1991). *Ministry to persons with AIDS.* Minneapolis, MN: Augsburg.

Peterson, E. A., & Nelson, K. (1987). How to meet your client's spiritual needs. *Journal of Psychosocial Nursing, 25*(5), 34–39.

Petty, J. (1997). Basic concepts of neoplastic disorders. In J. M. Black & E. Matassarin-Jacobs (Eds.), *Medical–surgical nursing: Clinical management for continuity of care* (5th ed., pp. 533–590). Philadelphia: W. B. Saunders.

Pullen, L., Tuck, I., & Mix, K. (1996). Mental health nurses' spiritual perspectives. *Journal of Holistic Nursing, 14*(2), 85–97.

Rice, R. (1996). Developing the plan of care and documentation. In R. Rice (Ed.), *Home health nursing practice, concepts and application* (pp. 41–60). St. Louis, MO: C. V. Mosby.

Roche, J. (1992, March). Spiritual care of the person with AIDS. *Health Progress*, 78–81.

Ross, L. A. (1994). Spiritual aspects of nursing. *Journal of Advanced Nursing, 9*(1), 437–439.

Russell, L. M. (Ed.). (1990). *The church with AIDS*. Louisville, KY: Westminister/John Knox Press.

Sandin, F. C. (1996). Walking through fire: Fostering faith in times of loss. *Journal of Christian Nursing, 13*(1), 23–26.

Sandys, S. (Ed.). (1993). *Embracing the mystery: A prayerful response to AIDS*. Collegeville, MN: The Liturgical Press.

Saylor, D. E. (1991). Pastoral care of the rehabilitation patient. *Rehabilitation Nursing, 16*(3), 138–140.

Schreiter, R. J. (1988). The faces of suffering. *New Theology Review, 1*(4), 3–14.

Schreiter, R. (1993). Trust. In M. Downey (Ed.), *The new dictionary of Catholic spirituality* (pp. 982–983). Collegeville, MN: The Liturgical Press.

Senior, D. (1995). Beware of the Canaanite woman: Disability and the Bible. In M. Bishop (Ed.), *Religion and disability: Essays in scripture, theology and ethics* (pp. 1–26). Kansas City, MO: Sheed & Ward.

Shelly, J. A. (1983). What are spiritual needs? In J. A. Shelly & S. D. John (Eds.), *Spiritual dimensions of mental health* (pp. 55–60). Downers Grove, IL: InterVarsity Press.

Shelly, J. A., & Fish. S. (1988). *Spiritual care: The nurse's role* (3rd ed.). Downers Grove, IL: InterVarsity Press.

Shelly, J. A., & John, S. D. (1983). *Spiritual dimensions of mental health*. Downers Grove, IL: InterVarsity Press.

Sherman, D. W. (2001). The perceptions and experiences of patients with AIDS: Implications regarding quality of life and palliative care. *Journal of Hospice and Palliative Nursing, 3*(1), 7–16.

Shoemaker, N. (1996). Getting to know the traveler: Mental health assessment. In V. B. Carson & E. N. Arnold (Eds.), *Mental health nursing: The nurse–patient journey* (pp. 273–302). Philadelphia: W. B. Saunders.

Shuler, P. A., Gelberg, L., & Brown, M. (1994). The effects of spiritual religious practices on spiritual well-being among inner city homeless women. *Nurse Practitioner Forum, 5*(2), 106–113.

Simsen, B. (1988). Nursing the spirit. *Nursing Times, 84*(37), 32–33.

Smeltzer, S. C., & Bare, B. G. (1996). *Brunner and Suddarth's textbook of medical–surgical nursing* (8th ed., pp. 17–24). Philadelphia: J. B. Lippincott.

Smith, T. (1997). Restorative and home health care. In P. A. Potter & A. G. Perry (Eds.), *Fundamentals of nursing: Concepts, process and practice* (4th ed., pp. 79–95). St. Louis, MO: C. V. Mosby.

Smith, W. J. (1988). *AIDS: Issues in pastoral care.* New York: Paulist Press.

Soeken, K. L., & Carson, V. B. (1987). Responding to the spiritual needs of the chronically ill. *Nursing Clinics of North America, 22*(3), 603–611.

Solimine, M. A., & Hoeman, S. P. (1996). Spirituality: A rehabilitation perspective. In S. P. Hoeman (Ed.), *Rehabilitation nursing: Process and application* (2nd ed., pp. 628–643). St. Louis, MO: C. V. Mosby.

Stoll, R. I. (1989). Spirituality and chronic illness. In V. B. Carson (Ed.), *Spiritual dimensions of nursing practice* (pp. 180–216). Philadelphia: W. B. Saunders.

Sunderland, R. H., & Shelp, E. E. (1987). *AIDS: A manual for pastoral care.* Philadelphia: The Westminister Press.

Swinton, J. (1997). Restoring the image: Spirituality, faith and cognitive disability. *Journal of Religion and Health, 36*(1), 21–27.

Taylor, C., Lillis, C., & LeMone, P. (1997). *Fundamentals of nursing: The art and science of nursing care* (3rd ed.). Philadelphia: J. B. Lippincott.

Taylor, E. J., Amenta, M., & Highfield, M. (1995). Spiritual care practices of oncology nurses. *Oncology Nursing Forum, 22*(1), 31–39.

Taylor, E. J., Highfield, M., & Amenta, M. (1994). Attitudes and beliefs regarding spiritual care. *Cancer Nursing, 17*(6), 479–487.

Taylor, E. J., & Mamier, I. (2005). Spiritual care nursing: What cancer patients and family caregivers want. *Journal of Advanced Nursing, 49*(3), 260–267.

Taylor, E. J., (2001). Spirituality, culture and cancer care. *Seminars in Oncology Nursing, 17*(3), 197–205.

Thomas, J., & Retsas, A. (1999). Transacting self-preservation: A grounded theory of the spiritual dimensions of people with terminal cancer. *International Journal of Nursing Studies, 36*(3), 191–201.

Thompson, M. (1994). Nurturing hope: A vital ingredient in nursing. *Journal of Christian Nursing, 11*(4), 11–17.

Tuck, I., Pullen, L., & Lynn, C. (1997). Spiritual interventions provided by mental health nurses. *Western Journal of Nursing Research, 19*(3), 351–363.

Turk, D., & Rudy, T. (1986). Living with chronic disease: The importance of cognitive appraisal. In J. S. McHugh & T. Vallis (Eds.), *Illness behavior: A multidisciplinary model* (pp. 309–320). New York: Plenum Press.

Ugarriza, D., & Fallon, T. (1994). Nurses' attitudes toward homeless women: A barrier to change. *Nursing Outlook, 42*(1), 26–29.

Ungvarski, P. J., & Matassarin-Jacobs, E. (1997). Nursing care of clients with altered immune systems. In J. M. Black & E. Matassarin-Jacobs (Eds.), *Medical–surgical nursing: Clinical management for continuity of care* (5th ed., pp. 614–651). Philadelphia: W. B. Saunders Company.

Vanier, J. (1975). *Be not afraid.* New York: Paulist Press.

Varcarolis, E. M. (1994). Alterations in mood: Grief and depression. In E. M. Varcarolis (Ed.), *Foundation of psychiatric–mental health nursing* (2nd ed., pp. 415–464). Philadelphia: W. B. Saunders.

Vash, C. L. (1994). *Personality and adversity: Psychospiritual aspects of rehabilitation.* New York: Springer.

Vernon, J. A. (1997). Basic human needs: Individual and family. In P. A. Potter & A. G. Perry (Eds.), *Fundamentals of nursing: Concepts, process and practice* (4th ed., pp. 478–495). St. Louis, MO: C. V. Mosby.

Virvan, D. (1996). The journey marked by homelessness. In V. B. Carson & E. N. Arnold (Eds.), *Mental health nursing: The nurse–patient journey* (pp. 1023–1038). Philadelphia: W. B. Saunders.

Wagner, C. D. (1996). Family needs of chronic hemodialysis patients: A comparison of perceptions of nurses and families. *ANNA Journal, 23*(1), 19–26.

Wagner, W. (1992). The voices on psychiatry: Inner tumult and the quest for meaning. In L. E. Holst (Ed.), *Hospital ministry: The role of the chaplain today* (pp. 151–162). New York: Crossroad.

Walgrove, N. J. (1996). Unique attributes of successful travelers: Personal strengths for the journey. In V. B. Carson & E. N. Arnold (Eds.), *Mental health nursing: The nurse–patient journey* (pp. 175–190). Philadelphia: W. B. Saunders.

Walsh, M. B., & Carson, V. B. (1996). Mind, body, spirit therapies. In V. B. Carson & E. N. Arnold (Eds.), *Mental health nursing: The nurse–patient journey* (pp. 487–502). Philadelphia: W. B. Saunders.

Warner-Robbins, C. G., & Christiana, N. M. (1989). The spiritual needs of persons with AIDS. *Family Community Health, 12*(2), 43–51.

Weaver, A. J., Flannelly, L. T., Flannelly, K. J., Koenig, H. G., & Larson, D. B. (1998). An analysis of research on religious and spiritual variables in three major mental health nursing journals, 1991–1995. *Issues in Mental Health Nursing, 19*(3), 263–276.

9 ✦ Spiritual Needs of Children and Families

We are made by relationships with other people.

CARLO CARRETTO
Summoned by Love (1978)

I n this chapter the spiritual needs of the ill child are identified and de-scribed through reports of the author's interactions with children liv-ing with such illnesses as cancer, including leukemia and lymphoma, and HIV infection. The spiritual needs of family members of both ill children and ill adults are also documented in data elicited through formal and in-formal interviews and observations. Patient and family data are supple-mented through interviews with nurses caring for ill children and their families. The first part of the chapter is directed toward the spiritual needs of the ill child in a variety of settings; the latter part explores the spiritual needs of the family, beginning with those of the new and expanding family at the time of childbirth and concluding with a discussion of family needs in terminal illness.

SPIRITUAL NEEDS OF THE CHILD

Perhaps no therapeutic intervention calls on the nurse's creative skills as much as that of providing spiritual care to an ill child. Children are unique and challenging in their varied developmental stages (Kenny, 1999); as fre-quently noted, a child is much more than a small adult. Children, espe-cially ill children, tend to be astoundingly straightforward in expressing their questions and concerns. They expect no less from their caregivers. Honesty and directness, to the degree possible and appropriate, is the most therapeutic approach for a nurse in the provision of spiritual care to an ill child.

Spirituality and the Child

Children! They are such a joy and such a mystery in our lives! Who can ever express sufficiently all that they are able to communicate, through gifts unknown to themselves. . . ? They make us understand something of the living God by the trust they show us.

ROGER OF TAIZE, 1990

The term *child* is broadly understood to refer to a young person from the developmental stage following infancy to the onset of adolescence; that is, from approximately 1 to 12 years of age. Moran (1997) identified the formal stages of growth and development as newborn (birth to 1 month), infancy (1 month to 1 year), toddlerhood (1 to 3 years), preschool age (3 to 6 years), school age (6 to 11 or 12 years), and adolescence (11 or 12 to 21 years of age) (p. 28). A child's trajectory of physical and psychological growth is accompanied by a parallel process of moral development (Kohlberg, 1984) and spiritual or faith development (Fowler, 1981).

In describing a child's moral development, Lawrence Kohlberg posited three phases of morality: the preconventional level (early childhood), the conventional level (later childhood to adolescence), and the postconventional level (adulthood). In brief, Kohlberg's schema suggests that the child progresses from an initial stage of simple acceptance of right and wrong, as identified through punishment or nonpunishment for an act; to the school-age phase of more abstract understanding of morality; and later, to the adolescent/adult stage, encompassing a societal view of right and wrong (1984).

James Fowler (1981) proposed a paradigm of spiritual development across the life span, labeled "stages of faith development" (discussed in chapter 3). Of Fowler's seven faith stages, three may be associated with the child's parallel physical and psychological development. Stage 2, intuitive–projective faith, is the period when the preschool child is influenced by the example of adults. During this period, God is often imagined as appearing similar to adult figures with whom the child interacts, and the child may imitate the religious practices of the family without really understanding the meaning. Many preschoolers, around age 5 or 6, can create their own prayers, and a number attend church services with the family. Stage 3, mythic–literal faith, occurs during the school-age period, as the child begins to internalize religious beliefs. The child understands and accepts a more sophisticated God from a monotheistic tradition and develops a conscience. Early school-age children pray and trust that prayers will be answered. Religious stories are often appreciated during this period, especially those describing biblical or religious heroes. Stage 4, synthetic–conventional faith, is developed during the adolescent period. The teen may begin to question some or all of the religious beliefs and practices of the family. Faith experiences occur outside of the home, and the adolescent begins to claim his or her own faith identity. Some teens become very involved in their faith and religious experience during the adolescent years; they may interact with other young people of similar religious belief as a significant peer group.

Burkhardt (1991) believes that children "live in their spirits more than adults," because they are less inhibited and more intuitive about spiritual matters (p. 34); she noted that while understanding the work of the developmental theorists is important, one should adopt a broad definition of spirituality in working with children (p. 34). Spirituality-related themes suggested by Burkhardt include the child's capacity for searching for meaning in life; a sense of relationship to "self, others, nature, and God or Universal Force"; and spirituality, viewed as the "deepest core" of the child's being (1991, p. 34). The comments of Anne Marie, a doctorally prepared pediatric nurse practitioner, reflect Burkhardt's perception related to a child's intuition:

> Working with children you have to have a very clear sense of your own spirituality, because they are very sensitive to the spiritual in others. You have to have a spirituality that projects total acceptance because, if not, the kids can read right through it; anything that's a facade or put on, they know it in a heartbeat. . . . In my nursing with children and families I have learned a lot about spiritual needs. I think some nurses are uncomfortable with spiritual care, to go into a 9-year-old's room and ask if he wants to talk about something religious. You just need to be open and give them the chance. They're not afraid of the hard questions, like "what's it like to die?" or "will I die?"; but you have to not be afraid to let them ask. Children will give you spiritual clues; you just have to pick up on them.

In exploring the spirituality of 40 children, ages 4 to 12, David Heller (1985) discovered differences in prayer styles among children from Jewish, Catholic, Protestant, and Hindu traditions. For example, whereas Baptist children reported being comfortable with silent devotion, both Catholic and Jewish children perceived prayer as associated with more formal religious ritual; Hindu children preferred chanting (p. 24). Psychologist Robert Coles offered poignant examples of differing religious beliefs of school-age children in his book *The Spiritual Life of Children* (1990). Coles identified four spiritual themes from his conversations with children of different traditions: Christian salvation, Islamic surrender, Jewish righteousness, and secular soul-searching. Mary, a 9-year-old Christian with whom Coles conversed, explained that Jesus "died so we will live forever" (1990, p. 203). Rita, a 10-year-old Muslim, asserted, "God is the one who made us, and He'll be the one to decide where we go" (p. 233). Joseph, a 12-year-old Jewish boy, explained, "We have the book, our Bible; it tells us what we should believe . . . a Jew is someone who lives the law" (p. 253). Finally, in examining the concept of secular soul-searching, Robert Coles spoke with 12-year-old Eric, who reported that although he did not belong to any church, he did sometimes "wonder" about things such as the existence of God (pp. 281–283).

The Ill Child and Religious Practices

For a child of any religious tradition who is experiencing illness, the ability to participate in religious devotions or practices, such as prayer, may provide a source of comfort and stability. Religious practices and beliefs can affect a child's health; illness may be interpreted in light of a child's religious understanding (Spector & Spertac, 1990, p. 58). The presence in a sickroom of devotional articles such as holy pictures, statues, crucifixes, crosses, or Bibles may provide a sense of security and stability during the disruption of usual life activities. For the preschooler who has a concrete concept of God as protector and father, simple bedtime prayers, such as "Now I lay me down to sleep, I pray the Lord my soul to keep," may help the child to feel more at ease during the night. The reading of a religious story or looking at images from a children's picture Bible can be comforting. If mealtime grace is usual in the family, this may be carried out in the sickroom. A preschooler, ill during a religious holiday such as Christmas, Easter, or Hanukkah, should be encouraged to participate in as many of the associated rituals as possible, to help maintain some sense of normalcy in the child's life.

In the case of an ill school-age child, use of a Bible or prayer book, if part of one's tradition, can be encouraged. A Jewish child may want to experience the lighting of Sabbath candles on Friday evening and have traditional passages from Hebrew Scripture read to him or her. The early school-age child can be encouraged to pray, but will, as noted earlier, expect to have prayers answered, so some counseling may need to be done around that issue. The older school-age child will have learned that prayers are not always directly answered; thus a discussion about the meaning of prayer will be helpful. Some school-age children find it important when ill to continue to participate in certain religious practices such as reception of the sacraments (Holy Eucharist and the Sacrament of Reconciliation), also. Special religious anniversaries, such as Christmas, Easter, Rosh Hashanah, Yom Kippur, Hanukkah, and Ramadan, may be very important to the school-age child, especially if participation in the associated worship rituals is usual in the family. Some reflections of the religious meaning of the celebrations may be brought into the child's sickroom, for example, the setting up of a small Christmas crèche or a menorah. These spiritual symbols can help the child cope with the frightening nature of an illness experience.

The ill adolescent may need spiritual counseling about the relationship of his or her sickness to the religious or spiritual meaning of life. During this developmental period, when the teen may question many of the tenets of organized religion, the young person might well question "why me?" in relation to an illness. The adolescent who has a strong commitment to his or her church and has experienced consistent participation in activities such as weekly Sunday school, church youth group, youth choir, or Bible study group may experience significant anxiety over not being able to participate in these activities, which are social as well as religious. Visits from an adolescent's peers in such a church group can provide support and comfort, as well as distracting the teen from the illness experience. Adolescence is also a time when young people cherish privacy. Teens often choose to keep their deepest and most treasured feelings to themselves. Thus, adolescents may "reject formal worship services, but engage in individual worship in the privacy of their rooms" (Wong, 1997, p. 472). It is important, even in illness, to allow for such periods of privacy, to the degree possible, for an adolescent patient.

Sometimes a very ill adolescent will request a church-associated ritual. Evelyna was a hospitalized 16-year-old from a Latin American country whose lymphoma was terminal. As a Catholic, Evelyna requested the sacrament of the Eucharist each day. One afternoon, after the chaplain, Sister Elizabeth, had administered the sacrament and offered a prayer, Evelyna looked up and said, "Sister, will you lay hands on me?" Because the "laying on of hands" is not a common practice in the Roman Catholic tradition, Sister Elizabeth was not certain what Evelyna desired, but wanted to honor her request. Several members of the family were present, so the chaplain asked that all gather around the bed with her and place their hands on Evelyna while God's blessing was sought. Especially in the case of an ill child, nurses and chaplains often have the opportunity to create small religious rituals appropriate to the sickroom setting and yet helpful in meeting the spiritual needs of the patient and the family.

Assessment of the Ill Child's Spiritual and Religious Needs

As to the question of whether a child is capable of having a serious rela-tionship with God, Judith Shelly (1982) noted that "stories abound of very young children who made serious and lasting commitments to God" (p. 12). Obviously a child's spiritual interests and concerns will vary greatly de-pending on age and the religious or denominational tradition of the fam-ily. Some broad measurement items reflective of religious tradition contained in a "family assessment interview" (Wong, 1997, p. 90) include identification of usual religious beliefs and practices, whether the family associates with a particular denomination or church, how religious beliefs influence the family's perception of illness, whether the family relies on re-ligious healers or remedies for illness, and who provides religious support for the family (e.g., clergy, relatives, or healers). Pediatric head nurse Judith Van Heukelem-Still (1984) wrote that, in assessing the spiritual needs of children, it is important not only to ask questions but also to observe the child for unusual behaviors such as nightmares or withdrawal from social activities (p. 5). She pointed out that the kind of visitors and cards a child receives may give some hint of whether spiritual influences and support are present (p. 5).

Spiritual assessment questions that Van Heukelem identified for an ill child focused on such topics as how the child behaves when frightened, who provides support in times of trouble, and what the child's understand-ing is of God and prayer (1982, p. 89).

A nursing diagnosis of spiritual distress can be identified for the ill child. Some defining characteristics of the diagnosis might relate to the child or family's lack of spiritual support or spiritual strength (Marlow & Redding, 1988, p. 78). Nursing interventions for a child reflecting spiritual distress may begin by encouraging the child to verbalize his or her feelings to a caring adult.

Spiritual Needs of the Acutely Ill Child

Pediatric nursing care, as defined by the American Nurses Association and the Society of Pediatric Nurses (1996), "focuses on helping children and their families and communities achieve their optimum health potentials" (cited in Ashwill, Droske, & Imhof, 1997, p. 11). Spiritual care of the pediatric patient is directed toward helping the child and family achieve and main-tain the greatest degree of spiritual health possible, in light of the present illness experience. As noted, in terms of assessment of spiritual need, the defining characteristics of spiritual health will vary according to the child's age, religious tradition, and the severity of the illness. Pediatric chaplain George Handzo advised that, regardless of religious background, one must be direct and frank in talking about spirituality with an ill child. "Children think a lot about faith and have more ability in theological reflection than most adults give them credit for" (1990, p. 17). Chaplain Handzo asserted that children have essentially the "same faith needs as adults"; they need to view God as one who will care for and support them, especially in times of crisis such as that of illness (1990, p. 18).

The child experiencing an acute illness, even if being cared for at home, may suffer psychosocial sequelae such as loneliness related to isolation from a peer group and interruption of school and school-related social activities (Melamed & Bush, 1985). For the older school-age child or adolescent, missing classes may cause not only a sense of alienation from peers, but also anxiety about future goals related to college and career. The adolescent may worry about "keeping up" with classes, even in the case of a relatively temporary condition. The ill teen whose schoolwork has been interrupted may feel some anger at God or at religious beliefs and question "Why me?" Spiritual counseling at such a time will allow the adolescent to verbalize frustration and potentially achieve a degree of peace and patience, a sense that ultimately all will be well.

For the young child who is acutely ill, spiritual care may be directed toward interaction with a parent or parents. Hashim was a 6-year-old Muslim child with acute lymphocytic leukemia; his father Mr. Mukti stayed with him almost continuously during a hospitalization, while his mother cared for the family's other children. On a first visit, the unit's chaplain, Elizabeth, asked Mr. Mukti if it would be acceptable, even though she was a Christian, to say a prayer for Hashim, who was receiving chemotherapy. Mr. Mukti responded, "Oh, yes, yes, we all worship the same God; you call him God; we say Allah! But He is the same God." This, and subsequent interactions with Hashim and Mr. Mukti gave Elizabeth the opportunity to discuss and learn more about Islam and the spiritual needs of a Muslim patient. One of Elizabeth's colleagues taught her a Muslim greeting in Arabic: *A salaam a le kum* (Peace be unto you). She asked Mr. Mukti if it would be appropriate for her to greet him and Hashim with the blessing when she visited. Mr. Mukti replied enthusiastically, "Oh, yes, that's wonderful. It means may you be filled with God's blessing. You can say the words when you arrive and when you leave and we will answer asking a blessing for you, *A le kum a salaam.*"

The Hospitalized Child

The hospitalized child is generally experiencing an acute illness or an acute exacerbation of a chronic condition. Such factors as the severity of illness, type of care unit (e.g., pediatric intensive care unit versus general pediatric care unit), previous hospital experience, and family support will influence the child's emotional and spiritual needs. Ashwill and Volz (1997) identified some universal stressors for the hospitalized child, however, including separation from family, fear of pain or physical injury, and fear of the unknown. Although the primary goal of a pediatric hospital unit is care of the ill child, parents, an important resource, also need attention (Hardgrove & Roberts, 1989; Leavitt, 1989). The spiritual care of the child should include spiritual support of the parents. In discussing spiritual ministry in a pediatric unit, Arnold (1992) asserted that pediatric ministry must include the entire family (p. 94). Because, Arnold noted, hospitalization of a child represents a crisis situation, needs are usually identified in spiritual language: "hope, trust, love and acceptance"; such needs may be met through the use of religious resources or simply by developing caring relationships with the child and family (p. 95).

Anna was a 13-year-old hospitalized for evaluation and staging of her escalating Ewing's sarcoma with metastasis; there was a question of surgery which would include a radical amputation of her right leg, including a hemipelvectomy. Anna's disease was progressing rapidly and known sources of chemotherapy had been exhausted. Anna relied on her own and her family's religious resources and demonstrated spiritual peace in her hope and trust in God; this was reinforced by hospital nursing staff and chaplains. Anna resisted the surgery, which physicians agreed had little chance of successfully alleviating the disease process; she decided to place her trust in God, fully aware that a physical cure might not happen. That was OK, Anna assured the staff, because, in her words, she was in a "win–win situation." She explained, "If God heals my body, then it will be wonderful and I can be a missionary and tell people about Him; but if He doesn't, then I will die and be with Jesus, so there's no way I can lose" (O'Brien, 1995, p. 141).

Spiritual Needs of the Chronically Ill Child

Childhood chronic illness is a long-term condition for which there is no cure, and which may affect the child's physical and psychological functioning. Statistics suggest that 10 to 15 percent of the pediatric population is chronically ill (Martin, 1997). Management of a child's chronic illness is complicated because of the necessity of family involvement in the provision of care (Johnson, 1985). A situation of childhood chronic illness may interfere in sibling relationships because parental attention is often heavily focused on the sick child. Although some non-ill siblings cope well, jealousy and emotional distress can occur for the well child (Holiday, 1989); the situation may thus engender feelings of guilt and inadequacy in the chronically ill sibling.

Fulton and Moore (1995) believe that the spiritual well-being of the school-age child with a chronic illness significantly affects the course of illness and treatment (p. 224). They described two nursing approaches to providing spiritual care as "therapeutic play," to generate understanding of the child's perception of spirituality vis-à-vis the illness experience; "bibliotherapy," employing such techniques as storytelling or journaling to help the child explore the meaning of life; and "use of self" in establishing rapport that may comfort the child and decrease anxiety associated with the illness and treatment (Fulton & Moore, 1995, pp. 228–231). The importance of providing devotional material to an older chronically ill child is described by a mother who reported that until her physically and cognitively disabled son's "beloved and much read Children's Bible" had recently fallen apart, he had carried it daily, attached to his walker (Cichon, 1995, p. 24).

Tony, an 18-year-old with recurrent lymphoma, was hospitalized for a course of chemotherapy. Although he talked mostly about sports with the nurses, his chaplain, Elizabeth, noticed a small worn Bible on the bedside stand. Tony's religious preference was listed on his chart simply as "Christian." As she was leaving the room one day, Elizabeth asked Tony if he would like her to read a passage from Scripture. Tony smiled and said, "Yes, that would be good. You pick something." Elizabeth chose a comforting passage about God's care from Matthew 6:25–30, commonly called the "lilies of the field" passage. "Therefore I tell you, do not worry about your life. . . . If God so clothes the grass of the fields . . . how much more will he not provide for you." Tony responded, "When I think like that, there really isn't anything to worry about. I get pretty scared about this cancer sometimes but when I put my thoughts to God, I know it's going to be OK. If God takes care of the birds and the flowers, He'll take care of me."

Spiritual Needs of the Dying Child

Like other ill children, the dying child's spiritual needs are reflective of age, spiritual or religious background, and degree of physiological and cognitive functioning. As a rule, the broad needs of dying children model those of dying adults; they desire comfort and freedom from pain, and the security that they will not be alone at the time of death (Martin, 1997, p. 414). These needs, Martin added, will be more acutely manifested in the school-age child and the adolescent (p. 414). Four of the most frequently occurring emotional reactions of dying children are "fear, depression, guilt and anger" (Winkelstein, 1989, p. 231). A school-age child, especially, may experience fear related not so much to the death itself but rather to the dying process. Children of this age may have witnessed the deaths of older family members or friends and are fearful of having to go through the pain and suffering they observed. The preschooler can feel guilty about dying, and leaving parents and siblings; he or she may feel responsible for the illness. The dying adolescent, while also experiencing some degree of fear and guilt, frequently goes through a period of depression and anger over the illness and impending death. As noted earlier, adolescence is the time of questioning spiritual and religious beliefs, as well as being the developmental stage when privacy is valued. Thus the dying adolescent may internalize and hide feelings of anger and depression for some time, resulting in an unexpected eruption of emotion as death nears.

To provide spiritual care to dying children, pediatric chaplain Dane Sommer (1989) advised that the caregiver become "theologically honest" (p. 231); that is, in order to help the child cope with suffering and death, nurses must be able to imagine their own deaths and admit that their personal faith may not provide satisfactory answers to the question, why? An exercise integral to most hospice training programs is imagining one's death and writing a personal obituary. A second requirement for those caring for dying children, identified by Chaplain Sommer, is to be able to "speak the language of children" and "enter into" the child's world (p. 231). The nurse must be sensitive to the age-related developmental stage of the child and also keep in mind that children can "see through" dishonesty and subterfuge quite easily; they find security in truth and directness, even if the information is painful. Caregivers must remember as well that a dying child who has experienced significant contact with the health care system may be very knowledgeable about his or her disease; such children expect information at a level of sophistication that may seem far beyond that warranted by chronological age. In an article presented in the *American Journal of Hospice and Palliative Medicine,* spirituality was identified as a key need in an empirically developed conceptual model of the needs of children with life-limiting conditions (Donnelly, Huff, Lindsey, McMahon, & Schumacher, 2005).

Pediatric oncologist Kate Faulkner (1997) offered some general suggestions related to caring for a dying child; these include being flexible in one's approach, being sensitive to the use of nonverbal communication, respecting the child's desire for privacy, and being "explicit and literal" in responding to questions about death (p. 69). These maxims are most appropriate for the provision of spiritual care. Regardless of a dying child's age and religious tradition, a nurse needs to employ the art as well as the science of nursing in approaching such difficult topics as spirituality and death. Perhaps the best advice is to let the child take the lead, through questions or comments; the nurse can then attempt to cross over, as it were, to the child's world, to that place where the dying child may feel alone. Thus the nurse can become friend and advocate, as well as spiritual caregiver.

Teresa, a baccalaureate-prepared pediatric oncology nurse, described the difficulty and the rewards of such nursing advocacy:

> In peds oncology, the most stressful time is around a child's death, and it's the most rewarding time also. It's a gifted experience to be with that child and family. It's a lot like being a midwife to send the child to God; but it hurts so much to lose them when you've become their friend and the family's friend. But it's a spiritual experience for the nurse and for the child. Sometimes you pray with them, sometimes you sing hymns with them, and then again, maybe you just hold them.

Teresa, a Christian, explained that, for her, if the dying child was from a religious family, it was sometimes easier to know how to give spiritual care. "I mean, you know there are certain prayers or rituals for a Christian or for a Jewish child." Teresa related a recent experience with a dying 8-year-old who did not believe in God and who asked her what would happen after death. She said, "I told him it would be like walking in a beautiful woods, a beautiful forest where there are all kinds of trees and flowers and birds, and everything will be really peaceful. And, that he will be happy and not ever be sick again."

Pam, a master's-prepared pediatric nurse, also described the rewards of providing spiritual care for dying children:

> I was raised Southern Baptist and that is generally my preference, although I also consider myself a born-again Christian. I would never impose my beliefs on anyone, especially a child, but I feel that I can discuss spiritual needs and assess children's needs, especially for the dying child. I have prayed with children, but sometimes maybe it's just listening and a hug. And in some instances I would call a

chaplain. . . . I have found the chaplains to be very good—excellent, in fact. It's just that sometimes you are the one who is there, who the child knows and will talk to. This is a special gift for you; it's real rewarding. I think spiritual care is definitely in the pediatric nurse's job description.

Certainly not to be neglected in the case of a dying child are the spiritual needs of the family, those of both parents and healthy siblings. As in caring for the child, a nurse will need to call on all of his or her own spiritual strength and experience in order to journey with a family during the predeath and death experience. Cook (1982) suggested, first, that one accept that the family members are probably "not totally rational" during this time (p. 125). Second, Cook advised that the family be encouraged to "continue to function as a family," and that family communication be fostered (p. 125). A parent of a dying child may express seemingly undue anger over a small "glitch" in the provision of hospital or hospice nursing care; this is related to the terrible frustration associated with the loss of parental control in protecting one's child. Nonjudgmental, caring support expressed by a nurse during such an outburst may go far in alleviating the parent's anxiety. The family may also experience internal disorganization during the terminal illness and death of a child. With the ill child receiving so much attention, well siblings can experience feelings of neglect and rejection. Well siblings may also feel guilty about being healthy while a brother or sister is suffering from catastrophic illness. A supportive nurse who welcomes the verbalization of fears and anxieties on the part of all members of the family can facilitate communication between parents and well children.

Camille, a pediatric oncology nurse with more than 22 years of experience, spoke articulately about the spiritual care and spiritual needs of the family of a dying child:

I think especially that nurses have to be careful not to be overzealous and impulsive with sharing their own spirituality, like saying, "this is God's will." The parents may be angry at God and not ready to hear that. Families accepting a terminally ill child is something they have to work through at their own pace; you don't want somebody anticipating that for you. Part of the art of nursing, the art of being human, is to determine where a person is spiritually. You want to embrace their needs and provide them empathy, but not overwhelm them. . . . You have to remember also that not everyone believes that there is a Divine Force guiding our lives, and so illness of a child can be totally overwhelming. You just have to try and be where that parent is at the time.

The first part of this chapter focused on the spiritual and religious needs of the ill child and the ill adolescent—in acute illness, in chronic illness, during hospitalization, and in the dying process. The discussion concluded with a reminder that in caring for an ill or dying child, one must not forget the spiritual needs of the family. The remainder of the chapter concerns the spiritual needs of the family of the ill adult, as well as those of the family of the ill child.

SPIRITUAL NEEDS OF THE FAMILY

The family is an important resource in the provision of spiritual care, not only for the sick child but for the ill adult as well. There are a number of understandings of the term *family* in contemporary society. Generally, the concept evokes an image of the basic nuclear family composed of two legally married parents and one or more offspring. Friedmann (1992) defined *family* as "two or more persons who are joined together by bonds of sharing and emotional closeness, who identify themselves as being part of the family" (p. 9). Today, however, there is a growing emergence of the single-parent family; for the single, unmarried individual, a number of persons belonging to such associations as church or friendship groups may be loosely described as family.

Families may be open, allowing members individuality and flexibility in role behavior, or closed and more rigid in terms of behavioral expectations (Dossey, 1988, p. 308). As social systems, families are said to have structure and function, including assigned roles, interactional patterns, and histories, each of which needs to be acknowledged in the planning of care (Turk & Kerns, 1985, p. 3). Some key functions of the modern family involve providing affection, companionship, security, a sense of purpose, socialization, and moral values (Reeder, Martin, & Koniak-Griffin, 1997, p. 46); additionally, the provision of shelter and material support and the maintaining of morale fall within the purview of family responsibilities (LeMone & Burke, 1996, p. 37). The family also plays an important role in managing its members' health: primary prevention in supporting a healthy lifestyle, secondary prevention related to decisions to treat illness symptoms, and tertiary prevention manifested by family support of a member's compliance with a prescribed therapeutic regimen (Danielson, Hamel-Bissell, & Winstead-Fry, 1993, p. 11).

The Family, Illness, and Spirituality

Because healthy families generally function as units, it is important to minister to the spiritual needs of the entire family when one member is ill or in need of support (Clinebell, 1991). Families faced with serious short-term or chronic long-term illness of one of the members can benefit greatly from spiritual support provided by friends, church members, or pastoral care providers both within or outside the health care system. Emeth and Greenhut (1991) noted that remaining connected with God or with spiritual beliefs "can be difficult in a health crisis" and observed that often one needs to "rely on the faith of others, to get through a difficult period" (p. 210). Thus, the nurse should welcome a family's presence as a resource in the provision of spiritual support; including family members in a religious ritual or prayer service may help them feel comfortable in sharing in the spiritual support and care of the ill person (Peterson & Potter, 1997, p. 452). Research has identified prayer and belief in God as being the most important coping strategies for a family dealing with illness (Friedmann, 1992, p. 331).

The family's particular spiritual or religious tradition and experience will, of course, direct the kind and degree of spiritual care and support that will prove helpful during an illness experience. For the family not of a religious tradition, spiritual care may consist simply of the presence and concern demonstrated by those providing the intervention. For the family whose members are or have been actively involved in a church or faith group, the religious prayers and practices of the community can be extremely comforting. A Jewish family may appreciate reading the Psalms or other passages found in the Jewish canon of Scripture; for the Muslim family, a passage from the Holy Qur'an can provide support and comfort; and for the Christian family, the Gospel messages of Jesus often provide hope and sustenance during times of illness.

The New or Expanding Family: Spiritual Needs in Childbirth and the Postnatal Experience

For the new or expanding family the childbirth experience can be a time of significant emotional stress, especially for the mother-to-be. Certain factors such as cultural background, social support, and maternal confidence may ameliorate the stress and pain associated with the birthing experience (Reeder, Martin, & Koniak-Griffin, 1997, p. 532). Spiritual support may also help in reducing anxiety and facilitating the labor and delivery process.

The childbirth experience itself may incorporate aspects of the family's spiritual or religious tradition. Callister (1995) recounted the story of an

Orthodox Jewish mother who gave thanks to God at the time of delivering a first-born son because of the belief that she is now "fulfilling the measure of her creation in obedience to Rabbinical law," and of a Mormon (Church of Jesus Christ of Latter Day Saints) mother who requested a blessing from her husband in the delivery room as she was about to give birth (p. 327). Callister asserted that nurses should provide the childbearing woman with an experience that respects the spiritual dimensions of her life (1995, p. 330).

A maternal–child health (MCH) nurse may diagnose spiritual distress in a new mother in the case of death of the neonate (Corrine, Bailey, Valentin, Morantus, & Shirley, 1992, p. 141) or following delivery of an infant with a disorder such as a congenital or genetic anomaly. Moderately severe neonatal conditions such as cleft lip and palate, talipes equinovarus (club foot), or hip dysplasia may be more or less distressing, depending on parental experience and expectations. More serious congenital or genetic anomalies, such as trisomy 21 (Down syndrome) or spina bifida, may be exceedingly traumatic for parents and siblings. Disorders such as anencephaly or Tay-Sachs disease have a devastating impact on the family. Obviously, the occurrence of any illness or anomaly in a newborn poses difficult spiritual and ethical questions for the family. Hardee (1994) raised the rhetorical question "Should severely impaired or handicapped newborns be allowed to die?" Findings from conversations with 10 intensive care nursery (ICN) nurses revealed three themes of concern in response to the question: the suffering of the newborn, the nurse's stress in caring for a suffering newborn, and the nurse's feelings of inadequacy in terms of ethical knowledge to confront such dilemmas (p. 28). Ultimately, response to this question will be guided by the nurse's personal spiritual and/or religious belief system.

In the provision of spiritual care to parents faced with a critically or terminally ill newborn, some suggested interventions are to attempt to include the entire extended family in the experience in order to engender support and affirmation for the parent or parents, to assist the family in facing the reality of the situation rather than retreating into denial or fantasy, and to try to create some meaningful and positive interaction with the newborn (Kline, 1991, pp. 89–91).

Spiritual Needs of the Family in Acute Illness

Families of acutely ill patients can be found both at home and in the hospital. Because of the unexpected and often sudden onset of an acute illness, or of an acute exacerbation of a chronic condition, families may be neglected and left to fend for themselves regardless of the setting. In a home care situation, where the family is more directly involved in a therapeutic regimen, spiritual support of extended family members and friends can be available and accessible; in the hospital a more formal type of spiritual care may be required. In the hospital setting, however, many families feel constrained by the institution's restrictions and schedules (Katonah, 1991). Most hospital and clinic waiting rooms abound with anxious family members in need of spiritual support. Some needs identified by the families of acutely ill persons include the desire for competent care, pain management, compassion, and extended family support in coping with the impact of the illness on their lives (Durand, 1993, p. xii). Additional needs perceived by the families of hospitalized acutely ill patients are information about changes in a patient's condition and honest answers to questions (Leavitt, 1989, pp. 266–267). Lynn-McHale and Smith (1993) described religion as an "additional support for families experiencing crisis" and considered addressing a family's spiritual and religious concerns as facilitating coping in an acute illness experience (p. 318).

Maria, the mother of Anna, a 13-year-old suffering from advanced Ewing's sarcoma with metastasis, spoke at length about the importance of spirituality in terms of personal faith and religious practices such as prayer and hymn singing for herself and for Anna:

> We are a very Christian family. I was saved when I was about 21 and ever since I have lived my life for Jesus. Anna has witnessed for Jesus too. I couldn't get through this without my faith. You know Anna has Ewings, one of the worst cancers you can get, and now she's relapsed so we just have to take each day at a time, each hour really! But we are putting the treatment in Jesus' hands; we are praying about it. . . . Anna has really gotten involved with the Church Youth; she has witnessed with them. They are a real support to her now. They come and pray with her. . . . I try to keep Anna up spiritually. Yesterday she had a "bone marrow" and we sang hymns and prayed through it to keep her spirits up. She's got a lot of faith; it's what gives her so much courage.

The Family in the Intensive Care Unit

Clark and Heindenreich (1995) identified spiritual well-being for the acutely ill patient experiencing intensive care as encompassing the support of caregivers, family members and friends, and religion and faith beliefs. The family of an acutely ill patient hospitalized in an intensive care unit (ICU) may spend long hours in waiting rooms, sometimes rarely leaving the hospital setting. This is a time when the arrival of a chaplain or nurse willing to provide spiritual care is generally welcomed unequivocally. Families need to verbalize their anxieties to someone with a caring heart as they attempt to face the severity of a loved one's illness (Niklas & Stefanics, 1975, p. 81). Families of ICU patients often express feelings of "helplessness" and "isolation" (Stromberg, 1992, p. 134) due to restricted visiting hours in a unit; the nurse or chaplain who is able to spend even a brief period of time with the family can become a bridge between the professional/technical aspects of the intensive care environment and the caring dimensions of the health care facility. Ultimately, spiritual support is reported to be a key dimension of family care in the ICU (Rukholm, Bailey, & Coutu-Wakulczyk, 1991).

Some spiritual care interventions for the family in a critical care setting might include giving information about the patient, environment, and staff, to the degree possible; encouraging the family members to verbalize their anxieties and concerns; suggesting some coping strategies for attempting to keep up with physical needs such as nutrition and sleep; and reinforcing the fact that the family's anxiety is normal in such a situation, with the suggestion of some possible coping strategies to reduce stress (Gillman, Gable-Rodriguez, Sutherland, & Whitacre, 1996, p. 15). The ICU nurse might also include patients' families in bedside discussions whenever acceptable and attempt to include family needs when developing a plan of care (Chesla & Stannard, 1997).

Karen, an ICU head nurse, explained how she had learned the importance of allowing critically ill patients' families to express their stressful emotions:

> My first experience with a family having a really hard time, I said something to the doctor like, "this patient is dying and the family is really upset. Could we have something to help calm them down a little bit?" Well, he got all over my case, and he said "They don't need sedation; they need ventilation." At first I couldn't figure it out, and then I thought, you know, he's right. So, if a family wants to scream and yell and lay on the floor or do whatever they need to do to let it out, let them do it. Let them express that anger and pain in whatever way they have to, at least for the time being. That's part of spiritual care as far as I'm concerned.

Spiritual Needs of the Family in Chronic Illness

Chronic illness may have periods of acute exacerbation, requiring intense medical care and perhaps even hospitalization. Because of the long-term nature of chronic illness, families may become very fatigued and frustrated in the process of providing care. The family of a chronically ill person must continually be alert to changes in the health of their loved one; thus, these families need "ongoing support from friends, health care providers and communities" (Gilliss, Rose, Hallburg, & Martinson, 1989, p. 289).

The syndromes identified as HIV infection and AIDS are, with the advent of more effective therapeutic regimens, now being described as chronic illnesses, although acute exacerbations of HIV-related cancer or opportunistic infections still occur and may be considered life threatening. Smith (1988) asserted that "AIDS is a family syndrome," which has an impact not only on the person infected with the virus, but also on all of the family members and friends with whom he or she "shares important relationships" (p. 135). The spiritual needs of the families of those living with HIV and AIDS may be complicated by the need for privacy related to the stigma some still associate with the conditions. Stigma and secrecy can isolate a family from usual support systems such as extended family members, friends, and church members (Perelli, 1991, p. 41). One mother commented, however, that in caring for her son, she was forced to tell certain people that he had AIDS, "because I needed their support, as did he, through prayers and physical help" (AIDS Ministry Program, the Archdiocese of Saint Paul and Minneapolis, 1991, p. 40). Despite all of the physical and psychosocial patient considerations associated with an HIV diagnosis, the family is also grieving and needs spiritual or religious support to assist in their own coping (Amos, 1988).

Cancer is another illness syndrome identified as a chronic condition with potentially life-threatening manifestations as well. Danielson, Hamel-Bissell, and Winstead-Fry (1993) believe that a family member's diagnosis of cancer can be "one of the most spiritually disabling events" that a family will ever experience (p. 357). Often, following such a diagnosis, both the patient's and the family's lives are disrupted because of a treatment regimen involving surgery and possible chemotherapy. The family needs significant support to facilitate coping with the myriad illness-related life changes (Sproull, 1992, p. 125).

In a study of 101 cancer patients and 45 parents of children with cancer, Spilka, Spangler, and Nelson (1983) discovered that spiritual and religious support was more important than psychological counseling; some activities appreciated were prayer, religious or spiritual reading, discussing church-related issues, spiritual counseling, and simply the presence of the spiritual caregiver (pp. 101–102). Raleigh (1992), in a study comparing 45 cancer patients and 45 patients with other chronic illnesses, found that overall the most important sources of hope were family, friends, and religion.

The significance of spirituality among 17 family caregivers of chronic dementia patients was revealed in nursing research conducted by Kaye and Robinson (1994). The investigators learned that the caregiver wives engaged in religious practices such as prayer and spiritual direction in coping with their spouses' illnesses and their own caring activities (p. 218). Based on their findings, the investigators recommended that nurses work with local churches that provide networks for such caregivers (p. 218).

Spiritual Needs of the Family Coping with a Terminal Illness

The spiritual needs of the family of an adult who has entered into the dying process are discussed in chapter 10. Here, a brief discussion of family needs in the predeath phase is presented; two case examples are drawn from the author's research with family members of persons in the later stages of AIDS.

In exploring the concept of nurse–family spiritual relationships among 11 hospice nurses and 12 bereaved families, Stiles (1990) identified five behaviors ascribed to nurses: being, doing, knowing, receiving and giving, and welcoming a stranger (p. 235). A nurse's way of being is sitting with and listening to the family; doing includes explaining, reassuring, and comforting; knowing involves sensitivity to the dying process; receiving and giving describes quality time spent between nurse and patient; and welcoming a stranger means inviting the patient's family to help prepare for the death (pp. 237–243). Wright (1997) asserted that listening to and being present to witness a terminally ill patient's and family's suffering is "the soul" of clinical nursing with families (p. 3). A veteran of 20 years of clinical work with families, Wright (1997) maintained that concern about a family's religious and spiritual beliefs has been one of the "most neglected" topics in family care. Yet, she asserted "the experience of suffering becomes transposed to one of spirituality as family members try to make meaning out of their suffering and distress" (p. 5).

Julia, the mother of 39-year-old Jonathan who was suffering from *Pneumocystis carinii* pneumonia as well as cytomegalovirus retinitis and other complications of advanced AIDS, spoke about the importance of spiritual care for herself and for her son:

> I can't tell everybody about this, but my pastor and some of the church members have been really kind and supportive; that helps so much. You really need God and the church at a time like this. Jonathan needs the support of prayers too. I've asked the pastor to pray. That's all we can do now but it's so comforting.

And Nora, whose 42-year-old son Matthew was also experiencing symptoms of advanced AIDS, asserted:

> It's only God and people's prayers that's getting me through this; they are holding me up. People have been sending prayers in cards and with phone calls. My wonderful priest is praying all the time. I don't know how I could survive without this spiritual support.

Nora admitted that sometimes she became angry with God over Matt's illness and questioned why, but she concluded, "Even when I was screaming at God, because you know, why, and why, and why? Even when I was angry with Him, I knew that God was crying with me" (O'Brien, 1992, p. 67).

Spiritual Needs of the Homeless Family

Only in recent years have texts dealing with topics such as family organization and family care begun to include the plight of the homeless family. Although families have been the last subcategory to be added to the American cadre of homeless persons, they are now considered to be "the most rapidly growing segment of the [homeless] population" (Friedmann, 1992, p. 109). Hatton and Droes (1997) reported that homeless families comprise "approximately 37% of the homeless population"; they added that in many situations family members have to split up to find accommodations at a shelter (p. 395). In McChesney's study of families living in shelters, four distinct types of homeless families were identified: "unemployed couples; mothers leaving relationships; AFDC [Aid to Families and Dependent Children] mothers; and mothers who have been homeless teenagers" (1992, p. 246).

Friedmann (1992) observed that studies exploring the effects of homelessness on families have identified myriad acute and chronic physical and mental health illnesses among family members, especially mothers and children (p. 161). In studying 250 homeless mothers and children, Menke and Wagner (1993) found that 22 percent of the children and 39 percent of the mothers were identified by the mothers as having at least one major health problem (p. 234).

Berne, Dato, Mason, and Rafferty (1993) developed a nursing model to circumscribe and address the health problems of homeless families. The key concepts of the paradigm include "individual and group factors," such as prior experiences and coping problems; "health promoting factors," including self-efficacy and self-esteem; "environmental factors," including stress and stigma; "health damaging factors," such as depression, anxiety, and low self-esteem; and "mediating factors," such as social support (p. 111). The model suggests that homeless families need to be empowered to develop self-esteem. Approaching the homeless families with empathy and respect, the authors asserted, "is pre-requisite to countering the stigmatizing attitudes that they face in other encounters with society" (p. 109). Two Robert Wood Johnson programs initiated during the past decade to alleviate some of the problems of homeless families are Health Care for the Homeless, which seeks to increase the availability and accessibility of health services for the homeless, and The Homeless Families Program, whose goal is to provide a variety of social services supportive of family well-being (Rog & Gutman, 1997, p. 209).

Providing spiritual care to homeless families, from a nursing perspective, will require all of the art, creativity, and spiritual strength a nurse can muster during a health care encounter. Because of the transient nature of the homeless, nurses may experience only brief and intermittent interactions with them. Because of the stigma and embarrassment of the homeless condition, parents seeking emergency or clinic care for themselves or their children may be shy about expressing their anxieties and concerns with a nurse caregiver; children, and especially teens, may also be reticent to discuss the pain associated with their homelessness.

An important strategy for the nurse is to provide a welcoming, accepting, and respectful environment for the homeless family seeking care. A compassionate and nonjudgmental attitude can go far in supporting the homeless client's fragile self-concept and may allow the opportunity for some spiritual sharing between client and nurse. If this occurs, the nurse may be able to guide the family in finding religious, and possibly some material, support to assist them in coping with the suffering associated with homelessness.

Migrant laborers comprise a unique population of families that are temporarily, or in some cases permanently, homeless. One group, the U.S. central stream migrants, who travel from south-central Texas through midwestern states engaging in seasonal farmwork, are predominantly Mexican American. Religious belief and practice is very important to this largely Catholic community. In the migrant workers' temporary housing, religious articles such as rosaries and holy pictures are proudly and prominently displayed (O'Brien, 1991). In a qualitative study of the health and illness beliefs and practices of a group of Mexican American migrant workers (described in chapter 3), a core category that emerged from the data analysis was labeled "sacred-ritualistic health attitudes and behaviors." This theme suggested that many health beliefs of the group were associated with religious practice. That is, health maintenance and health care were often supported by prayers and by the reverencing of such objects as medals and holy images. Migrant workers sometimes made pilgrimages to holy places to seek the intercession of certain saints or of the Virgin for the cure of illness or the preservation of health (O'Brien, 1982). The family unit is strongly united in the practice of their faith. Thus, the nurse caring for a homeless Mexican American migrant family must be aware of the importance of religious beliefs in relation to health/illness issues and must attempt to provide support for the family's spiritual tradition whenever possible.

Children and families have unique and important spiritual needs in dealing with illness and disability. For the young child as well as for the teen, the support of personal faith and religious practice can significantly mediate the suffering involved with an illness experience. Families of sick children and families of adults who are ill also need and benefit from spiritual care. Although the patient as the center of attention often receives much spiritual support and care, the patient's family members may be neglected or forgotten. Nurses have a prime opportunity to minister spiritually to children and to family members, especially during critical or terminal illness. Perhaps the most elusive category of families for the nurse to reach are those experiencing homelessness. The nurse must employ art and creativity in attempting to provide spiritual intervention for this fragile population.

REFERENCES

AIDS Ministry Program, the Archdiocese of Saint Paul and Minneapolis. (1991). *For those we love: A spiritual perspective on AIDS* (2nd ed.). Cleveland, OH: The Pilgrim Press.

American Nurses Association and the Society of Pediatric Nurses. (1996). *Statement of the scope and standards of pediatric clinical practice* (pp. 25–35). Washington, DC: American Nurses Publishing.

Amos, W. E. (1988). *When AIDS comes to church.* Philadelphia: The Westminister Press.

Arnold, J. (1992). The voices on pediatrics: Walking with children and parents. In L. E. Holst (Ed.), *Hospital ministry: The role of the chaplain today* (pp. 93–106). New York: Crossroad.

Ashwill, J. W., Droske, S. C., & Imhof, S. (1997). Introduction to pediatric nursing. In J. W. Ashwill & S. C. Droske (Eds.), *Nursing care of children: Principles and practice* (pp. 2–23). Philadelphia: W. B. Saunders.

Ashwill, J. W., & Volz, D. (1997). The ill child in the hospital and other care settings. In J. W. Ashwill & S. C. Droske (Eds.), *Nursing care of children: Principles and practice* (pp. 346–371) Philadelphia: W. B. Saunders.

Berne, A. S., Dato, C., Mason, D. J., & Rafferty, M. (1993). A nursing model for addressing the health needs of homeless families. In G. D. Wegner & R. J. Alexander (Eds.), *Readings in family nursing* (pp. 109–121). Philadelphia: J. B. Lippincott.

Burkhardt, M. A. (1991). Spirituality and children: Nursing considerations. *Journal of Holistic Nursing, 9*(2), 31–40.

Callister, L. C. (1995). Cultural meanings of childbirth. *Journal of Obstetrics, Gynecology, and Maternity Nursing, 24*(4), 327–331.

Carretto, C. (1978). *Summoned by love.* Maryknoll, NY: Orbis Books.

Chesla, C. A., & Stannard, D. (1997). Breakdown in the nursing care of families in the ICU. *American Journal of Critical Care, 6*(1), 64–71.

Cichon, K. K. (1995). Life with Noah: Growing toward wholeness through parenting a handicapped child. *The Journal of Christian Healing, 17*(4), 18–25.

Clark, C., & Heindenreich, T. (1995). Spiritual care for the critically ill. *American Journal of Critical Care, 4*(1), 77–81.

Clinebell, H. (1991). *Basic types of pastoral care and counseling.* Nashville, TN: Abington Press.

Coles, R. (1990). *The spiritual life of children.* Boston: Houghton Mifflin.

Cook, M. (1982). Ministering to dying children and their families. In J. A. Shelly (Ed.), *The spiritual needs of children* (pp. 117–129). Downers Grove, IL: InterVarsity Press.

Corrine, L., Bailey, V., Valentin, M., Morantus, E., & Shirley, L. (1992). The unheard voices of women: Spiritual interventions in maternal-child health. *American Journal of Maternal Child Nursing, 17*(3), 141–145.

Danielson, C. B., Hamel-Bissell, B., & Winstead-Fry, P. (1993). *Families, health & illness: Perspectives on coping and intervention.* St. Louis, MO: C. V. Mosby.

Donnelly, J., Huff, S., Lindsey, M., McMahon, K., & Schumacher, J. (2005). The needs of children with life-limiting conditions: A healthcare-provider-based model. *American Journal of Hospice and Palliative Care Medicine, 22*(4), 259–267.

Dossey, B. M. (1988). Relationships: Learning the patterns and processes. In B. M. Dossey, L. Keegan, C. E. Guzzetta, & L. G. Kolkmeier (Eds.), *Holistic nursing: A handbook for practice* (pp. 305–330). Rockville, MD: Aspen.

Durand, B. A. (1993). Preface: Determination of need. In S. L. Feetham, S. B. Meister, J. M. Bell, & C. L. Gillis (Eds.), *The nursing of families* (pp. ix–xiii). Newburg Park, CA: Sage.

Emeth, E V., & Greenhut, J. H. (1991). *The wholeness handbook: Care of body, mind and spirit for optimal health.* New York: Continuum.

Faulkner, K. W. (1997). Talking about death with a dying child. *American Journal of Nursing, 97*(6), 64–69.

Fowler, J. (1981). *Stages of faith: The psychology of human development and the quest for meaning.* San Francisco: Harper San Francisco.

Friedmann, M. M. (1992). *Family nursing: Theory and practice.* (3rd ed.), Norwalk, CT: Appleton & Lange.

Fulton, R. A., & Moore, C. M. (1995). Spiritual care of the school age child with a chronic condition. *Journal of Pediatric Nursing, 10*(4), 224–231.

Gilliss, C. L., Rose, D., Hallburg, J. C., & Martinson, I. M. (1989). The family and chronic illness. In C. L. Gilliss, B. M. Highley, B. M. Roberts, & I. M. Martinson (Eds.), *Toward a science of family nursing* (pp. 287–299). New York: Addison-Wesley.

Gillman, J., Gable-Rodriguez, J., Sutherland, M., & Whitacre, J. H. (1996). Pastoral care in a critical care setting. *Critical Care Nursing Quarterly, 19*(1), 10–20.

Handzo, G. F. (1990). Talking about faith with children. *Journal of Christian Nursing, 7*(4), 17–20.

Hardee, L. B. (1994). When a newborn cannot survive. *Journal of Christian Nursing, 11*(1), 16–18.

Hardgrove, C., & Roberts, B. M. (1989). The family with a hospitalized child. In C. L. Gilliss, B. M. Highley, B. M. Roberts, & I. M. Martinson (Eds.), *Toward a science of family nursing* (pp. 148–161). New York: Addison-Wesley.

Hatton, D. C., & Droes, J. M. (1997). The homeless. In J. M. Swanson & M. A. Nies (Eds.), *Community health nursing: Promoting the health of aggregates* (2nd ed., pp. 387–406). Philadelphia: W. B. Saunders.

Heller, D. (1985). The children's God. *Psychology Today, 19*(1), 11–17.

Holiday, B. (1989). The family with a chronically ill child: An interactional perspective. In C. L. Gilliss, B. M. Highley, B. M. Roberts, & I. M. Martinson (Eds.), *Toward a science of family nursing* (pp. 300–311). New York: Addison-Wesley.

Johnson, S. B. (1985). The family and the child with chronic illness. In D. C. Turk & R. D. Kerns (Eds.), *Health, illness and families: A life-span perspective* (pp. 110–154). New York: John Wiley & Sons.

Katonah, J. (1991). Hospitalization: A rite of passage. In L. E. Holst (Ed.), *Hospital ministry: The role of the chaplain today* (pp. 55–67). New York: Crossroad.

Kaye, J., & Robinson, K. M. (1994). Spirituality among caregivers. *Image: Journal of Nursing Scholarship, 26*(3), 118–121.

Kenny, G. (1999). Children's nursing: Assessing children's spirituality, what is the way forward? *British Journal of Nursing, 8*(1), 28; 30–32.

Kline, S. J. (1991). The voices on obstetrics: Participants and partners. In L. E. Holst (Ed.), *Hospital ministry: The role of the chaplain today* (pp. 79–91). New York: Crossroad.

Kohlberg, L. (1984). *The psychology of moral development.* San Francisco: Harper & Row.

Leavitt, M. B. (1989). Transition to illness: The family in the hospital. In C. L. Gilliss, B. M. Highley, B. M. Roberts, & I. M. Martinson (Eds.), *Toward a science of family nursing* (pp. 161–186). New York: Addison-Wesley.

LeMone, P., & Burke, K. M. (1996). *Medical–surgical nursing: Critical thinking in client care.* New York: Addison-Wesley.

Lynn-McHale, D. J., & Smith, A. (1993). Comprehensive assessment of families of the critically ill. In G. D. Wegner & R. J. Alexander (Eds.), *Readings in family nursing* (pp. 309–311). Philadelphia: J. B. Lippincott.

Marlow, D. R., & Redding, B. A. (1988). *Textbook of pediatric nursing* (6th ed.). Philadelphia: W. B. Saunders.

Martin, G. T. (1997). The child with a chronic or terminal illness. In J. W. Ashwill & S. C. Droske (Eds.), *Nursing care of children: Principles and practice* (pp. 394–417). Philadelphia: W. B. Saunders.

McChesney, K. Y. (1991). Homeless families: Four patterns of poverty. In M. J. Robertson & M. Greenblatt (Eds.), *Homelessness: A national perspective* (pp. 145–156). New York: Plenum Press.

Melamed, B. G., & Bush, J. P. (1985). Family factors in children with acute illness. In D. C. Turk & R. D. Kerns (Eds.), *Health, illness and families: A life-span perspective* (pp. 183–219). New York: John Wiley & Sons.

Menke, E. M., & Wagner, J. D. (1993). The health of homeless mothers and their children. In S. Feetham, S. B. Meister, J. Bell, & C. Gilliss (Eds.), *The nursing of families* (pp. 224–234). Newbury Park, CA: Sage.

Moran, M. (1997). Growth and development. In J. W. Ashwill & S. C. Droske (Eds.), *Nursing care of children: Principles and practice* (pp. 26–49). Philadelphia: W. B. Saunders.

Niklas, G. R., & Stefanics, C. (1975). *Ministry to the hospitalized.* New York: Paulist Press.

O'Brien, M. E. (1982). Pragmatic survivalism: Behavior patterns affecting low level wellness among minority group members. *Advances in Nursing Science, 4*(3), 13–26.

O'Brien, M. E. (1991). Reaching the migrant worker. In B. W. Spradley (Ed.), *Readings in community health nursing* (pp. 564–568). New York: J. B. Lippincott.

O'Brien, M. E. (1992). *Living with HIV: Experiment in Courage.* Westport, CT: Auburn House.

O'Brien, M. E. (1995). *The AIDS challenge: Breaking through the boundaries.* Westport, CT: Auburn House.

Perelli, R. (1991). *Ministry to persons with AIDS: A family systems approach.* Minneapolis, MN: Augsburg.

Peterson, V., & Potter, P. A. (1997). Spiritual health. In P. A. Potter & A. G. Perry (Eds.), *Fundamentals of nursing: Concepts, process and practice* (pp. 440–456). St. Louis, MO: C. V. Mosby.

Raleigh, E. D. (1992). Sources of hope in chronic illness. *Oncology Nursing Forum, 19*(2), 443–448.

Reeder, S. J., Martin, L. L., & Koniak-Griffin, D. (1997). *Maternity nursing: Family, newborn and women's health care* (18th ed.). Philadelphia: J. B. Lippincott.

Rog, D. J., & Gutman, M. (1997). The homeless families program: A summary of key findings. In S. L. Isaacs & J. R. Knickman (Eds.), *To improve health and health care 1997: The Robert Wood Johnson Foundation anthology* (pp. 209–231). San Francisco: Jossey-Bass.

Roger of Taize. (1990). *His love is a fire.* Collegeville, MN: The Liturgical Press.

Rukholm, E. E., Bailey, P. H., & Coutu-Wakulczyk, G. (1991). Family needs and anxieties in the ICU. *The Canadian Journal of Nursing Research, 23*(3), 67–81.

Shelly, J. A. (1982). Jesus and the children: A mandate to care. In J. A. Shelly (Ed.), *The spiritual needs of children* (pp. 11–16). Downers Grove, IL: InterVarsity Press.

Smith, W. J. (1988). *AIDS, living and dying with hope: Issues in pastoral care.* New York: Paulist Press.

Sommer, D. R. (1989). The spiritual needs of dying children. *Issues in Comprehensive Pediatric Nursing, 12*(1), 225–233.

Spector, R. E., & Spertac, A. M. (1990). Social and cultural influences on the child. In S. R. Mott, S. R. James, & A. M. Spertac (Eds.), *Nursing care of children and families* (2nd ed., pp. 53–75). New York: Addison-Wesley.

Spilka, B., Spangler, J. D., & Nelson, C. B. (1983). Spiritual support in life threatening illness. *Journal of Religion and Health, 22*(2), 98–104.

Sproull, A. (1992). The voices on cancer care: A lens unfocused and narrowed. In L. E. Holst (Ed.), *Hospital ministry: The role of the chaplain today.* New York: Crossroad.

Stiles, M. K. (1990). The shining stranger: Nurse–family spiritual relationships. *Cancer Nursing, 13*(4), 235–245.

Stromberg, R. (1992). The voices on coronary care: A confrontation with vulnerability. In L. E. Holst (Ed.), *Hospital ministry: The role of the chaplain today.* New York: Crossroad.

Turk, D. C., & Kerns, R. D. (1985). The family in health and illness. In D. C. Turk & R. D. Kerns (Eds.), *Health, illness and families: A life-span perspective* (pp. 1–22). New York: John Wiley & Sons.

Van Heukelem, J. (1982). Assessing the spiritual needs of children and their families. In J. A. Shelly (Ed.), *The spiritual needs of children* (pp. 87–97). Downers Grove, IL: InterVarsity Press.

Van Heukelem-Still, J. (1984). How to assess spiritual needs of children and their families. *Journal of Christian Nursing, 1*(1), 4–6.

Winkelstein, M. (1989). Spirituality and the death of a child. In V. B. Carson (Ed.), *Spiritual dimensions of nursing practice* (pp. 217–253). Philadelphia: W. B. Saunders.

Wong, D. L. (1997). *Whaley & Wong's essentials of pediatric nursing* (5th ed.). St. Louis, MO: C. V. Mosby.

Wright, L. M. (1997). Spirituality and suffering: The soul of clinical work with families. *Journal of Family Nursing, 3*(1), 3–14.

10 Spiritual Needs of the Older Adult

There is no such notion as retirement in terms of the purpose of God . . . God calls us to live life with Him as co-creators, co-workers in the reshaping and renewing of human history . . . and that calling is never completed until the day He calls us to live with Him.

JITSUO MORIKAWA, 1974
(cited in Seymour, 1995)

This chapter documents the spiritual needs of the frail or ill older adult. Data identifying spiritual needs were obtained through both structured and unstructured interviews and interactions with three groups of older persons living with illness; the study populations included chronically ill elders who are active, homebound elders, and elders residing in a nursing home. The elders experienced a multiplicity of illness conditions including congestive heart disease, hypertension, arteriosclerosis, arthritis, diabetes, and Alzheimer's disease. Interview data were also elicited from caregivers of the frail elderly. Nursing research has also documented the importance of nurses providing spiritual care to elders living both in the community (Castellaw, Wicks, & Martin, 1999) and in nursing homes (Hicks, 1999).

THE OLDER ADULT

Who are the elderly? Who are those individuals whom society labels "seniors," or "older adults"? Current definitions based on chronological age are changing as a result of the increasing longevity and functional ability of contemporary men and women. In a study to determine the preferred group descriptor of older Americans, the terms *mature, older,* and *senior* were the most frequently chosen adjectives; *aged* and *old* were the most disliked terms (Finley, 1989, p. 6). Demographic profiles identify persons as older adults if they have passed the age of 65. Individuals between 65 and 74 years of age are described as "young old"; those over 74 are identified as the "older elderly." Roen (1997) suggested, however, that the "young old" subgroup "may soon include people as old as 84" (p. 348).

Older adults are the most rapidly growing segment of the population. In 1991, the U.S. census identified 31 million Americans over the age of 65; Holland and McCurren (1997) estimated that the number will increase "to approximately 33.5 million by the year 2005" (p. 81). Presently the life expectancy of North American women is 78; and men, 71. The estimation for longevity by the year 2030 is 82.3 years for women and 75.4 years for men (Taylor, Lillis, & LeMone, 1997, p. 163). Twenty percent of the U.S. population will be over 65 by the year 2020; this group is anticipated to account for 70 percent of those who need "primary, acute, home and long-term nursing care" (Rice, Beck, & Stevenson, 1997, p. 27).

Tournier (1983) described the movement from adulthood to older age as one of the great turning points in life. Admittedly, certain potentially negative physiological and psychosocial changes accompany the aging process. Although each person ages differently, some common characteristics are physical changes in hair, skin, and teeth; impaired vision and hearing; lessened appetite; skeletal changes related to arthritis or osteoporosis; and lowered energy levels, among others. As a result of these physiological modifications, the older adult may experience social isolation, financial concern associated with the inability to work, and anxiety and depression related to worry about future health and health care issues. Despite this rather bleak chronology of negative factors associated with the aging process, Taylor, Lillis, and LeMone (1997) believe that the older adult can continue to carry out the usual activities of middle age as long as the pace is modified and rest periods are included (p. 59).

Heriot (1995) warned that for too long our society has viewed aging in depressing terms rather than seeking out the positive developmental processes than can occur despite the negative physical changes (p. 349). Some developmental tasks for the elder include the creation of a new self-image as an older person, learning to adjust to and find meaning in life despite physical impairments or decreasing energy levels, adapting to a simpler lifestyle necessitated by lowered or fixed income, and seeking to promote and maintain a high quality of life as an older adult (Lueckenotte, 1997, p. 573). It is possible for the older adult to move past his or her physical deficits and "find a sense of identity and worth in relationships, and in intellectual, artistic and spiritual pursuits" (Maltby, 1990, p. 101). As well as enjoying relationships with family and friends, some other strategies for aging well are cultivating a positive attitude toward life, choosing activities one enjoys, and maintaining a health regimen of diet and exercise (Hogstel, 1995).

More and more older adults, especially in the younger-old category, are remaining in the workforce or initiating second or third careers; many are also involved in full-time volunteer activities. Chronological age, of itself, should not be considered a disqualifier for maintaining a responsible place in society (Stagg, 1981, p. 11). Ultimately, Finch (1993) posited, the aging process may become a time of peace and joy during which the elder, no longer struggling with the challenges of career or ego, may be able to enjoy the beauties of loved ones and of nature in "wise tranquility" (p. 11). Wisdom is a spiritual gift that the older adult has to give to the world, a gift much needed in contemporary society.

THE SPIRITUALITY OF AGING

Even to your old age, I am, even when you turn gray I will carry you; I will carry you and will save you.

ISAIAH 46:4

Spiritual writers Henri Nouwen and Walter Gaffney, in their book *Aging: The Fulfillment of Life* (1990), described the aging process poignantly as a human experience "which overarches the human community as a rainbow of promises" (p. 19). Aging, the authors believe, "can lead us to discover more and more of life's treasures . . . aging is not a reason for despair but a basis for hope, not a slow decaying but a gradual maturing, not a fate to be undergone but a challenge to be embraced" (p. 20). Seymour (1995) also advanced the concept of viewing the aging process in a spiritual light, asserting that as one's physical strength weakens, the spiritual dimension of life may intensify. Supportive of that position is a quotation cited by Seymour from a 150-year-old volume, *Happy Talk Towards the End of Life*. "Is your eyesight dimmer? Then the world is seen by you in cathedral light. Is your hearing duller? Then it is just as though you were always where loud voices and footsteps ought not to be heard . . . Yes, for twilight and silence . . . old age makes us like daily dwellers in the house of the Lord" (p. 100).

Scholars of aging disagree as to whether the older adult becomes more or less involved in both spiritual and religious issues (Bianchi, 1995; Burt, 1992). Admittedly, some of the physical and psychosocial deficits of older age may hinder one's religiosity or religious practice; however, personal spirituality often deepens (Seymour, 1995). If an older person is relatively well, research has shown that religious practice may increase (Ainlay & Smith, 1984; Hunsberger, 1985; Markides, 1983). Membership in a church "is claimed by 73% of women and 63% of men older than 50 years, although fewer attend regularly" (Roen, 1997, p. 356); older adults tend to view the practice of religion as more important than do younger adults (Peterson & Potter, 1997). A church or synagogue may provide social networks for an older adult, as well as delineating a structure within which to live out one's spiritual beliefs. Some church groups may even facilitate health care for the older adult through the support of a parish nurse, as discussed in chapter 7.

David Moberg worried, however, that while many religious or faith communities have been concerned about meeting the physical needs of their elders, they may have neglected ministering to spiritual needs (1990, p. 18). Spiritual needs in the older adult are manifestations of the spiritual development associated with the aging process. As Bianchi pointed out, creatively dealing with the fact of one's mortality is a "major life task" (1995, p. 59), as well as a major faith task. The task can become central to finding meaning in life for an older adult. Boettcher (1985) believed that as an elder's physical and psychosocial world begins to shrink, "an inner expansion of awareness and spirit can develop" (p. 29).

In order to provide spiritual care to an older adult, it is important for the caregiver to have some understanding of the developmental faith tasks of aging (Maltby, 1990). One useful paradigm is that of James Fowler's (1981) stages of faith development (discussed in chapter 3). To explain the late adult era, the final two of Fowler's stages are appropriate: Conjunctive Faith, stage 5, and movement toward stage 6, Universalizing Faith. Stage 5, or Conjunctive Faith (midlife and beyond), is a time of attempting to look beyond rational explanations and seeing their limitations. In this stage, the older adult may look back on earlier religious beliefs and traditions, which may have been discarded, and begin to reincorporate them into current attitudes and practice. Fowler called this a "reclaiming or reworking of one's past" (1981, p. 197). He noted also that this is a time of "opening to the voices of one's deeper self," of one's "social unconscious" (p. 198). Previous prejudices toward people or religions can now be rejected and a new openness created. Despite this movement toward an attitude of justice for all, the individual in stage 5 may remain somewhat torn between preserving his or her own tradition and needs and a "more universal" caring (Koenig, 1994, p. 92).

Fowler's sixth stage, Universalizing Faith, occurring in the final years of life, is identified as "exceedingly rare." "The persons best described by it have generated faith compositions . . . inclusive of all being" (1981, p. 200). Persons in the sixth faith stage possess "enlarged visions of universal community," and generally tend to violate "usual criteria for normalcy" (p. 200). These persons are unequivocally committed to a vision involving justice and peace and are willing to sacrifice their lives in the cause (Koenig, 1994, p. 93). This final stage is similar to what has been labeled "mature religious faith," a time when one directs one's concerns away from self and toward the larger society (Koenig, 1994; Maitland, 1991; Payne, 1990).

SPIRITUALITY AND RELIGIOUS PRACTICE IN OLDER ADULTS

As an outgrowth of and support for one's spiritual development, religious practices may be very important to the quality of life of an older adult. The religious or faith tradition of the elder will direct the nature of specific practices. Studies of religiosity among elders have, however, identified certain practices common to a number of religious denominations. Some of these include prayer and meditation, church membership, participation in religious worship services, study of religious doctrine, and spiritual reading. Halstead (1995) also identified the use of religiously oriented videos, music tapes, and television programs as helpful to elders in practicing their religion (p. 416).

In a study of religious practice among 380 elders, Mull, Cox, and Sullivan (1987) found that 94 percent reported religion to be important in terms of their health and well-being. The well elders highly valued attendance at church or synagogue. For those who had greater physical disability, private religious practices such as prayer and watching religious TV programs became more important (p. 151). Religious practice can be seen as giving life to spiritual beliefs, providing an important spiritual support network for the older adult, and helping an ill elder to transcend physical or emotional suffering by internalizing a transcendent vision in terms of the meaning of life (Hall, 1985).

The common religious practice universally identified with most Western and Eastern religions is that of prayer. Despite diminishing physical health, persons of all religious beliefs tend to pray more during their senior years than at any other time in their lives (Finley, 1989). Prayer is a practice with many faces (different types of prayer are discussed in chapters 3 and 4). For a well elder, prayer may involve social interaction when engaged in during group worship services. For an ill or frail elder, private prayer or meditation can help alleviate feelings of loneliness or anxiety. For the confused or cognitively impaired older adult, traditional prayers learned in one's youth can sometimes be remembered and provide comfort. This is reflected in the comments of a chaplain with more than seven years of experience in ministering to nursing home residents. In justifying the inclusion of confused elders in religious rites, the chaplain asserted:

Even patients who are pretty much out of contact, they are still able to make the sign of the cross; they are still able to say prayers they learned when they were three or four years old. It [religion] is one of the things that goes last, as far as the memory is concerned; well, at least some basic tenets that they hang on to because they were so deeply ingrained. (O'Brien, 1989, p. 144)

Establishing a schedule for times of prayer during the day can be helpful for the newly retired person who may be somewhat "at loose ends"; the person can look forward to this time "not as a duty but as a time of joy and relaxation" (Coupland, 1985, p. 44). Spiritual writer Robert Wicks (1997) suggested that older adults might choose to engage in several types of prayer during the day, including both formal and informal prayers ("conversations with God"), religious reflections, "spiritual letter-writing," and creating of one's own parables (p. 22). Some comforting Psalms that an elder might pray are Psalm 23, "The Lord is my shepherd"; Psalm 25, prayer for guidance; Psalm 34, God as protector; Psalm 62, trust in God; Psalm 71, prayer in old age; and Psalm 121, God's support in trials (Hynes, 1989, p. 49).

SPIRITUALITY AND PHYSICAL DIMINISHMENT

Every age has its own beauty. Why be afraid of physical decline when the years bring deeper insight and greater gentleness of action.

BROTHER ROGER of Taize
(cited in Finch, 1993, p. 23)

When an elder's physical capacities are no longer functional at the level an individual may wish, a sense of inner comfort and peace may still be derived from spiritual beliefs and behaviors. Spiritual and religious practices such as meditation or silent prayer, or having a loving attitude toward others, may be part of a life plan even for the older old person afflicted with a multiplicity of physical deficits. In a study including 31 in-depth interviews with older adults whose health ranged from good to terminal illness, Hungelmann, Kenkel-Rossi, Klassen, and Stollenwerk (1985) found the concept of "harmonious interconnectedness" of relationships to constitute spiritual well-being. The core categories of spiritual well-being identified were "ultimate other," reflecting such concepts as belief and trust in God and religious practice; "other/nature," consisting of expressions of mutual love and forgiveness, and accepting and giving help; and "self," relating to accepting and valuing oneself (p. 150). The investigators reported that, for this population of elders, spiritual well-being represented a "state of peace and har-mony . . . linked to past experiences and future hopes and goals" (p. 151).

A nursing diagnosis of alteration in spiritual well-being or spiritual distress in an ill elder may be related to the individual's anger or frustration over an illness or disability. Chaplain Mary Brian Durkin, who ministers to patients on a rehabilitation unit, noted that a disabled patient's suffering was often associated with a negative attitude toward his or her condition (1992). For such a patient the provision of spiritual counseling and support can be a critical element in coping with illness and disability. Sister Mary Byrne (1985) asserted that for some ill elders "spiritual support is their great-est need"; she pointed out that emotional support is not adequate if an older person's problem is of a spiritual nature (pp. 30, 32).

SPIRITUALITY AND COGNITIVE DIMINISHMENT

Many older adults experience some degree of cognitive impairment as they progress through the aging process. Rice, Beck, and Stevenson (1997) re-ported cognitive impairment or senile dementia of the Alzheimer type (SDAT) in an "estimated 10.3% of those over 65," and that "the incidence may be as high as 48% in persons over 85 years of age" (p. 29). The authors posited that approximately 75 percent of nursing home residents have some cognitive impairment (p. 29).

The latter statistic was supported during the author's conduct of an exploratory case study of a 230-bed nursing home, labeled "Bethany Manor" (O'Brien, 1989). Because of the large number of Bethany Manor residents manifesting dementia symptoms, an attempt was made, through qualitative interview, to gain at least minimal understanding of their spiritual, physical, and emotional needs. Five dominant themes describing attitude and be-havior were derived from data elicited in interviews with a subsample of 24 moderately cognitively impaired residents. These concepts included con-formity, related to the residents' desire to please, especially the nursing home staff; privacy, which meant "minding one's own business" and limiting social interactions in the nursing home; activity, relating to activities of daily living in the nursing home, as well as visiting with staff and family; externality, a theme describing the fact that, according to their comments, some residents seemed to "live" in the worlds of family and friends outside of the nursing home; and reminiscence, or telling stories of one's life, even as far back as childhood (O'Brien, 1989, pp. 37–39). Some hints as to a resident's spiritu-ality did emerge in the data, for example, remarks about God, prayer, or at-tendance at church as a child. One woman commented, "When you look at the handicaps all the people here have, I say God's been good to me" (p. 39); another long-term resident asserted, "I have been brought up as a Christian and my belief is a great support to me now" (p. 47).

As pointed out by Sharon Mooney, "The effect of Alzheimer's disease on spirituality, or on a person's relationship with God, is an area that has not been studied extensively" (2006, p. 9). Thus, Mooney has explored "ways to help dementia patients remember God"; one suggestion was the use of "rituals" associated with a patient's faith tradition. Mooney explained, "For the present generation of older adults with progressive dementia, the importance of rituals as a means of enhancing some degree of orientation to reality, calming emotions and decreasing agitated physical behavior should not be underestimated" by nurses caring for these patients (p. 9).

SPIRITUAL CONCERNS OF THE OLDER ADULT

Loneliness

Loneliness can be a significant problem for the older adult (Fischer, 1995; Lotito, 1993; Normille, 1992). This is related to the onset of both physical and psychosocial deficits. Such deficits may cause the older person to become distanced from a faith or worship group. Restriction in ambulation can hinder an elder's religious practice in terms of attendance at church or synagogue worship services; impairment in sight and hearing may cause an elder to be sensitive about participating in faith group activities where such a limitation might be noticed. Elders may also retreat from church activities as a result of fatigue or depression associated with the aging process. For the elder not of a religious tradition, loneliness may relate to isolation from former work and friendship or volunteer groups, such as clubs and charitable organizations.

An older adult may take a number of steps to alleviate loneliness, such as making a conscious effort to get out, if able physically. Many churches today have special programs and groups for elders only; these can be social or may involve volunteer activities (Finley, 1989). Also, a number of community programs encourage the participation of the elderly who are mobile. For the homebound elder, church groups and some hospitals have projects such as Senior Connection, through which the ill older person can stay connected by phone to others in the area.

Although loneliness is a phenomenon experienced at some time and to some degree by virtually everyone, the loneliness of the older adult is unique in that it often grows out of loss (Valentine, 1994). An elder's loneliness can be the result of multiple losses: physical (isolation related to disabling health deficit), emotional (deaths of family and friends), social (loss of work-related relationships), financial (inability to travel or participate in social activities due to a fixed income), or spiritual (loss of ability to participate in religious worship services).

Although steps can be taken to alleviate an elder's loneliness, spiritual literature on the concept advises that "aloneness need not be a negative experience": "On the contrary, the emptiness of feeling alone can open one's heart, and make one more perceptive of the presence of God" (Deeken, 1986, p. 41). After a life filled with activity, work, family, and social activities, seniors may find that their aloneness provides a time of peace and quiet joy. For those elders, rather than bringing loneliness, the period of retirement from active work is welcomed as a spiritual journey, a preparation for the transition to eternal life.

Uncertainty of the Future

For the older adult, especially one experiencing illness, uncertainty of the future can be the source of much anxiety. The elder may have already witnessed the lingering illnesses and deaths of relatives or friends, each loss raising anew the specter of one's own mortality. Central concerns for the older adult generally are focused on economics (financial security or lack of security in the later stages of life) and autonomy (being able to care for oneself in illness or having some control over the kind of care received). Associated fears are those related to the possibility of future loneliness and cognitive impairment. The comments of a 77-year-old nursing home resident reflect such uncertainty. "I just don't know about the future. You work hard all your life, but in the end you never know. It's a worry, I'll tell you that for sure."

Some older adults, however, especially those with a spiritual or religious perspective on life, express little fear of the future. An 83-year-old nursing home resident described her present life as satisfactory. "I'm at peace and I hope to die here. I have reached a good age. God has been good to me. The things that could make me wonder about things, worry me, are lost. Death doesn't frighten me" (O'Brien, 1989, p. 45).

SPIRITUAL NEEDS OF THE OLDER ADULT

Hammer (1990) identified the spiritual needs of the older adult as relating to the carrying out of religious practices such as grace before meals, Scripture reading, and prayer; for the older or frail elderly, some contact with a former church or faith group is important (pp. 3–4). Forbis (1988) advanced a broader understanding of spiritual need among older adults, identifying such activities as listening to music, reading poetry, and verbalizing fears and anxieties, as well as prayer and spiritual reading (p. 159). Forbis warned that an ill elder who had strong religious beliefs may be fearful of express-ing doubts or anxieties to family or friends; such an individual may, however, share these concerns with a nurse who does not have the same expectations as significant others (p. 158).

A key spiritual need of the older adult, regardless of whether the elder identifies with a particular religious tradition, is the ability to find meaning in the aging process (Blazer, 1991). Although this can be the most difficult task of aging in the face of multiple physical, psychological, social, and fi-nancial losses, it is also the most challenging dimension of an elder's spiri-tual journey. Closely linked to this faith task of aging is the need to confront the prospect of death and the dying process. Although those who adhere to a religious tradition generally fear death less than those with no particular religious belief, the prospect of coping with the dying process causes anxi-ety in most older adults (Berggren-Thomas & Griggs, 1995). In the face of terminal illness, specific spiritual needs for trust, hope, and forgiveness most frequently manifest in an older adult. Related to these needs is the desire for reminiscence, which may help the elder to put present anxieties into the perspective of an entire lifetime.

Trust

Trust, a concept that was defined broadly in chapter 7 as being related to a sense of security in one's future, can be greatly tested during the later stages of the aging process. Fear of the unknown associated not only with death and the dying process but also with the concept of an afterlife poses a great threat to trust in the older adult (Swift & Rench, 1991). The religious elder who has lived according to the tenets of his or her tradition may more easily main-tain trust by reflecting on the rewards identified for the faithful. An older adult who does not subscribe to any particular religious belief system will need to draw on personal philosophical beliefs about the meaning of life and one's own contribution to society for support.

Hope

Hope, or the expectation of a positive outcome in the future, is closely linked to trust, especially for the elder from a religious background. Hope is strengthened by an older adult's adherence to strong religious and moral values (Fischer, 1988; Lenarz, 1988; Lotito, 1993). Hope may be more difficult for an ill elder who no longer feels in control of his or her life or future activities. Through a qualitative study to explore the meaning of hope among 12 older adults, Gaskins and Forte (1995) identified hope-related themes related to such factors as health, relationships, material resources, positive emotions, giving service, and reminiscing (p. 19). The most significant and frequently identified theme, however, was that of spirituality. "All of the [study] participants spoke of the important role spirituality played as a source of hope" (p. 19). The authors admitted that all elders in the study identified with a faith tradition, and thus the spirituality theme was often associated with religious practice and belief; hope was, for others, however, described as "having a moral creed for living one's life" (p. 20). And in a study of hope among 94 chronically ill elders residing in a long-term care facility, Beckerman and Northrop (1996) found the most important sources of hope to be faith, relationships, self-esteem, and the ability to give to others. Hope engenders in an elder the spirit to find meaning and joy in life and to maintain a positive sense of self-worth amid diminishing physical and psychological capacities.

Forgiveness

Perhaps the most frequently identified spiritual need for the older adult, especially in the face of serious or terminal illness, is the desire to give and to receive forgiveness. It is rare to find any person, especially one who has lived to elder years, who is not able to acknowledge some attitude or behavior for which he or she would wish forgiveness. The individual from whom the elder desires forgiveness may not be aware of the elder's need; the concern may totally reside in the heart and conscience of the one seeking forgiveness. The other important dimension of the concept relates to an older person's need to extend forgiveness to a person who in the elder's perception has done harm. To give and receive forgiveness are tasks not easily accomplished. Both, noted Fischer (1995), involve "a long and complex process of healing" (p. 127). Much emotional baggage related to old hurts, both given and received, may be deeply ingrained in the elder's persona; they are not easily let go of (Finley, 1989). It is important to remember, also, that desiring to forgive or accept forgiveness does not erase the memories; what forgiveness may accomplish is to "humanize" and incorporate a memory into an elder's current "self-understanding" (Maitland, 1991, p. 160). Healing occurs as the forgiving or forgiven elder reframes his or her self-image and is able to make peace with the past (Bozarth, 1995).

Reminiscence

Another need for the older adult, and one closely linked to giving or receiving forgiveness, is the need for reminiscence. As an individual reviews his or her life story, the need for forgiveness may emerge. There are also many other positive aspects to the act of reminiscence. First, an elder may be strengthened in dealing with present concerns and anxieties by remembering and reidentifying past coping skills used in dealing with stressful experiences. An elder may come to recognize that he or she has "endured beyond [the] ability to endure" (Seymour, 1995, p. 104). This can be a very beneficial memory in terms of facing the unknown future. The process of reviewing past life accomplishments can also serve to suggest what tasks an elder might still undertake, and what legacies can be left (Erikson, 1995, p. 14). In this way, reminiscence may serve as the catalyst for initiating a new career in later life or for helping the older adult to complete some partially finished tasks or activities. Additionally, an elder who reminisces as a social activity with family or friends can offer hard-earned wisdom as a gift to loved ones.

SPIRITUAL NEEDS IN LONG-TERM CARE

Long-term health care for the elderly involves providing "comprehensive, continuous care for older adults in diverse settings" (Collins, Butler, Guelder, & Palmer, 1997, p. 59). These settings include the elder's home or the home of relatives, retirement communities, assisted care facilities, and skilled care nursing homes. The care populations consist of active elders with chronic illness, the homebound elderly, and elders in need of skilled nursing home care. In discussing the need to "revolutionize" long-term care, Patricia Emery, RN, MS, a nursing home director, commented, "Only two populations in this country still face routine and/or permanent institutionalization— convicted felons and the elderly" (2006, p. 16). Some of the positive suggestions for change identified by Emery are "to explore placing control back in their (the elderly) hands" and "allowing them to participate in the decision making processes of life" (p. 22). This can be accomplished, Emery adds, "by providing a *home*, a sanctuary, a healing environment, where elders experience life and growth" (p. 22).

In a nursing study to explore the relationship between spiritual well-being and positive quality of life, the author conducted both structured and open-ended (conversational) interviews with three populations of older adults: mobile elders living with chronic illness, homebound elders, and nursing home residents (O'Brien, 1997). All study participants were over the age of 65 years. The sample group consisted of 38 mobile elders, 4 older adults who were homebound, and 10 nursing home residents. Data elicited from all three groups reflected a strong association between spiritual well-being, evaluated by a Spiritual Assessment Scale (O'Brien, 1997)—which measures personal faith, religious practice, and spiritual contentment/distress—and quality of life, evaluated in terms of hope (Miller Hope Scale, Miller & Powers, 1988; adapted 1997) and life satisfaction (Life Satisfaction Index-Z, Wood, Wylie, & Sheafor, 1969).

Qualitative data generated through open-ended, conversational interviews (Spirituality and Religiousness Interview Guide, O'Brien, 1997) also demonstrated the presence of hopefulness and life satisfaction among elders with a high degree of personal faith, involvement in religious practice, and lack of spiritual distress, that is, a strong sense of spiritual well-being. Data reflecting spiritual and religious characteristics of chronically ill elders—active elders living with chronic illness, homebound elders, and nursing home residents—are discussed relative to each subcategory.

Active Elders Living with Chronic Illness

Census data for 1989 revealed that 70 percent of men and 77 percent of women over 65 had one or more chronic illness; 81 percent of the men and 90 percent of the women were chronically ill by the age of 80 (Sapp & Bliesmer, 1995, p. 4). In an ethnographic study of spirituality among 12 chronically ill elders ranging in age from 65 to 89 years, Young (1993) identified recurrent themes of "hope, comfort, strength and well-being" as related to spiritual beliefs. The concept of hope was associated with trust in the existence of an afterlife, comfort and strength were derived from an elder's belief in God, and well-being was related to the sense of God's love and care provided both in the present and after death (p. 299). Koenig (1994), who also explored the spiritual needs of physically ill elders, described specific concerns such as the need for meaning and hope, the need for belief in transcendence, the need for spiritual support, the need to carry out religious practices, the need for a feeling of self-worth, the need for love, the need to trust in God, and the need to give to others (pp. 284–291). Ill elders, Koenig asserted, need to be not only prepared for death and the dying process, but also supported "in the life they have remaining" (p. 294).

In the author's study of spiritual well-being and quality of life (O'Brien, 1997) among 38 active (non-homebound) chronically ill elders, participants ranged in age from 67 to 96 years; 30 were female and 8 were male. Thirty-five persons were white and three were African American. Fifty percent of the group had some college education. Twenty-three of the elders were Roman

Catholic, fourteen were Protestant, and one was Jewish. Seventy-eight percent of the chronically ill elders attended church at least once a week. Chronic illness conditions included such diagnoses as rheumatoid arthritis, hypertension, cardiomyopathy, asthma, osteoporosis, peptic ulcer, and diabetes mellitus. A number of the study participants also reported multiple diagnoses such as congestive heart failure, arthritis, and hearing loss; hypertension, arthritis, and glaucoma; and hypothyroidism and coronary artery disease.

Although, as noted, the association between spiritual well-being and positive quality of life was strong overall, certain individual scale items revealed interesting findings. Hope, as a concept, was rated high among the group; however, seven of the study participants disagreed with Miller Hope Scale item 4 ("I have energy to do what is important to me"), and over half of the group, 22 (57.8 percent), agreed moderately rather than strongly with the statement. And, although most elders responded negatively to the Life Satisfaction Index-Z item 3 ("This is the dreariest time in my life"), 16 respondents or 42 percent of the group also disagreed with Life Satisfaction Index-Z item 5 ("These are the best years of my life"). One 72-year-old woman penciled in the comment, "These are not the best years of my life, but they're good!" Several respondents commented on item 14 in the Spiritual Assessment Scale ("I am helped to communicate with God by spiritual reading or thinking about religious things"). For example, an 84-year-old woman admitted that because of failing eyesight, reading had become a problem.

The author's analysis of qualitative data elicited in interviews with the 38 chronically ill elders revealed five dominant themes reflecting spiritual well-being among the group: trust, comfort, joy, acceptance, and peace. Trust was associated with the constancy of God's protection, especially during difficult times. Comfort was defined as a sense of well-being received from prayer and spiritual reading, especially the reading of Scripture. Joy was seen as deriving from personal faith beliefs, religious practices, and the support of one's church. Acceptance was related to patience in the face of pain and suffering and faith that God would provide needed support. Peace was achieved in facing death; this was frequently associated with an elder's perception of having lived a "good life," as he or she understood the concept.

Trust

Mrs. Daly, an 88-year-old Roman Catholic diagnosed with congestive heart disease and arthritis, expressed great confidence in God. "I can always count on God to help me in my times of need. My trust in Him affects my whole life; he gives me strength to take part in senior citizen's programs. My belief in God makes me feel great, knowing that He is there watching over me every day, giving me time to spend with my daughter and my grandchildren. I'm healthy and happy. God is very good to me."

Mrs. Kelly, an 81-year-old Catholic who was somewhat more ill with cardiovascular disease, also verbalized trust in God. "I feel as though all my life God has been standing by me. He has always watched over me and helped me get through the pain." Mrs. Kelly added, "But more importantly God showed me how to find love."

Comfort

Mrs. Ann Johnson, an 89-year-old Baptist diagnosed with heart disease and arthritis, described the comfort she received from religion and religious practices. "I pray and am at peace. God and I have a relationship that comforts me. I talk to Him when I am lonely or in need or thankful. My trust in God is part of my everyday life. . . . My faith in God got me involved in my church and the people in my church are the bright spot in my life, so I guess God has been a great comfort in my life."

Sixty-five-year-old Miss Smith, a Christian suffering from rheumatoid arthritis, reported comfort from spiritual reading. "I read from a religious book, *My Daily Bread,* which I find very comforting, especially in times of illness or sadness in my life. It keeps me remembering that God will never send me crosses heavier than I can bear."

Joy

Mrs. Davis, a 65-year-old Presbyterian with cardiac disease, described the joy her spirituality and religious practice brought to her life. "I know that I am in God's hands; He is looking out for me and that is a joy. Another thing that brings me a lot of happiness is that I attend Sunday school and church every Sunday. I have been with the same people in Sunday school for almost 29 years. These friends are very dear to me and we help each other in rough times; they are my church support."

Sixty-seven-year-old Mrs. Flaherty, a Catholic suffering from cardiomyopathy, reported, "My joy is from my love of God which affects my everyday relationships with people. Although I can lose my temper sometimes, I try to be true to my faith and be loving and share the joy with people in my life."

Acceptance

Mr. Anderson, a 70-year-old diagnosed with a brain tumor, spoke about the importance of his Lutheran beliefs and practices in helping him accept his illness. "I know God cares for us in times of sickness. I pray and talk to Him and know that He hears me. He may not always answer the prayers the way I would like Him to do, but He knows what is best for me. I am at peace in my relationship with God. I trust in His Son, Jesus Christ, and know Him as my Lord and Savior. He has given me an inner peace to accept whatever happens, whatever my illness situation may be." Mr. Anderson explained that his church, the Evangelical Lutheran Church of America (ELCA), provided much support. "It gives me strength to deal with my illness. We are a community of believers, and God gives us the assurance that He is with us in time of need, and that He will heal us." Mr. Anderson concluded, "He is a caring and healing God. We are in His hands. Who could ask for anything more?"

Roman Catholic Mrs. Doherty, an 86-year-old suffering from arthritis, observed, "I feel at great peace in my relationship with God. I have been able to accept pain and put difficult times in perspective because I feel that God allows things to happen for a reason. I just trust that God will be watching over me no matter what happens. So in that way I can accept whatever happens."

Peace

Miss Mahoney, a 75-year-old Catholic and a cancer survivor also suffering from congestive heart failure, described the meaning of peace in her life. "I truly am at peace right now. I completely feel at peace in my relationship with God; I always have. There are hard times when you are struggling, but that does not take away your peace, your faith in God. I am at peace about death too; I'm not afraid to die. I know that God will be with me then, as always."

Seventy-eight-year-old Mrs. Pearson, diagnosed with coronary artery disease, explained that as a member of the Baha'i faith, her peace was related to having lived well. "I don't exactly have a relationship with God as in the sense of a 'relationship.' Baha'i's believe that God is all around us. But I do feel at peace with God, because I have led a good life. I honor God every day."

The Homebound Elderly

Chronically ill elders who are homebound or nonmobile and living in assisted care facilities may have significant spiritual needs related to the physical and psychosocial sequelae of their conditions. The physical and emotional pain associated with being homebound requires a depth of faith and spirituality (Burghardt, 1991), as well as spiritual maturity, which Birren (1990) interpreted as the elder's ability to focus on transcendent spiritual values, while still appreciating religious experiences of the past (p. 42).

In studying 26 Protestant, Catholic, and Jewish homebound elders, Brennan (1994) found that personal spirituality was described as giving "meaning and purpose to life" (p. 96). Brennan's study participants understood the difference between the concepts of religion and spirituality, yet perceived them to be interrelated; many described using prayer as a coping mechanism. A specific need expressed by more than half of the study group was the "desire to be able to discuss their spiritual beliefs and feelings with others, especially in times of crisis" (p. 96).

Four homebound elders interviewed for a study of spiritual well-being and quality of life (O'Brien, 1997) ranged from 75 to 91 years of age; all were female and were wheelchair or walker restricted. Three of the women were white and one was African American. Two members of the homebound subgroup were Roman Catholic, one was Mennonite, and the other was a member of the Church of Christ; all were unable to attend worship services because of physical disability. Their illness conditions included rheumatoid arthritis, diabetes and post-polio syndrome, hypertension and cardiovascular disease, and congestive heart failure and hypertension. Quantitative measures for this group revealed a strong relationship between spiritual well-being and positive quality of life.

Qualitative data elicited from the homebound elders reflected one unifying theme that might be described as *confident prayer*; that is, all four study participants spoke about the depth of their faith and trust in God related to their prayer practices and the prayers of their families and church members. Mrs. Allen, an 83-year-old Mennonite diagnosed with diabetes and post-polio syndrome, described herself as almost totally disabled, yet she displayed a strong faith. "I pray to God daily; He's on my mind all the time. I rely on God and on my church in hard times. God is very accessible. I'm very much at peace in my relationship with God." The remarks of 91-year-old Mrs. McCarthy, a Catholic with multiple diagnoses of congestive heart failure, coronary artery disease, and hypertension, who lives in an assisted care setting, reflected a similar theme. "I believe in God who watches out for me in times of sickness and health. I feel at peace with God; I pray to Him every day and I know He will take me when He is ready." Mrs. McCarthy added, "When I'm sick I also count on the prayers of my family and my church."

Mrs. Clark, an 82-year-old homebound member of the Church of Christ who was diagnosed with diabetes and hypertension, reported that although she could not get out to attend church services, she prayed all the time. "I pray and I know that God is taking care of me in all my trials and tribulations, and I will come out better in the end. I believe that no matter what happens God will be with me. You can trust God all the time." Mrs. Clark also commented on the importance of the prayer support of others. "My family members are all of the same religion and they pray for me, and we pray for each other. Being a Christian has helped keep us together, to keep God in the middle of everything."

Mrs. O'Connell, a 75-year-old Catholic who is wheelchair bound because of arthritis, described the peace she received from prayer. "I do feel at peace when I pray; it affects all the activities of my day. It gives me a positive attitude about things. I pray every day and trust in God and the Blessed Mother to get me through."

Nursing Home Residents

The term *nursing home* is broadly understood as describing a facility that "provides twenty-four hour skilled nursing care at an intermediate [i.e., non-hospital] level" (Simmons & Peters, 1996, p. 7). Data obtained in 1984 identified 19,100 nursing homes with approximately 1.6 million beds; this statistic reflected "a 22% increase over the previous ten years" (Millsap, 1995, p. 99). Presently almost 20 percent of older old adults (over 80) reside in nursing homes, and by the year 2030, the number is expected to triple (Koenig, 1994, p. 353).

Some characteristics of a contemporary nursing home population include average age in the 80s; most widowed or single; women in 3:1 proportion to men; many having some degree of dementia and/or arthritis or cardiovascular disease; many experiencing impaired vision or hearing, or both; and most requiring assistance with activities of daily living (Holland & McCurren, 1997, p. 97). Data from an urban nursing home with approximately 230 residents revealed a population physical profile heavily laden with such diagnoses as arteriosclerotic heart disease, diabetes mellitus, hip fracture, osteoporosis, arthritis, Parkinson's disease, Alzheimer's disease, and senile dementia (O'Brien, 1989, pp. 22–23).

The multiplicity of health deficits experienced by current nursing home residents requires skill and ingenuity in care planning, including that of spiritual ministry. Malcolm (1987) believed that nurses must work at developing "creative spiritual care" for elderly nursing home residents; she suggested that although usual care plans place symptoms of dementia under a psychosocial need heading, these aspects of an elder's personality may also be "interwoven with the spiritual" (p. 25).

Some religious rituals appropriate for the responsive nursing home resident include Baptism (for one who has never experienced the sacrament earlier in life), Communion (according to the resident's religious tradition), Anointing of the Sick, and celebrations of religious feast days (Simmons & Peters, 1996, pp. 76–83). For the seriously physically or cognitively impaired resident, Simmons and Peters noted that these rituals may be adapted and modified to meet the elder's condition. Many nursing homes are formally affiliated with a particular religious denomination, so the worship services and rites of that tradition may be central to the home's activities; however, arrangements are generally made for religious ministry to residents of different traditions.

The 10 nursing home residents who participated in the author's recent study of spiritual well-being and quality of life (O'Brien, 1997) ranged in age from 71 to 98 years; eight were female and two were male. Eight of the nursing home residents were African American and two were white; three of the group were married. Group members had been living in the nursing home from four months to five years; all were wheelchair bound. Five of the nursing home residents were Roman Catholic, two were Baptist, one was Seventh Day Adventist, one was Pentecostal, and one was a Jehovah's Witness. Their collective diagnoses included peripheral vascular disease, bilateral knee replacements, cerebral vascular accident, rheumatoid arthritis, congestive heart disease, diabetes, blindness, right-sided paralysis, and fractured hip.

Quantitative data demonstrated a strong relationship between spiritual well-being and positive quality of life among the group. Interestingly, all of the nursing home residents agreed with the Miller Hope Scale item 4 ("I have energy to do what is important to me"). One might speculate that this group of wheelchair bound nursing home residents had modified their expectations in terms of those activities for which they perceived energy to be required.

Three dominant themes were derived from qualitative data elicited in interviews with the nursing home group: faith in God and religious beliefs despite illness and disability, and acceptance of nursing home life; devotion, relating especially to private religious practices such as prayer and Scripture reading; and spiritual contentment, or a sense of peace in relation to where the elder is on his or her spiritual journey.

Faith

Mrs. Jackson, an 81-year-old Baptist resident who had experienced bilateral knee replacements, described a powerful faith. "I do believe in God; He gives me strength to do everything I need to do. He has blessed me so in my life; I am able to go on because of Him. Sometimes the road is rough; not everything is smooth. Sometimes it's hard to be in a nursing home. There are some bumps and some knocks but Jesus will be right beside you." Mrs. Jackson added, "I don't ever feel far away from God regardless of what happens. I read the Twenty-third Psalm in the Bible, you know, 'Yea, though I walk through the valley of the shadow of death, I will fear no evil for Thou art with me.' It just makes you forget anything that might have happened."

The remarks of Mrs. Earhardt, a 76-year-old Seventh Day Adventist resident with peripheral vascular disease, also reflected a strong faith. "I have faith in God, a relationship with God, and when I get stressed out or something happens to me, the Lord always makes a way for that to ease over. Then the stress leaves me and the breath of God comes back in me. My faith is everything to me; if the effect of God didn't work in me, I couldn't make it. There is no way that I could make it without the Lord. I might as well just hang it up and forget it." Mrs. Earhardt concluded, "Faith in God means everything. If you don't have faith in God, you don't have faith in anybody. There is no one I look up to but Jesus. If you believe in His word, He will answer you."

A male nursing home resident, Mr. Martin, an 82-year-old bilateral amputee and member of a pentecostal church, the Church of God in Christ, explained his faith. "Faith is having a personal relationship with Jesus. I believe that to be a child of God, you have to be born again of the Spirit. You can go to Jesus and tell Him anything and He will listen to you. And according to His will, He will grant you what you ask."

Devotion

Mrs. Meehan, an 87-year-old Catholic resident who was recovering from a stroke, described her religious devotion. "I try to stay very close to God through my prayers and church services. Many times I have talked to God; I talk with my God every day, a lot of times a day. I also go to Mass here in the chapel every day and I have a spiritual advisor who I talk to. And I have my rosary too that I say for my family who have gone to God, and for my friends."

An 88-year-old Jehovah's Witness resident, Mrs. Jensen, also recovering from a stroke, spoke especially about the importance of Scripture reading. "I'm at peace with God because I believe deeply in Him through the Bible. I read the Bible every day and I've come through with flying colors. Scripture gives comfort in Jesus. I am a Jehovah's Witness and we believe deeply in Jesus Christ. Jehovah is our great God. I find him in my Bible."

Spiritual Contentment

Seventy-two-year-old Mrs. Annie Smith, a Baptist nursing home resident with hypertension and stroke sequelae, described the contentment brought about by her spiritual and religious beliefs. "I believe in God and in His Son Jesus who care for me in times of trials and tribulations. God is such a consolation to me. And I am content and very confident that I will be taken care of in any matter. I think I've lived according to His commandments and I feel that God directs me in things I have done in my life, so I'm at peace." Mrs. Smith concluded, "I am in constant prayer with God, and I pray day and night or anytime that I feel I need to."

Mrs. Loughlin, a 98-year-old with multiple cardiovascular conditions and a Catholic, also reflected spiritual contentment in her remarks. "I'm at peace at this time in my life. I can't go to church anymore, but I get to the chapel here. I say my rosary in the evening for all my relatives and I pray for the people here. Most of my life God has answered all of my prayers. He is the power and the glory and the strength of my life. And I don't ever feel far away from Him, so I'm very happy here." Mrs. Loughlin concluded, "I thank God for all the lovely privileges I've had in my life; my home, and my family, and some of the beauty of the world. I realize that if it is God's will that I live a little longer then its OK, but if it is not, then He will take me home to Glory."

Overall findings from the author's study of spirituality and quality of life among three groups of elders—active elders living with a chronic illness, homebound elders, and nursing home residents—revealed the presence of spiritual values including faith, hope, trust (confidence), joy, acceptance, peace (contentment), and devotion (commitment to prayer for self and others) among the study participants. These study data documenting the spiritual and religious beliefs and practices, as well as the needs, of ill elders are supportive of James Fowler's (1981) final faith stages in which the older adult seeks a deepening of his or her own spiritual life as well as expressing concern over the needs of the larger society.

SPIRITUALITY AND QUALITY OF LATER LIFE

The quality of life for an older adult depends greatly on the personal spirituality supporting the elder's perception of his or her current life stage. As has been demonstrated in this chapter, some of the physiological and psychosocial literature presents a rather bleak picture of life and functional ability for an elder; the older a person becomes, the more forbidding the image seems to be. On the other hand, spiritual and religious writing has affirmed the journey of aging as encompassing a time of peace and fulfillment; a "time to be eagerly awaited and warmly embraced" (Sapp, 1987, p. 133). The truth, for most older adults, probably lies somewhere between these two extremes. Certainly there is a greater risk of physical deficit as one ages. Oppenheimer (1991) believed, however, that "realism does not require that we should anticipate all these ills" (p. 43). Some future problems may be prevented by heeding health/illness-related precautions. And, if unexpected health deficits occur, the use of established coping skills, especially those of a spiritual or religious nature, can greatly mediate the negative impact of the condition. As Oppenheimer concluded, some future suffering can be "circumvented"; other suffering needs to be "faced."

In nursing research to explore the meaning of quality of life among residents of a long-term care facility, Aller and Van Ess Coeling (1995) identified three themes descriptive of the concept; these include "ability to communicate with others," "ability to care for self," and "ability to help others" (p. 23). The latter theme also reflects well Fowler's (1981) final stages of faith development, Conjunctive Faith and Universalizing Faith, in which an older individual's social conscience takes precedence over the needs of self; the desire to reach out to others becomes primary. As one of Aller and Van Ess Coeling's elder study respondents commented, "Quality of life, to me, is not only self-betterment, but the betterment of others (1995, p. 23).

A study of 71 elders residing in a nursing home revealed that quality of later life was decidedly subjective. An 88-year-old resident in relatively good physical and mental health admitted that she did not want to do "much of anything" at this point in her life. "I made up my mind I am at the end of my rope. You do sort of get that notion. I have felt I really don't have any incentive to live" (O'Brien, 1989, p. 44). An 83-year-old woman, however, compared her quality of life to that of more seriously disabled residents. "You feel sorry for them. Of course, you say to yourself: 'There but for the Grace of God, go I!' I wake up in the morning and say, 'Thank God, I've got another day.' I mean it" (p. 44).

Contemporary elder adults are living longer and functioning better than ever before. Although obviously some physiological and psychosocial deficits accompany the aging process, a strong personal faith and participation in religious practices can greatly enhance an elder's quality of life.

Chronically ill older adults living in a nursing care facility, as well as those living at home, may enjoy significant spiritual well-being in their later years. The aging adult may take comfort in the wisdom of Brother Roger of Taize who observed:

> *Every age has its own beauty. Why be afraid of physical decline when the years bring deeper insight and greater gentleness of action.*

> (Cited in Finch, 1993, p. 23)

While some older adults are able to maintain a significant degree of physical and psychological health well into their later decades of life—even to the eightieth and ninetieth years—others are struck by illness and disability as aging occurs. For some, the disease processes are diagnosed as progressive and ultimately terminal, thus placing the individual in an end-of-life status—some well before their anticipated time of death.

The following chapter addresses the spiritual needs of adults facing the end of life. While specific identification of when an ill person is, in fact, at the end of life is ambiguous and difficult to determine, some guidelines reflective of an end-of-life status are presented and discussed. Several research studies, reflective of the spiritual needs of end-of-life patients, are included to illustrate nursing care needs and suggest possible nursing interventions.

REFERENCES

Ainlay, S. C., & Smith, D. R. (1984). Aging and religious participation. *Journal of Gerontology, 39*(3), 357–363.

Aller, L., & Van Ess Coeling, H. (1995). Quality of life: Its meaning to the long-term care resident. *Journal of Gerontological Nursing, 21*(2), 20–25.

Beckerman, A., & Northrop, C. (1996). Hope, chronic illness and the elderly. *Journal of Gerontological Nursing, 22*(5), 19–25.

Berggren-Thomas, P., & Griggs, M. J. (1995). Spirituality in aging: Spiritual needs or spiritual journey. *Journal of Gerontological Nursing, 21*(3), 5–10.

Bianchi, E. C. (1995). *Aging as a spiritual journey.* New York: Crossroad.

Birren, J. E. (1990). Spiritual maturity in psychological development. In J. Seeber (Ed.), *Spiritual maturity in the later years* (pp. 41–53). New York: The Haworth Press.

Blazer, D. (1991). Spirituality and aging well. *Generations, 15*(1), 61–65.

Boettcher, E. (1985). Linking the aged to support systems. *Journal of Gerontological Nursing, 11*(3), 27–33.

Bozarth, A. R. (1995). *Lifelines: Threads of grace through seasons of change.* Kansas City, MO: Sheed & Ward.

Brennan, Sr. M. R. (1994). *Spirituality in the homebound elderly.* Doctoral dissertation, The Catholic University of America. Ann Arbor, MI: UMI.

Burghardt, W. J. (1991). Aging, suffering and dying: A Christian perspective. In L. S. Cahill & D. Mieth (Eds.), *Aging* (pp. 65–71). London: Conciliam.

Burt, D. X. (1992). *But when you are older: Reflections on coming of age.* Collegeville, MN: The Liturgical Press.

Byrne, Sr. M. (1985). A zest for life. *Journal of Gerontological Nursing, 11*(4), 30–33.

Castellaw, L. S., Wicks, M. N., & Martin, J. C. (1999). Spirituality in white older women with arthritis. *Graduate Research Nursing, 1*(1), 1–9.

Collins, C. E., Butler, F. R., Guelder, S. H., & Palmer, M. H. (1997). Models for community-based long-term care for the elderly in a changing health system. *Nursing Outlook, 45*(2), 59–63.

Coupland, S. (1985). *Beginning to pray in old age.* Cambridge, MA: Cowley.

Deeken, A. (1986). *Growing old and how to cope with it.* San Francisco: Ignatius Press.

Durkin, M. B. (1992). A community of caring. *Health Progress, 73*(8), 48–53.

Emery, P. (2006). Building a new culture of aging: Revolutionizing long-term care. *Journal of Christian Nursing, 23*(1), 16–24.

Erickson, R. M. (1995). *Late have I loved thee: Stories of religious conversion and commitment in later life.* New York: Paulist Press.

Finch, A. (Ed.). (1993). *Journey to the light: Spirituality as we mature.* New Rochelle, NY: New City Press.

Finley, J. (1989). *The treasured age: Spirituality for seniors.* New York: Alba House.

Fischer, K. (1988). Hope never ends: God's promise to the elderly. *Journal of Christian Nursing, 5*(4), 32–35.

Fischer, K. (1995). *Autumn gospel: Women in the second half of life.* New York: Paulist Press.

Forbis, P. A. (1988). Meeting patients' spiritual needs. *Geriatric Nursing, 9*(3), 158–159.

Fowler, J. W. (1981). *Stages of faith: The psychology of human development and the quest for meaning.* San Francisco: Harper.

Gaskins, S., & Forte, L. (1995). The meaning of hope: Implications for nursing practice and research. *Journal of Gerontological Nursing, 21*(3), 17–24.

Hall, C. M. (1985). Religion and aging. *Journal of Religion and Health, 24*(1), 70–78.

Halstead, H. L. (1995). Spirituality in the elderly. In M. Stanley & P. G. Beare (Eds.), *Gerontological nursing* (pp. 415–425). Philadelphia: F. A. Davis.

Hammer, M. L. (1990). Spiritual needs: A forgotten dimension of care. *Journal of Gerontological Nursing, 16*(12), 3–4.

Heriot, C. J. (1995). Developmental tasks and development in the later years of life. In M. Stanley & P. G. Beare (Eds.), *Gerontological nursing* (pp. 349–356). Philadelphia: F. A. Davis.

Hicks, T. J. (1999). Spirituality and the elderly: Nursing implications with nursing home residents. *Geriatric Nursing, 20*(3), 144–146.

Hogstel, M. O. (1995). Mental health wellness strategies for successful aging. In M. Stanley & P. G. Beare (Eds.), *Gerontological nursing* (pp. 17–27). Philadelphia: F. A. Davis.

Holland, B. E., & McCurren, C. (1997). Aging. In J. M. Black and E. Matassarin-Jacobs (Eds.), *Medical–surgical nursing: Clinical management for continuity of care.* (5th ed., pp. 81–104). Philadelphia: W. B. Saunders.

Hungelmann, J., Kenkel-Rossi, E., Klassen, L., & Stollenwerk, R. M. (1985). Spiritual well-being in older adults: Harmonious interconnectedness. *Journal of Religion and Health, 24*(2), 147–153.

Hunsberger, B. (1985). Religion, age, life satisfaction, and perceived sources of religiousness: A study of older persons. *Journal of Gerontology, 40*(5), 615–620.

Hynes, M. (1989). *The ministry to the aging.* Collegeville, MN: The Liturgical Press.

Koenig, H. G. (1994). *Aging and God: Spiritual pathways to mental health in midlife and later years.* New York: The Haworth Press.

Lenarz, M. A. (1988). In the dark: A nurse struggles to give hope to the elderly. *Journal of Christian Nursing, 5*(4), 30–32.

Lotito, F. A. (1993). *Wisdom, age and grace: An inspirational guide to staying young at heart.* New York: Paulist Press.

Lueckenotte, A. G. (1997). Older adult. In P. A. Potter & A. G. Perry (Eds.), *Fundamentals of nursing: Concepts, process and practice* (pp. 568–593). St. Louis, MO: C. V. Mosby.

Maitland, D. J. (1991). *Aging as counterculture: A vocation for the later years.* New York: The Pilgrim Press.

Malcolm, J. (1987). Creative spiritual care for the elderly. *Journal of Christian Nursing, 4*(1), 24–26.

Maltby, T. (1990). Pastoral care of the aging. In H. Hayes & C. J. van der Poel (Eds.), *Health care ministry: A handbook for chaplains* (pp. 98–104). New York: Paulist Press.

Markides, K. S. (1983). Aging, religiosity, and adjustment: A longitudinal analysis. *Journal of Gerontology, 38*(5), 621–625.

Miller, J., & Powers, M. (1988). Development of an instrument to measure hope. *Nursing Research, 37*(1), 6–10.

Millsap, P. (1995). Nurses' role with the elderly in the long-term care setting. In M. Stanley & P. G. Beare (Eds.), *Gerontological nursing* (pp. 98–106). Philadelphia: F. A. Davis.

Moberg, D. O. (1990). Spiritual maturity and wholeness in later years. In J. Seeber (Ed.), *Spiritual maturity in the later years* (pp. 5–24). New York: The Haworth Press.

Mooney, S. F. (2006). When memory fails: Helping dementia patients remember God. *Journal of Christian Nursing, 23*(1), 6–14.

Morikawa, J. (1974, September). American Baptist news service, Division of communications. *Aging without apology: Living the senior years with integrity and faith.* Valley Forge, PA: Judson Press.

Mull, C. S., Cox, C. L., & Sullivan, J. L. (1987). Religion's role in the health and well-being of well elders. *Public Health Nursing, 4*(3), 151–159.

Normille, P. (1992). *Visiting the sick.* Cincinnati, OH: St. Anthony Messenger Press.

Nouwen, H. J., & Gaffney, W. J. (1990). *Aging: The fulfillment of life.* New York: Doubleday.

O'Brien, M. E. (1989). *Anatomy of a nursing home: A new view of resident life.* Owings Mills, MD: National Health Publishing.

O'Brien, M. E. (1997). Spiritual well-being and quality of life in chronically ill elders. Unpublished study funded by Research Grant-in-Aid, The Catholic University of America, Washington, DC.

Oppenheimer, H. (1991). Reflections on the experience of aging. In L. S. Cahill & D. Mieth (Eds.), *Aging* (pp. 39–45). London: Conciliam.

Payne, B. (1990). Spiritual maturity and meaning-filled relationships. In J. Seeber (Ed.), *Spiritual maturity in the later years* (pp. 25–39). New York: The Haworth Press.

Peterson, V., & Potter, P. A. (1997). Spiritual health. In P. A. Potter & A. G. Perry (Eds.), *Fundamentals of nursing: Concepts, process and practice* (pp. 440–455). St. Louis, MO: C. V. Mosby.

Rice, V. H., Beck, C., & Stevenson, J. S. (1997). Ethical issues relative to autonomy and personal control in independent and cognitively impaired elders. *Nursing Outlook, 45*(1), 27–34.

Roen, O. T. (1997). Senior health. In J. H. Swanson & M. A. Nies (Eds.), *Community health nursing: Promoting the health of aggregates* (2nd ed., pp. 347–386). Philadelphia: W. B. Saunders.

Sapp, S. (1987). *Full of years: Aging and the elderly in the Bible and today.* Nashville, TN: Abington Press.

Sapp, M., & Bliesmer, M. (1995). A health promotion/protection approach to meeting elders' health care needs. In M. Stanley & P. G. Beare (Eds.), *Gerontological nursing* (pp. 3–12). Philadelphia: F. A. Davis.

Seymour, R. E. (1995). *Aging without apology: Living the senior years with integrity and faith.* Valley Forge, PA: Judson Press.

Simmons, H. C., & Peters, M. A. (1996). *With God's oldest friends: Pastoral visiting in the nursing home.* New York: Paulist Press.

Stagg, F. (1981). *The Bible speaks on aging.* Nashville, TN: Broadman Press.

Swift, H. C., & Rench, C. E. (1991). *Life, fulfillment and joy in the sunset years.* Huntington, IN: Our Sunday Visitor Publications.

Taylor, C., Lillis, C., & LeMone, P. (1997). *Fundamentals of nursing: The art and science of nursing care* (3rd ed.). Philadelphia: J. B. Lippincott.

Tournier, P. (1983). *Learn to grow old.* Louisville, KY: Westminister/John Knox Press.

Valentine, M. H. (1994). *Aging in the Lord.* New York: Paulist Press.

Wicks, R. J. (1997). *After 50: Spiritually embracing your own wisdom years.* New York: Paulist Press.

Wood, V., Wylie, M., & Sheafor, B. (1969). An analysis of a short self-report measure of life satisfaction: Correlation with later judgments. *Journal of Gerontology, 24*(2), 465–469.

Young, C. (1993). Spirituality and the chronically ill Christian elderly. *Geriatric Nursing, 14*(6), 298–303.

11 ▨ Spiritual Well-Being and Quality of Life at the End of Life

Just like the clay in the potter's hand, so are you in my hand.

For the person at or near the end of life, the words of the Old Testament prophet Jeremiah can be deeply comforting; they express the idea that one is held firmly, yet tenderly, in the hands of the Divine Potter who both created and cares for all His people. In a small volume entitled *The Nurse's Calling*, I devoted an entire chapter to interpreting the meaning of Jeremiah's potter's story for practicing nurses (O'Brien, 1991). I believe that, because nurses like to be "in control"—in fact, need to be in control to a degree in caring for our patients—we find the concept of being like "clay" in the hands of a "potter" somewhat difficult to accept.

The same can probably be said for most persons in our contemporary society. We all like to be in control of our lives, our environment, and certainly our health, as much as possible. In regard to our health, many of us spend a great deal of time and energy on such things as exercise programs, shopping for nutritious foods and supplements, and participating in numerous other health promotions or health-enhancing activities.

When, however, a person is faced with a life-threatening, terminal illness, when one accepts the fact of being at or near the end of human life, loss of control becomes a lived and living reality—a living reality that can be both frightening and depressing. But it is precisely at this point in one's life journey that Jeremiah's account of his visit to the "Potter's House" can come alive:

> The word came to Jeremiah from the Lord: Come, go down to the potter's house, and there I will let you hear my words. So I went down to the potter's house, and there he was working at his wheel. The vessel he was making of clay was spoiled in the potter's hand and

he reworked it into another vessel, as seemed good to him. Then the word of the Lord came to me: Can I not do with you . . . just as this potter had done? says the Lord. Just like clay in the hands of the potter, so are you in my hand." (Jeremiah 18:16)

A plethora of literature in recent years has documented the relationship between personal faith beliefs, associated with a variety of religious denominations, and positive coping with illness and disability. An ill individual's personal faith, supported by scripture such as the Jeremiah passage cited above, can be both consoling and strengthening. This is particularly true in cases of serious or life-threatening illness.

There is still, however, minimal research documenting the relationship between spiritual well-being or strong faith beliefs and positive quality of life in persons facing the end of life. In an attempt to understand better the spiritual concerns and needs of the terminally ill, three studies were carried out exploring the concepts of spiritual well-being and quality of life at the end of life. Both quantitative and qualitative data reflecting the importance of spiritual well-being in enhancing overall coping and quality of life were collected from persons at or near the end of their lives. These studies are entitled "Spiritual Well-Being at the End of Life: An Experiment in Parish Nursing," "Meeting Spiritual Needs of Elders Near the End of Life," and "The Relationship Between Spiritual Well-Being and Quality of Life in Older Adults at the End of Life."

SPIRITUALITY AT THE END OF LIFE

Your fear of death is but the trembling of the shepherd when he stands before the King whose hand is to be laid upon him in honor.

Kahlil Gibran

Myriad definitions of "end of life" may be found, although most authors admit to ambiguity and vagueness in attempting to define the concept. Hamilton (2001) suggests that "end of life care can be defined as medical and other supportive care given to a person during the final six months of life" (p. 74). This statement is immediately followed, however, with the question, "But how do we know which are the final six months?" (p. 74). Other authors have suggested that end of life may be defined as from as long as two years prior to death. Ultimately, Hamilton concluded that "Given the difficulty of predicting when and by what process death will come, end-of-life can best be defined . . . as that care which the health care team provides in what they think could be the final days, weeks or months of the patient's life" (p. 74).

The National Institutes of Health "State of the Science Conference Statement on Improving End-of-Life Care" (2004) noted "the evidence does not support a precise definition of the interval referred to as end-of-life or its transitions" (p. 3). The statement added, "There is no exact definition of end of life; however, the evidence supports the following components: (1) the presence of a chronic disease(s) or symptoms or functional impairments that persist but may also fluctuate; and (2) the symptoms or impairments resulting from the underlying irreversible disease require formal (paid, professional) or informal (unpaid) care and can lead to death. Older age and frailty may be surrogates for life-threatening illness and comorbidity; however, there is insufficient evidence for understanding these variables as components of end of life" (p. 3).

A significant amount of contemporary literature suggests the existence of a strongly positive relationship between spirituality (relating to one's relation with the transcendent) and religiousness or religiosity (relating to the practice of one's religious faith) and coping with end of life and the death experience. Harold Koenig, in discussing the role of religion and spirituality at the end of life, observed that "it is often religious faith and support from (a) spiritual community" that gives individuals facing the end of life "greater control over the dying process" (2002, p. 20). Koenig added, "Rather than trying to control everything, faith allows them to give up the need for control and instead to trust that God will control their circumstances based on God's love, wisdom, and unique knowledge about their situations. They say, 'It's all about letting go and letting God, not hanging on and holding tight to that which on this earthly plane is passing away'" (p. 20).

Spirituality and End-of-Life Care

In a survey of 861 critical care nurses, the purpose of which was to obtain suggestions on ways to improve end-of-life care, spiritual needs did not emerge as a major theme; however, several suggestions were at least indirectly related to the topics of spirituality and religion. These suggestions were the building of a "chapel in the intensive care area for the use of patients' families and hospital staff," creation of a "small walking garden," and the idea that no patient should die alone. "Every patient needs to have someone present with them at the moment of death—to touch them, speak to them, to let them know it's okay to go" (Beckstrand, Callister, & Kirchoff, 2006, p. 41). Under "Miscellaneous findings," the authors also noted a suggestion for "more involvement from ancillary personnel such as pastoral staff" (p. 42).

The critical care nurses' suggestion for "presence" at the time of death is in fact considered a "spiritual caregiving strategy" by Young and Koopson and Father Joseph Driscoll. Young and Koopson note that "health care providers can provide spiritual care of the dying by dealing with spiritual issues from the individuals' and families' perspectives . . . (one) way is to listen to individuals who have a desire and a need to discuss the experience" (2005, pp. 174–175). Father Driscoll observes, "Spiritual care is so much more than religious care. Spiritual care discovers, reverences, and tends the spirit—that is, the energy, or the place of meaning and values—of another human being" (2001, p. 334).

In describing spirituality and end-of-life care as "a time for listening and a time for caring," Christina Puchalski, M. D., cited a survey poll in which end-of-life patients stated that "they wanted warm relationships with their providers, to be listened to, to have someone to share their fears and concerns with, to have someone with them when they are dying, to be able to pray and to have others pray for them" (2002, p. 290). Puchalski concluded, "We need to listen to the dying . . . and be with them, for them. The process of dying can be a meaningful one—one that we can all embrace and celebrate rather than fear and dread" (p. 294).

Finally, palliative care nurse Polly Mazanec asserts that "spirituality can be especially significant in end-of-life care, offering the patient a way to find meaning and purpose in dying as in life" (2003, p. 55). Mazanec also cites the importance of religious rituals for some end-of-life patients. "Spiritual or religious practices (customs) and rituals (more formal ceremonies) often play important roles . . . at a time of transition in one's life. For example, a Roman Catholic ritual known as Anointing of the Sick might be performed for a seriously ill person. Considered 'a sacrament of healing,' it's intended to bring the recipient physical and spiritual strength and to convey God's grace. A Muslim family might request that immediately after death, the patient's body be turned to Mecca, their holiest city" (2003, p. 55).

The following three nursing studies on spiritual well-being at the end of life, illustrate well the above themes related to the importance of being present and listening to persons at the end of life; helping them to "let go and let God"; supporting such faith-related practices as reverence, religiousness (religious practice), and devotion; helping patients achieve spiritual peace; and supporting such concepts as "the gift of life" and "the spirituality of community."

SPIRITUAL WELL-BEING AT THE END OF LIFE: AN EXPERIMENT IN PARISH NURSING

The overall purpose of this study was to explore selected correlates of spiritual well-being and quality of life among a population of persons at or near the end of life, as well as to test the impact of parish nursing intervention on spiritual well-being and quality of life at the end of life. Although initial sample criteria for seriously ill study participants did not include their being at or near the end of life, approximately 75% of the study population fit that criteria. Of the 45 participants entered into the study, 31 (69%) resided in nursing homes or assisted care facilities, and 39 subjects or 87% of the group were over the age of 70 (40% were 70 to 79; 29% were 80 to 89; and 18% were 90 to 96).

The conceptual model undergirding the research was the "Middle Range Theory of Spiritual Well-Being in Illness" (chapter 4).

The research method consisted of a quasi-experimental, pre-test, post-test design, including a correlational dimension. Methodological triangulation was also employed in data collection; both quantitative and qualitative tools were used to measure key variables in the study.

Sample

Of the 45 cognitively alert adults who agreed to participate in the study, all except one were at or nearing the end of life. The study sample consisted of those individuals who were able and willing to respond to nursing intervention to enhance spiritual well-being, as well as to participate in data collection activities.

Variables/Instruments

Three quantitative tools and one qualitative tool were used to assess the variables of spiritual well-being and quality of life (operationalized in terms of hope and life satisfaction) prior to and following parish nursing intervention.

- The Spiritual Assessment Scale (SAS) (O'Brien, 2003a, chapter 3) is a 21-item Likert-type scale that measures spiritual well-being overall and uses three subscales that assess **personal faith, religious practice** and **spiritual contentment.**
- The Miller Hope Scale is a 15-item tool that measures hope in terms of such issues as meaning of life and attitudes toward the future. This

instrument was abbreviated for a more fragile end-of-life population with permission of the author, Dr. Judith Miller (Miller and Powers, 1988).
- The Life Satisfaction Index-Z is a 13-item scale designed to measure satisfaction with life among elder adults (Wood, Wylie, & Sheafor, 1969).
- The qualitative tool is an investigator-developed instrument called the Spiritual Well-Being Interview Guide (O'Brien, 2003a).

The SAS established reliability and validity. Reliability, using Cronbach's alpha, was again established with the study population. All statistics were calculated at time 1 (T1) prior to the parish nursing intervention and at time 2 (T2) following intervention. The SAS total scale measured spiritual well-being as T1: 0.94, T2: 0.92. For subscales, **personal faith** was T1: 0.95, T2: 0.94; **religious practice** was T1: 0.86, T2: 0.76; and **spiritual contentment** was T1: 0.77, T2: 0.87.

The Spiritual Well-Being Interview Guide explores, in narrative responses, the concepts of personal faith, religious practice, and spiritual contentment. Content validity was established by a panel of experts in the area of spiritual well-being and chronic illness.

A demographic data form was used to collect data on the potentially mediating variables of severity of illness (degree of disability), age, gender, religious orientation, religiosity (religious practice) as well as other demographics, including diagnosis, to provide a sample population description.

Nursing Intervention

Following collection of baseline data, a nursing intervention plan was designed and carried out to enhance spiritual well-being and quality of life; each intervention was tailored to the specific spiritual and/or religious needs of the study participant. The experimental parish nursing intervention plan was carried out in context of at least three visits to the study participant, following initial data collection, and prior to post-intervention (outcome) data collection. At the time of baseline data collection, the parish nurse assessed the study participant's spiritual needs; a broad intervention plan to be carried out over the next three visits was developed. The interventions differed somewhat based on such variables as a study participant's degree of disability, spiritual beliefs, and/or personal coping style; this, however, represents the norm in contemporary parish nursing intervention. For example, if the study participant was able to read, and had a spiritual history of Bible reading, he or she may have wished to discuss appropriate passages with the parish nurse. If a study participant had impaired vision, the nurse read a relevant scripture passage to the participant, then initiated discussion of the content.

Some study participants desired the nurse to pray with them; others wished to reminisce about their past lives or speak about the imminence of death and dying with the parish nurse. Several study participants requested that the nurse arrange for specific pastoral care intervention, such as administration of church sacraments, if they had not been receiving such spiritual ministry. In sum, the primary focus of the parish nursing intervention at or near the end of life was to allow the ill person the opportunity to receive whatever spiritual support or comfort he or she needed as death approached.

It should be pointed out that the parish nurse, who visited as a representative of the church and was also a spiritual companion, was also vested with the roles of educator, advocate, referral agent, and counselor. Thus, the nursing intervention visits sometimes included listening to and guiding the study participants in regard to a variety of issues related to their illness or disability. These activities also supported and strengthened the spiritual well-being of the person nearing the end of life.

As was noted in the final report of the study, "Because of the diversity of spiritual needs and concerns among study participants, as well as myriad physical deficits and disabilities, the parish nursing visits varied somewhat in terms of process and content; this was expected for, as with any intervention in the area of spiritual well-being, the nurse cannot plan precisely what will occur as the nurse–patient interaction evolves. Nevertheless, significant findings, both quantitative and qualitative revealed the positive impact of parish nursing intervention on the study participants' spiritual well-being and quality of life" (O'Brien, 2001, p. 11).

Analysis

Quantitative analysis was carried out using appropriate parametric procedures for both correlational and pre-post intervention data such as Pearson's *r* multiple regression analysis and paired *t*-test. Although quantitative tools established reliability and validity, reliability scores were again calculated on quantitative tools (overall scale scores and subscales) using Cronbach's alpha procedure. Qualitative data were content analyzed to identify and describe dominant themes that emerged idiosyncratic to the data.

Study Findings

Quantitative data analysis "revealed significant positive increases in study variables following the parish nursing intervention . . . as revealed by evaluation of the paired *t*-test data. Paired *t*-tests were computed for all scales. There were statistically significant differences; that is positive increases on all three instruments: The Spiritual Assessment Scale overall (t 0.44 = 5.23, p 0.0005); the three subscales for personal faith (t 0.44 = 3.86, p 0.0005), religious practice (t 0.44 = 3.41, p 0.001), and spiritual contentment (t 0.44 = 4.80, p 0.0005); the Miller Hope Scale (t 0.44 = 2.68, p 0.010); and the Life Satisfaction Inventory-Z (t 0.44 = 2.12, p 0.040). In sum, following the parish nursing intervention, the study participants had a greater sense of spiritual well-being, more hope and a higher degree of life satisfaction than at the initiation of the study" (O'Brien, 2003b, p. 221).

There were also significant positive correlational relationships between the key variables of spiritual well-being and quality of life as measured by hope and life satisfaction.

Following the nursing interventions, qualitative data were also collected and analyzed. From these data, five dominant themes reflecting spiritual well-being emerged including *reverence, faithfulness, religiousness, devotion,* and *contemplation.* (Specific details of the study design, analyses, and conclusions may be found in *Parish Nursing: Healthcare Ministry Within the Church* [O'Brien, 2003, pp. 213–284]).

Significance

This study was of significance to nursing on three fronts: spirituality in nursing, parish nursing, and end of life. **Spirituality in nursing** is an important dimension of the holistic health care paradigm that gives attention to body, mind, and spirit. **Parish nursing** is a newly recognized subfield of nursing. Finally, it addressed nursing's contemporary concern with the quality of life of those who are near or at the **end of life**.

Data from both clinical nursing practice and nursing research reveal that sick persons who manifest spiritual well-being cope significantly better with illness and disability than those who do not. Even as physical deficits increase, a strong sense of spiritual well-being promotes a perception of hope and comfort for the person nearing the end of life. The Joint Commission on Accreditation of Healthcare Organizations (JCAHO) mandates, in its regulations, attention to the spiritual needs of those who are being treated in health care settings. In February 1998, with publication of the *Scope and Standards of Parish Nursing Practice*, the newly created subfield of parish nursing was formally acknowledged by the American Nurses' Association Congress on Nursing Practice. However, minimal research currently documents the impact of parish nurses' interventions on the spiritual well-being of their patients; this is especially true in terms of the parish nurse's intervention with persons at or near the end of life.

MEETING SPIRITUAL NEEDS OF ELDERS NEAR THE END OF LIFE

Following the parish nursing intervention study described above, an interpretive phenomenological study of 15 chronically ill elders (ages 65 to 82 years) near the end of life was carried out. The study sample consisted of five Roman Catholics; four persons who identified themselves broadly as "Christian"; three individuals who were Baptist; and three who were Presbyterian, Episcopalian, and Unitarian respectively.

The study aim was to identify through open-ended interviews the lived experience of spirituality and/or religious practice, and specifically of spiritual needs, at or near the end of life. Nursing interventions to meet specific spiritual needs were then implemented, as needed, by the parish nurse.

Ultimately, five nursing diagnoses related to spiritual well-being were identified and appropriate nursing interventions initiated; the nursing diagnoses were spiritual alienation, spiritual anxiety, spiritual anger, spiritual loss, and spiritual peace.

> **Spiritual alienation** was evidenced by perceptions of being distanced from God; of feelings of lack of peace in terms of God's care and comfort.
>
> **Spiritual anxiety** was demonstrated by verbalization of fear of God or lack of trust in God's mercy and forgiveness.
>
> **Spiritual anger** was reflected in an individual's sense of frustration or outrage at God for real or perceived pain and sufferings in his or her own life or that of a loved one.
>
> **Spiritual loss** was manifested by feelings of no longer being loved by God, often related to a decrease in former spiritual peace.
>
> **Spiritual peace** was determined by a study participant's perception of trust, joy, and security in the love, mercy, and compassion of God.

(O'Brien, 1982, pp. 106–107; O'Brien, 2006, pp. 30–32; details of the study design, analysis, and findings may be found in the article "Parish

Nursing: Meeting Spiritual Needs of Elders Near the End of Life," O'Brien, *Journal of Christian Nursing, 23*[1], 28–33).

SPIRITUAL WELL-BEING AND QUALITY OF LIFE IN OLDER ADULTS AT THE END OF LIFE

The overall purpose of the study was to explore the relationship between spiritual well-being and quality of life among a population of ill elders at or near the end of life. A limitation of the earlier referenced study "Spiritual Well-Being at the End of Life: An Experiment in Parish Nursing" related to the religious élan of the private foundation funding the work; that is, it was mandated that all of the study participants belong to one religious denomination, that of the funding institute. As noted, however, statistically significant relationships between spiritual well-being and quality of life were found among the study population, as well as the five dominant themes reflective of spiritual well-being that emerged from content analysis of qualitative data: reverence, faithfulness, religiousness, devotion, and contemplation.

The present study differed from the parish nursing intervention study in four ways.

(a) Designation of a correlational rather than an experimental design
(b) Broadening of the sample to include persons of all religious faiths and/or spiritual belief systems
(c) Replacement of two previously used measures of quality of life with the McGill Quality of Life Questionnaire (MQOL) developed for end-of-life research
(d) Exploration of two additional potentially mediating variables: symptom severity and social support

Two investigator-developed tools were used to measure the latter two variables: The Geriatric Severity of Physical Symptoms Scale (GSPSS) and The Geriatric Social Support Scale (GSSS). Content and construct validity were established on all research instruments.

Aim

The specific study aim was to examine the relationship between spiritual well-being and quality of life in ill elders at or nearing the end of life. Also explored were the effects of potentially mediating variables such as physical symptom severity, social support, and selected demographic variables.

Conceptual Framework

The conceptual model undergirding the research was the "Middle Range Theory of Spiritual Well-Being in Illness (chapter 4), the core component of which is "the concept of finding spiritual meaning in the illness experience" (O'Brien, 2004, p. 39). Quality of life was understood according to the McGill end-of-life conceptualization, which includes focus on physical, psychological, and existential well-being. Spiritual well-being was described as encompassing an individual's positive attitudes toward his or her personal faith, religious practice, and spiritual contentment.

Method

The research included a correlational design, also employing the concept of methodological triangulation. Both quantitative and qualitative tools were used to measure key variables in the study.

Sample

The sample consisted of 22 ill, yet cognitively alert, elders, 65 years or older, at or nearing the end of life, who were physically able and willing to participate in data collection activities.

Instruments

Four quantitative tools—the Spiritual Assessment Scale (SAS) (O'Brien, 1999; 2003); the McGill Quality of Life Questionnaire (MQOL) (Cohen, 2001); the Geriatric Severity of Physical Symptoms Scale (GSPSS) (O'Brien, 2004); and the Geriatric Social Support Scale (GSSS) (O'Brien, 2004)—were used to assess the variables of spiritual well-being and quality of life, as well as mediating variables of symptom severity and social support. A demographic data form was employed to assess the additional potentially mediating variables of age, gender, religious orientation, marital status, education, and frequency of church attendance.

Following collection of quantitative data, a qualitative tool, the Spiritual Well-Being Interview Guide (SWBIG) (O'Brien, 2003a) was used to explore the study participants' perception of key study variables expressed in narrative form.

Procedure

Study participants were accessed from several urban nursing home/ assisted care facilities. After appropriate informed consent procedures had been carried out, quantitative data were collected using the above noted standardized tools. Following completion of response to the standardized tools, a tape-recorded open-ended interview was conducted with all study participants, employing the identified interview guide to focus the discussion. Because of the fragile nature of the study participant population, i.e., ill elders at or near the end of life, data collection was conducted in two sessions, if needed, in order not to unduly fatigue participants.

Protection of Human Subjects

Study participants, who had signed the informed consent form were carefully reminded that they could withdraw from the study at any time or refuse to answer any questions without penalty. It was not anticipated that study questions would cause emotional discomfort; however, if a study participant became fatigued or distressed during questioning, the interview was to be immediately terminated and supportive counseling provided. This did not occur. Study participants' confidentiality was assured; data were kept in a locked file and tape recordings destroyed following transcription and analysis.

Data Analysis

Quantitative and qualitative analyses were carried out using appropriate descriptive and interpretive procedures in order to identify patterns of thought and behavior among the study participants.

Significance and Relationship to Future Research

Both previous research and clinical experience have documented relationships between spiritual well-being and positive coping with illness and/or quality of life in chronically ill persons (O'Brien, 2003; Koenig, 1999). However, little research has been done to explore these relationships among older adults at or near the end of their lives. This study was designed to achieve the following goals:

   a) Expand the investigator's previous research in the area
   b) Establish reliability of several investigator-developed quantitative tools for use with a population of elders at or near the end of life

c) Explore use of the investigator-developed middle range conceptual model A Model of Spiritual Well-Being in Illness for use to undergird research with older adults at or near the end of life.

Note: It is recognized that there may appear to be some conceptual overlap related to the variables of "symptom severity" and "quality of life" (the McGill Questionnaire contains several items dealing with "recent troubling symptoms"). However, the investigator-developed Geriatric Severity of Physical Symptoms Scale (GSPSS), was created to provide a measure of overall (global) and persistent severity of physical symptoms that might significantly mediate the correlational relationship under investigation, as well as interact with the quality of life questions relating to immediate physical symptoms (i.e., problems within the last two days prior to the time of interview).

Study Findings

Quantitative Findings

The study participants, as noted earlier, consisted of 22 elders at or near the end of life. Those participating in the research were suffering from a variety of illnesses and disabilities; most individuals identified at least two health problems and a number had as many as five or six. This, of course, was to be expected considering that the study sample consisted of a population of elders at the end of life. Some of the disease conditions and/or disabilities reported included arthritis, diabetes, cardiovascular disease, congestive heart failure, hypertension, chronic obstructive pulmonary disease, lung cancer, prostate cancer, osteoarthritis, esophageal cancer, emphysema, glaucoma, heart arrythmias, loss of hearing, loss of vision (cataracts), memory loss, and depression.

One case example of an end-of-life elder experiencing multiple illnesses and disabilities and being treated with myriad therapeutic remedies was Frances, an 84-year-old widow living in an assisted care facility. Frances's diagnoses included altered cardiac status secondary to hypertension, hypothyroidism, osteoarthritis, left mastectomy secondary to breast cancer, mitral valve prolapse, endocarditis, atrial fibrillation, syncopal episodes resulting in frequent falls, subdural hematoma (evacuated), and gastro-esophageal reflux disease (GERD).

Frances's routine medications consisted of Synthroid, 100 mcq qd; Colace, 100 mg bid; Prilosec, 20 mg qd; Lopressor, 25 mg bid; Fosamax, 70 q wk; calcium, 600 mg+D qd; Lipitor, 10 mg qhs; Detrol LA, 4 mg qhs; and Extra Strength Tylenol, 2 q 6hrs PRN.

The study group, which consisted of 18 women and 4 men, reported a variety of religious affiliations including 5 Protestants, 13 Roman Catholics, 1 Jewish person, 1 Quaker, and 2 individuals who did not claim any specific religious affiliation. Ages ranged from 70 years to 94 including 1 person who was 70 years of age, 2 who were between 71 and 74, 4 who were 76 to 79, 7 persons who were between 80 and 85, 3 who were between 86 and 89, and 5 individuals who were between 90 and 95.

Nine of the study participants had attended high school including 5 who attended for two years and 4 who completed a four-year program. The other 13 individuals had attended college including 7 who attended two to four years and 6 who had masters or doctoral degrees in a variety of subjects. Five research participants were single and the other 17 were widowed.

The frequency of being able to attend formal worship services depended on a number of factors such as the physical condition of the study participant, availability of services at the nursing home or assisted care facility (study participants were living in a variety of health care facilities), and desire. In general, 3 individuals reported attending some kind of worship service daily, and 3 attended more than once a week; 5 attended services once a week; 2, once a month; 5, several times a year; and 3 study respondents admitted that they never attended any formal worship services.

Descriptive quantitative findings revealed specific patterns of response on each of the study tools. In responding to the Geriatric Severity of Physical Symptoms Scale (GSPSS), most study participants admitted to pain at least sometimes; this was generally associated with disease conditions such as arthritis or osteoarthritis. Fatigue associated with such diagnoses as congestive heart failure or cancer also was a predominant theme. Difficulty walking was associated with progressive arthritis or age-related vertigo; and difficulties in seeing and hearing were related, respectively, to age-related hearing loss and vision loss from such conditions as glaucoma and cataracts. In some persons, these losses were corrected through the use of glasses and hearing aids. Some age-related memory loss was also admitted to by many study participants.

In responding to the Geriatric Social Support Scale (GSSS), a number of end-of-life persons identified little if any social support from family or friends. This was associated with the fact that, for many, their significant others' lives had already been claimed by age-related illness conditions. The study participant was the last member of his or her support system left alive.

Responses to the Spiritual Assessment Scale (SAS) revealed that most study participants had fairly strong personal faith beliefs and a high degree of spiritual contentment. The lower scale scores elicited by the SAS subscale "Religious Practice (RP)" were associated with lower response on the specific items dealing with belonging to a church and participating in worship services. Many individuals decried the fact that they could no longer drive and thus get out to church on their own. Some of the health care residential facilities had weekly or biweekly in-house worship services; others were limited in that regard. Another "religious practice" item on which study group members scored lower was the item asking if one had a "spiritual friend or companion." In some cases, it was reported that pastors and/or church members visited frequently; for many, not at all.

On the McGill Quality of Life Questionnaire (MQOL), the weakest response from the study group was to the item "I feel that I have control over my life." Obviously, living in a nursing home or assisted care facility greatly decreased an individual's personal sense of control. Despite this response, a large number of study participants responded very positively to the question that asked if "the past two days" had been a "gift." Many reported that, on waking or sometime during the day, they thanked God for "still being here" or "for another day of life." Despite a multiplicity of physical and psychosocial deficits, persons at the end-of-life frequently wanted to remain alive as long as possible.

The above themes are also reflected in the qualitative study data presented later in this chapter.

Finally, there was a strongly positive correlation between the key study variables of spiritual well-being and quality of life. Those study participants who scored higher on the SAS (measuring spiritual well-being), including the subscales that measured personal faith, religious practice, and spiritual contentment, also reported a more positive quality of life as measured by the McGill Quality of Life Questionnaire (MQOL). Those persons who perceived a greater degree of social support (GSSS) also scored higher on the SAS and the MQOL. The severity of physical symptoms, as evaluated by the GSPSS did not seem to affect the study participants' spiritual well-being and quality of life significantly.

Qualitative Findings

Six dominant themes related to spiritual well-being emerged from content analysis of open-ended interviews with study participants; these themes included **the gift of life; spiritual comfort, which included subcategories companionship of God, faith and prayer, and devotional practices; religious reminiscence; spiritual pain; death awareness; and spirituality of community.**

The Gift of Life

The comment that life was a "gift" or "blessing" was a recurring theme related to spiritual well-being elicited from the population of elders at or near the end of life who responded to the Spirituality and Religiousness Interview Guide. Interestingly, although most reported no fear of death and, in fact, suggested that they were simply waiting to be "called by the Lord" or "go to God," study participants still expressed a sense of gratitude for their lives; some reported feeling "blessed to still be here."

Ninety-four-year-old Sarah, who had severe osteoporosis and difficulty walking and seeing, observed, "I am so blessed; life is a gift from God. Oh, I trust in God; others are so much worse off than I."

Seventy-two-year-old Eliza, who was wheelchair bound with a degenerative spinal condition as well as heart disease, commented, "I'm so grateful to have my mind and my hearing. Lord, I'm grateful that I'm part of your little gang down here and I don't have to holler out: 'what's that, again?' Life is a gift and I'm never alone. God will take care of me. Some people just hate being here (nursing home) but I feel privileged that there's a place like this. I can't think of anything more precious in my life than letting God do the controlling. I realized that peace was not going to be what Eliza wanted but what God wanted."

Robert, an 84-year-old with cardiovascular disease, emphasized, "I feel that my life has been a gift and that God's not finished with me yet! The gift I appreciate most is my ability to pray; daily Mass, the Stations, the Rosary, personal prayers; all are increasingly meaningful to me. That is my number one gift in life. That makes my day and alongside it, I still have my wits about me. I can listen to people and make sense of what they are saying. And make some sense in what I am saying. The ability to converse and to share thoughts, to share views and talk about world events." Robert concluded, "They also serve who only stand and wait. I offer each day to God. I'm in a waiting position."

Finally, Anna, a 79-year-old woman suffering from heart failure, arthritis, and osteoporosis, asserted, "Every day is a gift!" She showed the researcher a holy card that stated, "Old age leads to Him and old age will touch me only as He wills." Anna added, "I like the sense of being more available to people than before I retired. I'm more connected to people; there's more sharing."

Spiritual Comfort

A second theme that emerged very strongly in study participant interviews was the spiritual comfort brought about by the individuals' awareness of the companionship of God, their faith beliefs and personal prayer life, and their participation in devotional practices such as attending worship services, reading spiritual books, and/or looking at religious statues and pictures.

Companionship of God

Eighty-seven-year-old Martha, a widow whose husband had long suffered from Alzheimer's disease and who herself had myriad illnesses and disabilities related to vision, hearing, and walking, unhesitatingly stated, "God is my life! I have a beautiful relationship with God. God understands me. I don't say the rosary but I'm never without them, if I was I'd be frantic. I think God would like it because I try to do things for others." Martha added, "I memorize prayers so that I can sit outside on the bench and say them and people won't say: 'Oh, she's praying again': 'Remember O most compassionate Virgin Mary.'"

Ada, a 73-year-old heart disease patient who got around in an electric wheelchair, explained her perception of the constant companionship of God. "I'm never alone. God will always take care of me. His dying on the Cross with open arms. He will forgive everybody. God is just waiting for all of us. The only control I want over my life is what God wants me to be doing every day."

Faith and Prayer

Teresa, a 91-year-old widow suffering from high blood pressure and heart disease and taking multiple medications, asserted emphatically, "I don't know how I could live without my faith in God; that's my anchor. The least little problem I turn to Him. Every night and morning when I get up I kneel down and say the prayer: 'Look down upon me good and gentle Jesus while before thy face I humbly kneel and, with burning soul, pray and beseech thee to fix deep in my heart lively sentiments of faith, hope and charity and true contrition for my sins. Amen.'" Teresa concluded, "I pray every day for my family. Oh, I couldn't live without my faith in God."

Elizabeth, a 79-year-old widow with multiple illnesses including diabetes and heart disease, described her faith and her prayer life. "I pray the rosary. I go to the chapel. I feel so sad for others who don't have faith in God. I don't worry. I talk to God in my own words. God always takes care of me. I know that God loves me; that's my faith."

Rachel, an 86-year-old widow with crippling osteoarthritis, noted, "I pray all the time. I really talk to God. If I'm having a bad day I see people who are so much worse off than I am. I say my rosary and I know how many

'Our Fathers' and 'Hail Marys' it takes to get down the path outside. I trust God but I'm a little afraid of the future." Rachel explained her fear and her prayer, "I pray to God: 'Please God let me die before my mind goes' because I think that's terrible when people are in the last stages of Alzheimer's."

Robert, an 84-year-old single man with arthritis and heart disease, described the importance of his faith and prayer life in the midst of illness. "My sensitivity to pain is modified by my faith. I carry the Cross with Jesus. Without faith my life would be unlivable! God has been very good to me. I've been blessed in more ways than I can express." Robert added, "I feel that I'm making a contribution because I pray for people and I carry crosses."

Finally, 79-year-old Alice described how growing older had changed her prayer life. "Since I have reached the 'golden years,' my morning starts with a 'Thank You' to God for another day of life. When I look back on my life, I realize that I never prayed enough. I pray to God every day to help me accept my pain from arthritis in my knees and in my hips. I pray for my grandchildren who have a rare disease and I pray for my daughter and son-in-law. And, when God takes me, I pray to God that I will go to heaven so that I can see my mother and father."

Devotional Practices

Eighty-seven-year-old Camille, a 30-year insulin-dependent diabetic with congestive heart failure, hypertension, and advanced arthritis, described herself as a "loner." "I don't mingle," she asserted. Camille did, however, report that her devotional faith practices were very important in her life. "I believe God is watching over me. If I feel down I go and sit in the chapel and I feel better. I say my rosary every day. I pray many times during the day. I just look up and say 'Thank you, Lord, for my blessings. Thank you, Lord, that I'm still here.'"

Rita, an 84-year-old widow with multiple illnesses and disabilities including cardiac arrythmias, hypertension, arthritis, glaucoma in both eyes, and past hip and knee surgeries, spoke about the value of spiritual reading and having religious articles in her room. "I get a little magazine with religious stories and I love it; the stories all end up with God. They all have a spiritual point." Rita also proudly showed off her statue of the Infant Jesus and described the joy of having it in her room to look at.

Another octogenarian, 86-year-old Jeanette, pointed out the crosses hanging on her lampshade that her granddaughters had sent and added, "I have a rosary that my daughter got at the Vatican."

Seventy-seven-year-old Katherine, suffering from emphysema and lung cancer, admitted, "I don't know what I'd do if I didn't believe in God."

She explained that watching religious TV programs was very comforting to her. "Watching EWTN (Eternal Word Television Network) gives me support and strength."

Religious Reminiscence

Reminiscence of past life events in general occurred a great deal during open-ended study interviews. Sometimes the "remembering" simply dealt with family occasions or social highlights in an individual's past life. Frequently, however, the reminiscence took on a spiritual tone.

Carolyn, an 87-year-old Quaker suffering from a variety of illnesses including arthritis, bowel dysfunction, and hypothyroidism, reminisced about the joy of her Quaker Meeting experiences. "I wouldn't want to be anything else. We gathered together and waited on the presence of God. I don't like all the 'ups and downs' of the Catholic and Protestant services. I liked a silent meeting with God." Carolyn continued, "We did occasionally sing. I found peace at a 'Gathered Meeting.' We gathered strength from just being together."

Frank, a 67-year-old with chronic lung disease and emphysema who had difficulty breathing, reminisced about the importance of his Church in his life. "It's (emphysema) a constant battle but I lean on God. God put me in this for a reason. I talk to God; I always have and it makes me feel better. I do believe there is a God (repeated several times). Sometimes I like to just sit and meditate in the Chapel; I like the silence. My Church, St. Peter's, was like that; I'm going to be buried in St. Peter's cemetery. That's where my ashes will be. My Church was everything to me so it's important that I have the 'Last Rites' of the Church. That's why I came here (nursing home). It makes me not afraid of the future."

Several other study participants related how they were taught about religion from their parents, especially their mothers. One example was Rebecca, an 87-year-old Jewish widow suffering from angina, arthritis, and diabetes. "My mother taught us a lot about Judaism. We always kept a Kosher household. Her parents raised her in a Kosher household in Russia. She taught us to believe in God and that God will take care of the future. I keep a Star of David from her in my home and it's 41 years old."

Spiritual Pain

A few of the study participants described experiences of spiritual pain, sometimes related to occurrences in their own lives, sometimes to those in the lives of their children or relatives, and occasionally having to do with organized religion.

Rebecca noted sadly that her two daughters had married "outside the faith." "It really shook up me and my husband" but, she added, "I had to accept it if I didn't want to lose my daughters and their husbands are wonderful boys. If there is something special going on in the Synagogue, they will put on yarmulkes and go."

Eighty-seven-year-old Camille reported, "My son was always raised to go to church but he married a girl who was not Catholic and they don't go to church. That makes me very sad and I pray they'll come back to the church."

Eighty-seven-year-old Rita commented, "It hurts me a lot because I have two great-nieces who are not baptized and I worry about that a lot. I pray for them and for the family and that is comforting."

Michael, a 77-year-old widower with prostate cancer and numerous other illnesses, spoke about his disillusionment with his former Church. "I'm not much of any religion now. I only go to church at Christmas. I get depressed and my eyes are not too good. I still have one friend at the church and I get their newsletter but I've become uncertain about the existence of God. Going to church does not impact my life at all." When Michael was asked if he prayed, he responded "No!" He then added, "I'm sorry to upset your statistics!"

Rachel, at 86, noted, "I'm afraid that over the years I've gotten cynical about the church and that hurts. My family doesn't go to church; my husband doesn't go either. I've become disillusioned with the church because my pastor never came to visit me even though I went to his church for over 40 years. My boys were altar boys and I sat right up front every week but he never even came to see me. Now I take a walk outside and talk to God instead of going to church."

Marta, an 82-year-old widow with cardiovascular disease and osteoporosis, spoke about her struggles with joining and quitting a variety of Christian Churches related to weakness in the pastors and congregations. She described leaving one parish community by saying, "Not one member of that church ever consoled me (after her husband's death) so I left. I was so disillusioned with churches and religion." Marta now describes herself as a "secular humanist" and reported that she visited the headquarters of the "American Humanist Society" in Washington, DC, and gets their magazine once a month. Marta added, "It's (humanist society) not a faith group; it's just a way of life."

Death Awareness

Eighty-seven-year-old Rebecca spoke about the imminence of death. "One of my best friends is in the final stages of Alzheimer's and my other best friend has emphysema and can't come to visit me anymore. There is a 90-year-old here who is always talking about death and I say: 'Ruth, God hasn't called you yet, you have to wait your turn.'" She added, "All our turn is coming at this age."

Ninety-year-old Martin, who was experiencing severe hypertension, heart disease, and glaucoma, observed, "After my wife died the day before Christmas, suddenly I didn't know if God was with me or not or if I would die soon. I don't know if there's a hereafter but I imagine she's with God. I talk to her but unfortunately (laughs) she doesn't talk back."

An 82-year-old single woman described a family experience as taking away her fear of death. "I'm not afraid of death. My cousin who was like a sister to me died at 49 of cancer. I knew that if she could do it, I could do it."

An 80-year-old woman with severe diabetes stated calmly, "I ask God sometimes: 'I want to go to be with you.'"

An 86-year-old commented, "I would like to die in my sleep. As long as I'm mentally alert, I'm fine but I'm afraid of Alzheimers."

Spirituality of Community

A number of study participants, even though suffering from many personal illnesses and/or disabilities, expressed spiritual satisfaction in reaching out to others less fortunate than themselves. This was possible because the end-of-life study group resided in health care facilities, either nursing homes or assisted care residences. An example of the spirituality of community in one facility was reflected in an anecdote related by Mary, an 87-year-old widow who had diagnoses of diabetes, congestive heart failure, hypertension, osteoporosis, a past fractured pelvis, glaucoma in both eyes, and who had frequent dizzy spells necessitating her use of a walker. Mary reported that she attended daily Mass because it "makes me feel my life is worthwhile."

Mary gave the following example of the spirituality of community. "I keep to myself mostly but I want to tell you about something that really made me feel good. I was in the chapel one morning when Sister Ann approached me and asked me if I would take Tim to the dining room. He is only about 50 years old but blind and he has to use a cane to go anywhere. I did so and since then we talk to each other often about God. When I am at Mass with him I am very impressed with his gentleness and how he knows all the prayers."

At the conclusion of the open-ended study interviews, many respondents reported that they had truly enjoyed the interview process and the opportunity to reflect on spiritual and religious beliefs as related to the quality of their lives. One study participant, Ruth, called her interviewer three months after their first meeting to request a follow-up visit. Ruth, an 82-year-old widow with cardiovascular disease and osteoporosis, asked for a second visit because, she commented, "Talking . . . gave me comfort." "I've been a worrier all my life," Ruth said and suggested that her anxiety may be related to a kind of spiritual "testing" she was to undergo. She is not sure about the existence of God but admitted that she prays "if there is a God."

This chapter has presented both literature and nursing research supporting a positive relationship between spiritual well-being and quality of life for persons at or near the end of life. The research was undergirded by the author's newly developed middle-range theory of spiritual well-being in illness, which practicing nurses and nurse researchers may use to guide their work with seriously ill patients (see chapter 4). The theory evolved from the author's previous research and practice with both chronically and terminally ill persons. The multiple studies, three of which are included in this chapter, well validate the usefulness of the theory of spiritual well-being in illness to guide the assessment of a person's spiritual and/or religious concerns and needs at the end of life.

REFERENCES

Beckstrand, R. L., Callister, L. C., & Kirchoff, K. T. (2006). Providing a "good death": Critical care nurses' suggestions for improving end-of-life care. *American Journal of Critical Care, 15*(1), 38–45.

Cohen, S. R. (2001). McGill Quality of Life Questionnaire. Quebec, Canada: Royal Victoria Hospital (personal communication; permission to use tool).

Driscoll, J. (2001). Spirituality and religion in end-of-life care. *Journal of Palliative Care, 4*(3), 333–335.

Gibran, K. (1980). *The Prophet.* New York: Alfred A. Knopf.

Hamilton, J. B. (2001). The ethics of end-of-life care. In B. Poor and G. P. Poirrier (Eds.), *End of Life Nursing Care* (pp. 73–103). Sudbury, MA: Jones and Bartlett Publishers.

Koenig, H. G. (1999). *The healing power of faith: Science explores medicine's last great frontier.* New York: Simon and Schuster.

Koenig, H. G. (2002). A commentary: The role of religion and spirituality at the end of life. *The Gerontologist, 42,* 20.

Mazanec, P. (2003). Cultural considerations in end-of-life care: How ethnicity, age and spirituality affect decisions when death is imminent. *American Journal of Nursing, 103*(3), 50–58.

Miller, J., & Powers, M. (1998). Development of an instrument to measure hope. *Nursing Research, 37*(1), 6–10.

National Institutes of Health. (2004). State-of-the-science conference on improving end-of-life care. December 6–8, 2004. Bethesda, MD: National Institutes of Health.

O'Brien, M. E. (1982). The need for spiritual integrity. In H. Yura and M. Walsh (Eds.), *Human needs and the nursing process* (pp. 87–115). Norwalk, CT: Appleton Century Crofts.

O'Brien, M. E. (1991). *The nurse's calling: A Christian spirituality of caring for the sick.* Mahwah, NJ: Paulist Press.

O'Brien, M. E. (2001). *The gift of faith in chronic illness.* Washington, DC: The Catholic University of America. Final report submitted to the Our Sunday Visitor Institute, Huntington, Indiana.

O'Brien, M. E. (2003a). *Spirituality in nursing: Standing on holy ground.* (2nd ed.). Sudbury, MA: Jones and Bartlett Publishers.

O'Brien, M. E. (2003b). *Parish nursing: Healthcare ministry within the church.* Sudbury, MA: Jones and Bartlett Publishers.

O'Brien, M. E. (2004). *A nurse's handbook of spiritual care.* Sudbury, MA: Jones and Bartlett Publishers.

O'Brien, M. E. (2006). Parish nursing: Meeting spiritual needs of elders near the end of life. *Journal of Christian Nursing, 23*(1), 28–33.

Puchalski, C. M. (2002). Spirituality and end-of-life care: A time for listening and caring. *Journal of Palliative Medicine, 5*(2), 289–294.

Wood, V., Wylie, M., & Sheafor, B. (1969). An analysis of a short self-report measure of life satisfaction. *Journal of Gerontology, 24*(2), 465–469.

Young, C., & Koopsen, C. (2005). *Spirituality, health and healing.* Thorofare, NJ: Slack Incorporated.

12 Spiritual Needs in Death and Bereavement

By faith that Abraham obeyed when he was called to set out for a place . . . that was an inheritance given to him, and he set out not knowing where he was going.

HEBREWS 11:8

In this chapter the spiritual needs of the dying are explored. Also identified are the family's spiritual needs related both to the death and to the bereavement experience. The author obtained empirical data through observation and informal interviews with dying patients and their families, as well as with their professional nursing caregivers.

THE SPIRITUALITY OF DEATH AND DYING

Death is defined physiologically as occurring "when an individual has sustained either (1) irreversible cessation of circulatory and respiratory functions, or (2) irreversible cessation of all functions of the entire brain, including the brain stem" (President's Commission for the Study of Ethical Problems in Medicine, 1981, p. 1). From a theological perspective, death is conceptualized as "the final point of a human person's individual history . . . the decisive act of human freedom in which the person can either accept or reject the mystery of God and thereby put the final seal on his or her personal history and destiny" (Hayes, 1993, pp. 272–273). The spiritual understanding of death is undergirded by an individual's religious belief, that is, faith tradition. In Judaism, attitudes toward death vary both within and among specific traditions: Orthodox, Conservative, Reform, and Reconstructionist. In general, however, Judaism places great value on life as God's gift; there may be uncertainty about the existence of an afterlife (Grollman, 1993; Neuberger, 1994). Christian spirituality views death and dying in terms of the Gospel message of Jesus. Jesus' death provides a model for His followers who accept their sufferings in hope of the eternal reward He promised. For Jesus, death was not an ending but the beginning of eternal life with His Father (Kinast, 1993). Similarly, the Islamic perception of death incorporates the belief that an eternal life is part of God's plan (Esposito, 1990); the death of a loved one is considered only a "temporary separation" (Neuberger, 1994, p. 36).

The study of death and of the dying process teaches us much about the prevailing culture's attitude toward living (Moller, 1990). Historically, a number of theories of death and dying have been advanced; perhaps the best known is Kübler-Ross's, which describes the stages of denial, anger, bargaining, depression, and acceptance (1969). Angelucci and Lawrence (1995) developed a more contemporary nursing schema: "Health Promotion During the Dying Experience." This model includes cognitive-perceptual factors, such as perceived control and perceived benefits of preparing for dying; modifying factors, such as demographics, cultural influences, and social support; and health-promoting behaviors (p. 405). An important dimension of nursing support included in Angelucci and Lawrence's model is concern for meeting the patient's spiritual needs. This is seen as a significant element in promoting quality of life for the dying person (p. 412).

In discussing the "spirituality of dying," Chaplain Sharon Burns pointed out that to provide holistic care for a terminal patient, medicine and religion must work together (1991). Chaplain Burns views spirituality as the "life principle" of a person's being and asserted that when the body is ill or dying, the spirit must be affected. An important facet of dealing with the spiritual dimension of dying is the introduction of reminiscence and reconciliation, that is, of allowing the patient to review his or her life and to accept the past as well as the present and future (Burns, 1991, p. 50). In this way, the dying person can integrate spiritual beliefs about the meaning and purpose of life with personal experiences and find comfort and consolation in legacies to be left.

In a similar vein, Derrickson (1996) described the spiritual work of the dying process as including the tasks of remembering, reassessing, reconciling, and reuniting. Remembering relates to reminiscence or a life review through which one can recognize the goodness of life, reassessing is the act of redefining personal worth, reconciliation means healing damaged or broken relationships, and reuniting refers to combining the material and spiritual elements of the person and the world (pp. 14–21). As well as engaging in a life review, some other specific tasks that comprise the "work" of dying are conversing with family and friends, which provides the opportunity to say what needs to be said, and giving and receiving forgiveness when needed (Kalina, 1993, pp. 36–38).

Kalina (1993) also identified spiritual signs that death is imminent, such as detachment from material goods; less tolerance for the mundane in conversation and preference for more times of silence; detachment from concern about appearance; and finally, detachment from relationships as the person recognizes that the end is near (pp. 45–46).

How a person dies can reveal a great deal about how he or she lived. So also, the spirituality manifested in death and in the dying process reflects the personal spirituality of the dying person. For a dying individual who adheres to the tenets of a religious denomination that professes belief in an afterlife, the dying process can represent a joyful transition to a better state, a place where the good acts of one's life are rewarded and sins are absolved. For the person who believes that existence of both body and spirit cease with physical death, the dying process may represent a fearful experience, especially if the individual has not fulfilled desired life goals and ambitions. Spiritual care will need to be carefully planned so as to be relevant to the prevailing spiritual and religious beliefs of the dying patient and his or her family. Many deaths occur in the hospital, nursing home, or hospice setting. With changes in the contemporary health care system, however, more and more terminally ill individuals will die at home. Thus, the provision of spiritual support for patient and family may fall to the home health care or parish nurse, as well as to hospital, hospice, or nursing home nursing staff.

SPIRITUAL NEEDS IN THE DYING PROCESS

The dying process is unique to each person; a multiplicity of demographic, physical, psychosocial, and spiritual values may influence and mediate the experience. Such factors as age, gender, marital status, religious tradition, socioeconomic status, diagnosis, coping skills, social support, and spiritual belief, especially as related to the meaning of life and death, can influence one's management of the dying process. Despite the uniqueness of the individual, however, some universal needs are identified for most dying persons. These include the need for relief from loneliness and isolation, the need to feel useful, the need to express anger, the need for comfort in anxiety and fear, and the need to alleviate depression and find meaning in the experience (Kemp, 1995, pp. 11–16). Kenneth Doka (1993b) posited three broadly circumscribed spiritual goals of the dying person: "(1) to identify the meaning of one's life, (2) to die appropriately, and (3) to find hope that extends beyond the grave" (p. 146). The search for the meaning of life represents an attempt to bring together the dying individual's experiences, activities, and hoped-for goals and outcomes; dying appropriately refers to dying in the manner that the individual finds most acceptable; and finding hope that extends beyond the grave relates to the dying person's peace and trust in his or her concept of an afterlife (pp. 146–148). If a dying person is unable to find purpose and meaning in life, he or she may experience guilt from the perception of aspirations unfulfilled (Featherstone, 1997). Other spiritual needs of the dying person identified in the nursing literature include the need for forgiveness and love (Conrad, 1985), for self-acceptance, and for positive relationships with others, including, for some, relationship with God or a deity (Highfield, 1992).

Although the physical and psychosocial needs of the dying may be more readily identified by overt emotional or physical symptoms, spiritual needs can be more difficult to assess. Because one's spiritual and religious beliefs are personal, symptoms of spiritual distress may not be openly displayed and thus may be neglected in the planning of care for a dying patient (Charlton, 1992). Such lack of attention to spiritual needs is not acceptable, however, for nurses attempting to provide holistic care during the dying process (Stepnick & Perry, 1992).

Dealing with spiritual needs of the dying, identified as a central task of caring for the terminally ill, is not easy (Katz & Sidell, 1994). The spiritual needs of a dying person with no formal religious affiliation can be particularly problematic; the individual may "agonize over life and death issues . . . asking 'why me?' questions" (p. 120). However, a religious person facing death may also raise such questions depending on his or her spiritual maturity and experience. Frequently these concerns arise when the dying person is young and has not yet achieved his or her desired life goals. For the nurse caring for such a dying patient, therapeutic intervention may include dealing with the major spiritual issue of anger at God and/or organized religion.

In a study of 40 patients, 20 dying of lung cancer and 20 of heart failure, qualitative interviews elicited data reflecting both spiritual need and spiritual well-being (Murray, Kendall, Boyd, Worth, & Benton, 2004). Some of the spiritual needs identified included "expressions of frustration, fear, hurt, doubt or despair, feeling isolated and unsupported, feeling useless . . . and feeling of losing control" (p. 41). Some signs of spiritual well-being were having hope, goals and ambitions, social life and place in community retained, feeling valued, coping with and sharing emotions, being able to practice religion and finding meaning" (p. 41). Ultimately the authors concluded that "patients with life-threatening illness, even if still on 'active treatment' need help to cope with the prospect of dying, well before the terminal stage" (p. 44).

Tim, a 37-year-old terminal cancer patient, explained the importance of resolving spiritual issues prior to his impending death. "I guess it's like they say about 'no atheists in fox holes.' Well I'm in more than a foxhole. I need to get things together with myself and God before I go. I'm praying, and a pastor's been coming by to see me. I guess you don't think about all this until it gets near the end, but it's time now; it's definitely time."

SPIRITUAL SUPPORT IN DEATH AND DYING

Dying patients and their families cope with impending death in a variety of ways, depending on such factors as the age of the patient, the severity of the illness, the patient's religious beliefs, and cultural norms and values. One of the most frequently observed dilemmas is the fluctuation between acceptance and denial of the immediacy of death. Helping dying patients and families to manage the tension between these two attitudes is a key role of the spiritual caregiver (Joesten, 1992). One of the best ways of providing spiritual support in this situation is to allow the patient and family to verbalize their feelings; for a dying person "one of the greatest spiritual gifts" a nurse can give is to listen (Burns, 1991, p. 51).

Nursing literature subscribing to the concept of holistic care points out repeatedly that nurses must include spiritual support as part of the therapeutic regimen for the dying client (Conrad, 1985; Hittle, 1994; Taylor & Amenta, 1994). Some researchers have suggested also that if a nurse is to master the ability to assess and meet the spiritual needs of dying patients, he or she must engage in a personal spiritual journey in the process (MacDonald, Sandmaier, & Fainsinger, 1993; Praill, 1995; Price, Stevens, & LaBarre, 1995). It is impossible for a nurse to undertake the work of therapeutic spiritual support of patients without some understanding and acceptance of his or her own beliefs and attitudes about such issues as spirituality, religion, end-of-life decisions, and the existence or nonexistence of an afterlife. Olson (1997) believes that the "nurse's own spirituality will be reflected in the choice of interventions selected" (p. 132). This may be correct to a degree. The situation can be problematic, however, if nurse and patient have serious divergence in spiritual or religious beliefs and behaviors. The nurse must be comfortable and secure enough in his or her own spirituality and/or religious beliefs to remain open to differing spiritual or religious attitudes and needs on the part of the dying patient.

Some broad areas of spiritual nursing care for dying persons include assisting the patient to find meaning in life, hope, a relationship to God, forgiveness or acceptance, and transcendence (Kemp, 1995, p. 45). Five specific spiritual interventions for dying patients that fall within the purview of the nurse are praying, facilitating the presence of loved ones, allowing the dying person time to share, assisting in the completion of unfinished tasks, and assuring that the dying person has been given "permission" to die (Olson, 1997, p. 133). Nurses caring for dying patients should also attempt to identify the presence of spiritual pain, which may be manifested in terms of "the past (painful memories, regret, failure, guilt); the present (isolation, unfairness, anger); the future (fear, hopelessness)" (Eisdon, 1995, p. 641). Hospice research has documented the fact that spiritual care of dying patients falls within the scope of nursing practice (Hermann, 2001). Assessment of spiritual needs may be complex in end-of-life care (Sheldon, 2000); however, the provision of spiritual care in death and dying have been shown to enhance nurses' personal spirituality (Highfield, Taylor, & Amenta, 2000). A nursing theory recommended to support the provision of spiritual care for the terminally ill is the humanistic theory of Paterson and Zderad (Vassallo, 2001).

Stepnick and Perry (1992) offered a plan to guide nurses in providing effective spiritual care to dying patients, employing a model of the transitional phases of dying. They believe that, although patients may have different beliefs and levels of spiritual maturity, they share some common characteristics and needs as death approaches (p. 18). Based on Kübler-Ross's phases of denial, anger, bargaining, depression, and acceptance (1969), some suggested nursing strategies include listening and assuring trust, being nonjudgmental about anger, being sensitive to the pain of the bargaining stage, keeping communication open, and preparing the dying patient for what to expect in terms of the end stages of illness (pp. 19–23).

Brian, a master's-prepared psychiatric–mental health nurse, spoke about how he drew on his own spiritual journey in caring for dying patients:

> I hope that I always carry the motto of my former religious community [of nursing brothers], "Christ impels me," to my work with dying patients. Now I haven't done a good job of that every day of my life, I assure you; I'm an "earthen vessel" too. But nursing, for me, is a vocation; and I have always felt very privileged to work with patients in the last chapter of their lives on earth. It's such a rewarding experience. It's a tremendous privilege of being there, of ministering to the dying person.
>
> There was this patient and I was holding one of her hands and her daughter was holding the other, and it was like we were saying: "It's OK, you can let go." And then her daughter asked me to say a

prayer, and I just sort of incorporated some ideas, like "you are sur-
rounded by people who love you, and whenever you're ready to go,
you can go to God. He's waiting for you." . . .

When the patient dies, you think of what that person has given
to you, and how their spirit will live on in you, and that's very special,
very gifting.

Maggie, a hospice nurse, spoke about the importance of using touch
to calm the anxieties of her patients entering the death experience:

I will frequently reach out and touch a dying person physically; it's
so important when they're scared. I don't think people are afraid to
die; they are afraid of the process of dying. It's the loneliness, the
isolation, the abandonment, the fear of people not wanting to touch
them or care for them. . . . What is most fearful is the unknown in the
dying process. Are they going to be in pain; are they going to feel
loved; is their family going to be there? And then, what happens
after? I think we nurses are good about giving physical attention to
dying patients, and even psychosocial, but we're afraid to talk about
the spiritual, about the fact that maybe they feel abandoned or forsaken by God. As caregivers, I think we shy away from that. But I've
learned that it's really important that people are supported in whatever they feel comes after life, and in their concept of God.

Palliative Care

The World Health Organization (1990) defined palliative care as "the active
total care, by a multi professional team, of patients whose disease is not responsive to curative treatment. Control of pain, of other symptoms, and of
psychological, social and spiritual problems is paramount. The goal of palliative care is achievement of the best quality of life for patients and their
families" (p. 1). Palliation essentially relates to the acts of relieving suffering
and restoring peace to those who cannot be cured (Doyle, 1984). Palliative
care focuses on immediate quality rather than length of life (Olson, 1997) and
integrates physical, psychosocial, and spiritual care in its therapeutic plan
(Katz & Sidell, 1994). Palliative care may be carried out in a variety of settings:
a hospital, a nursing home, a hospice, or a patient's home. In addition to
providing symptom relief and support of positive quality of life, palliative
care as an emerging subspecialty of health care also includes promoting the

dying person's independence as much as possible, facilitating communication between collaborating care agencies, supporting families and staff during the bereavement period, and influencing care through education and research in the area (James & MacLeod, 1993, p. 6).

Spiritual or religious beliefs may influence both the choice and the practice of palliative care for a dying person (Hamel & Lysaught, 1994). Hamel and Lysaught explained that in palliative care patients' religious beliefs may affect decisions about death and dying by "(a) helping to shape [their] worldviews, (b) giving form to their particular beliefs, (c) giving rise to moral principles and rules, and (d) shaping community character and dispositions" (p. 61). For the dying person whose life history has been consistent with the worldview, beliefs, and moral principles central to his or her religious tradition, a sense of peace and security related to end-of-life decisions will usually be demonstrated; the support of the individual's religious community is also generally evident. In such a case the palliative care interventions should be consistent with the religious tradition of the dying patient. The caregiver should attempt to "build on" the existing beliefs of the patient and support the faith tradition that has provided comfort and sustenance in the past (Murray & Lyall, 1994).

Hospice Care

The concept of palliative care was initiated primarily in concert with the hospice movement in Europe and the United States. The first modern nursing hospice of note, St. Christopher's, was founded in Sydenham, England, in 1967, under the direction of Dame Cicely Saunders, M.D. The goal of St. Christopher's founder was to provide compassionate and loving care for those who were dying (Saunders, 1981, 1983).

During the medieval period a *hospice* was considered a place of hospitality for pilgrims on a journey, a stopping off place for travelers. The modern nursing hospice may also be described as a "way station" or "place of transit"; here, however, individuals are helped "to live fully in an atmosphere of loving kindness and grace" as they experience the process of natural death (Stoddard, 1978, p. 10). The goal of providing care and a place for the "weary traveler" to find "rest and safety" has not really changed from medieval times (Cohen, 1979). Most patients are indeed battle scarred and weary by the time they arrive at the hospice seeking relief. The central philosophy of hospice care emphasizes the fact that the outcome will be death, not prolongation of life; thus the care focus is in "comfort not cure" (Kirschling & Pittman, 1989, p. 1).

Hospice care in the United States is generally considered to have begun with the Hospice of New Haven project associated with Yale University, initiated in the mid-1970s. Nurses caring for those with terminal illness, especially nurses whose personal spirituality espoused the Judeo-Christian tradition, eagerly received the hospice message of compassionate care; for those caregivers the hospice concept was a direct reflection of the Scriptural admonitions to provide loving and sensitive care to those who are ill and in need of comfort. In hospice care, the nurse has the opportunity of reflecting a concept that Chaplain Trevor Hoy (1983) believes "lies at the heart" of spiritual care of the dying, and which is expressed in the Twenty-third Psalm: "Yea, though I walk through the valley of the shadow of death, I will fear no evil; for thou art with me" (p. 177). Hoy's position was supported by that of hospice chaplain Ted Harvey (1996) who described the two central concerns of spiritual care for the dying as relating to the patient's emotional well-being and his or her relationship with God (p. 41).

The modern hospice concept refers to either a facility or a program that supports the dying person's spiritual and religious beliefs and goals (Franco, 1985, p. 80). Related to the complexities of the changing health care system in this country, hospice chaplain Richard Grey (1996) suggested that the contemporary hospice mission and identity needs clarification. To that end, Grey proposed a psychospiritual care paradigm within which all hospice personnel can situate their particular activities, yet share in the common element of compassionate care. The National Hospice Organization Standards and Accreditation Committee developed a set of hospice service guidelines, which include policies related to admissions and discharge; levels of care; staffing, including a chaplain to provide spiritual care; services; and treatment (The National Hospice Organization, 1996b). A Hospice Code of Ethics has also been created, the first precept being "to remain sensitive to and be appreciative of the ethnic, cultural, religious and lifestyle diversity of clients and their families" (The National Hospice Organization, 1996a, p. 76).

Five palliative care physicians conducted an open-ended qualitative study to assess hospice patients' attitudes toward the discussion of religious and/or spiritual topics with their doctors. From the study data, four dominant themes emerged: "1) treating the whole person, 2) treating with sensitivity, 3) favorable attitudes toward religious or spiritual discussions with doctors, and 4) no preaching" (Hart, Kohlwes, Deyo, Rhodes, & Bowen, 2003, p. 160). The physicians concluded that they were not expected to be "spiritual advisors" for their patients but that many patients did feel positive about speaking about spiritual issues with their doctors (p. 160).

Several nursing studies have explored the prevalence of spiritual care in the hospice setting. Millison and Dudley (1992), in surveying 117 hospice directors in three states, found that many nonclergy hospice personnel were providing spiritual care by listening to patients, teaching meditation or guided imagery, and referring patients to clergy. These authors also found that hospice personnel are a spiritual group, and that those who identified themselves as more spiritual "found greater satisfaction in their hospice work" (p. 63). In a chart review of home visits to 37 hospice care patients, Reese and Brown (1997) discovered that spirituality and death anxiety were the most commonly discussed topics between patients and caregivers.

Laurie, a hospice nurse for five years, spoke about the concepts of death anxiety, spirituality, and caring, as experienced with some of her patients:

> The patients are afraid when they are in the dying process, of what the end will be like; some use their faith to help but even still they can be afraid of the unknown. That's when I think the nurse's caring is so important. Caring is hard to define. I think it's the ability to show compassion, to be able to touch someone. To just sit and listen, especially to their spiritual concerns and feelings and not to be critical or judgmental, to be with the flow of the moment. Time is such a commodity for people who are dying; it's so important to listen to people who are dying. That's spiritual caring I think.

RELIGIOUS PRACTICES ASSOCIATED WITH DEATH AND DYING

For a dying person, religious practices can provide an important dimension of spiritual support and comfort. Even if an individual has become alienated from a religious denomination or church, a terminal illness may be the catalyst for return to the practice of one's faith. This was clearly reflected in the comments of a 47-year-old male patient in the advanced stages of cancer. "I hadn't gone to my church for years; I don't know why. I just stopped going. But lately I've started up again, and I've been reading the Bible. When I die I want to have a church burial and be buried in a Christian cemetery; that's a big thing with my family."

Although the nurse caring for dying patients cannot be knowledgeable about the death-related beliefs and practices of all religious faiths, some familiarity with those of the major Western and Eastern traditions may provide a starting point for the provision of spiritual support. Having some idea of the theological positions and religious practices of different groups may assist the nurse in developing a relationship with a dying person and an empathetic and caring attitude (Head, 1994, p. 310). Anglican priest David Head (1994) believes that such knowledge on the part of a care provider will allow a dying patient to express spiritual or religious concerns more freely, without fear of being misunderstood (pp. 311–312). Ultimately, as noted in chapter 5, the best nursing approach to providing spiritual care to a dying person is to request information about religious beliefs and practices directly from the patient or family.

Western Traditions: Judaism, Christianity, and Islam
Judaism

Attitudes toward death for the Jewish patient may vary according to identification with a particular subgroup of Judaism: Orthodox, Conservative, Reform, or Reconstructionist. A Jewish person's approach to the dying process will also be influenced by his or her belief or nonbelief in the existence of an afterlife. Some Jews, especially those of the Orthodox tradition, do not subscribe to the concept of eternal life; they may, however, believe that faithful Jews will be resurrected when the Messiah comes. Some believe that one's good deeds in this life live on in the memories of family and friends. In Judaism, life is highly valued as a gift of God; all efforts to continue a productive life are supported. Thus, facing death may represent an ending of something precious. As Rabbi Julia Neuberger (1994) explained, "It is not so much uncertainty about the afterlife which causes a problem, but the emphasis put on the here and now" (p. 13).

A Jewish person who is dying, especially an Orthodox Jew, will generally receive visits from friends and synagogue members, because the duty to visit the sick is considered a *mitzvah* or good deed in Judaism. Some contemporary synagogues have established formalized groups called *Bikkur Cholim* societies, whose express purpose is to visit and minister to those who are ill; *Bikkur Cholim* members receive training from their synagogues in how to work with the sick. These individuals may also be present at a Jewish person's death and will offer prayers or readings from the Psalms, if desired by the patient or family.

After death occurs, synagogue members from the Jewish Burial Society may come to prepare the body of an Orthodox patient; no action should be taken by hospital or hospice personnel until it is determined whether this will occur. It is also customary that, after death, a Jewish person be buried within 24 hours; an exception may be made for the Sabbath. The formal ritual prayer of mourning, the *kaddish*, may be recited by a rabbi or family member; cremation and autopsy are avoided. After the burial has taken place, the important task of mourning is initiated. This involves friends and relatives of the deceased visiting at the family's home, or sitting *shiva* for the next seven days. This mourning period provides the grieving family with the support and care of those close to them and to the deceased person during the time immediately following death. Following *shiva*, 30 days of mourning, *sh-loshim*, continues; during this time the family may resume usual activities but avoids formal entertainment (Grollman, 1993).

Christianity

Three major subgroups within the Christian tradition are the Eastern Orthodox Churches, Roman Catholicism, and Protestantism; in addition, a number of other faith groups are identified as followers of Christ. Virtually all Christian traditions believe in eternal life, as promised in the Gospel message of Jesus. Thus, for the devout Christian, although the dying process can raise anxieties in terms of possible pain and suffering, death itself is viewed as a positive transition to a life with God and to one's eternal reward. Protestantism, which relies on the concept of salvation, trusts that faith will bring the believer into a better world (Klass, 1993). Older adult Christians sometimes express a desire for God to come and "take them home."

As death approaches, the majority of Christian patients and their families welcome a visit from a priest or minister; the pastoral visitor may be from the family's church or can be a hospital or hospice chaplain. These ministers will generally pray and read a Scripture passage with the dying person and their family. Eastern Orthodox Christians, Roman Catholics, and some Episcopalians may request an anointing or the "Sacrament of the Sick" prior to death; they may also wish to make a confession of sins and receive the sacraments of Penance and of Holy Eucharist (Holy Communion). A priest or family member may cross the arms of the Eastern Orthodox patient after death, situating the fingers to represent a cross.

After death occurs, most Christians will have a period of "viewing" of the body, sometimes called a "wake"; this ritual, which provides the opportunity for friends and family to call, takes place from one to three days after the death, in either the family home or a funeral home. A priest or minister may offer prayers periodically during the viewing. Christian burial services vary according to denomination. Eastern Orthodox, Roman Catholic, and some Episcopalian (Anglo-Catholic) Christians attend a funeral Mass of Requiem for the deceased prior to interment in a church cemetery. Although Mass is still the norm for the Catholic funeral, emphasis is now placed on life rather than death, and the central theme is resurrection; the priest celebrant wears white rather than black vestments. This changed focus, from grieving the death to hope in God's love and trust in the resurrection, indicates "a more healthy biblicism and pastoral practice" (Miller, 1993, p. 42). Other Christians participate in funeral or memorial services of their denominations; some families prefer a private service conducted by a minister in the home. The latter may be desired if cremation is chosen and no formal trip to the cemetery is planned.

Private memorial services are also the norm for the deceased who did not adhere to any conventional religious tradition. As Irion (1993) pointed out, a dying "secularist" also has a spiritual need to find meaning and purpose in life and in death (p. 94). The secular humanist usually places a high value on life and life accomplishments; these may be remembered and honored at a nonreligious memorial service.

Islam

The devout Muslim, like the Christian, views death as representing a spiritual transition to eternal life with Allah (Renard, 1993). Although a terminally ill Muslim may fear the dying process related to possible suffering, the concept of death itself is accepted as the will of Allah. Thus, excessive grieving of death by a Muslim may be considered inappropriate and represent a contradiction of Allah's plan. The death of a loved one should be viewed as only a temporary loss (Neuberger, 1994, p. 36). Islam, like Christianity, holds a belief in "resurrection of the body, final judgement and assignment to heaven or hell" (Kemp, 1995, p. 58).

As death approaches, family members or a Muslim minister, an imam, may read a passage from the Holy Qur'an to comfort the patient and family. The dying Muslim may wish to face Mecca, in the East, and ask forgiveness of Allah for sins. After death occurs, members of the family frequently wish to prepare the body through ritual washing and wrapping in a white cloth. After the body is prepared, the deceased may be laid out in a position facing Mecca.

Burial rites for a Muslim patient can vary, but generally interment takes place in a Muslim cemetery 24 hours after death.

Eastern Traditions: Hinduism, Buddhism, and Confucianism

Hinduism

Hinduism, as described in chapter 5, consists of a number of related Indian religious traditions, all of which are centuries old. Although a pantheon of lesser gods is associated with Hinduism, as demonstrated in Indian temples and holy places, most devout Hindus believe in the existence of one supreme being or deity. The many less powerful gods and goddesses are considered to be forms or derivatives of the one deity, with power and interest in specific areas of one's life.

The concept of reincarnation or rebirth influences the dying Hindu's attitude toward death; death itself is viewed as union with God. How one has lived in this world is influential in how one might return in the next life; this concept is referred to as karma.

Hindu patients often prefer to die at home where they can be more certain of the presence of a priest (Green, 1989a). A Brahmin priest, who performs the death rites, may tie a string or cord around the dying person's neck or wrist which should not be removed; prayers are also chanted by the priest. Following a Hindu's death, the funeral is usually carried out within 24 hours, and cremation is the traditional ritual.

Buddhism

Buddhism, founded by Gautama Siddhartha, differs from most other major religious traditions in that the Buddhist does not accept the existence of God or of a Supreme Being; Buddhists do, however, acknowledge the presence of a multiplicity of individual gods who are involved and interested in the lives of the Buddhist. Devout Buddhists live according to the "eightfold path" of right belief, right intent, right speech, right conduct, right endeavor, right mindfulness, right effort, and right meditation (Kemp, 1995, p. 60). The ultimate goal of the Buddhist is to reach the interior state of Nirvana or inner peace and happiness; this is achieved after having lived according to the eightfold path.

The Buddhist's attitude toward death is also influenced by belief in the concept of rebirth; death is accepted as a transition and as part of the cycle of life. A Buddhist monk may chant prayers at the death of a devout Buddhist in order to provide peace of mind at the point of death (Green, 1989b). An important dimension of the dying process for a Buddhist is to remain conscious in order to be able to think right and wholesome thoughts (Kemp, 1995). The deceased is generally cremated after death.

Confucianism

Confucianism is the tradition founded by the ancient Chinese scholar and philosopher, Confucius. Confucianism places great emphasis on respecting the memories and the contributions of one's ancestors. Elaborate death and burial rituals allow the bereaved to formally express grief and bring "continuity with the past and with tradition" (Ryan, 1993, p. 85). Ryan (1993) reported that in the Confucian tradition a person is taught to live life in such a way that after death good memories of the deceased may be honored (p. 86). The fate of the deceased in an afterlife depends on the quality of his or her natural life; it is also important that the deceased be properly honored by relatives after death. This relates to a strong belief in a "continuity of life after death" (Neuberger, 1994, p. 48).

The Confucianist's funeral may be an elaborate ritual, its complexity reflecting the status of the deceased. A carefully crafted coffin may be purchased by the family prior to death so that the dying person will know that he or she will be well honored at the burial rites.

SPIRITUALITY AND THE RITE OF BURIAL

The burial rite provides important spiritual support for the family and friends of a deceased person. The planning of one's own funeral or memorial service may provide comfort for the dying person. In contemporary society, as chronically ill persons live longer and are able to anticipate death, they often become involved in the planning of their burial rites. During the early period of the AIDS epidemic in this country, with many gay men not only anticipating their own approaching deaths but also experiencing the deaths and burial rites of friends, planning the memorial service became a central activity of the dying process. As one 45-year-old man suffering from advanced Kaposi's sarcoma humorously commented, "I've put so much into the plans for my memorial service, it's beginning to resemble the coronation of a king." Despite the humor of the patient's remark, he nevertheless admitted that creating the memorial service plans was very comforting, observing, "This way I don't have to worry about my family having to deal with this when they are grieving my death."

As Rando (1988) pointed out, burial rites help families confront the death of a loved one and begin the grieving process (p. 261). The funeral provides an opportunity for meeting the spiritual, psychological, and social needs of the bereaved (Raether, 1993, p. 214). Some specific therapeutic benefits of the bereavement ritual include confirming the reality of death; acknowledging the loss; providing an opportunity to express feelings; remembering and validating the life of the deceased; accepting the changed relationship with the deceased; supporting family and friends; and, in the case of religiously oriented funerals, placing the meaning of life and death in a religious/philosophical context (Rando, 1988, pp. 266–269).

Burial rites can also be helpful to nurse caregivers who wish to formally terminate relationships with patients who have died. In one clinical research facility, nurses worked extensively with dying children, most of whom returned home to a different geographical location for death and burial; thus, staff requested that the hospital chaplain periodically conduct pediatric memorial services to provide nursing staff the opportunity for formal farewells to the deceased children.

SPIRITUALITY AND THE BEREAVEMENT EXPERIENCE

The body of literature dealing with the post-death period includes the terms *bereavement, grief,* and *mourning;* these are sometimes used interchangeably, all being understood as describing the physical and psychosocial experience of loss following the death of a loved one. Rando (1988) defined grief as "the process of experiencing the psychological, social and physical reactions to [one's] perception of loss" (p. 11). Mourning, derived from the Greek "to care," is described as "an emotion that results from the universal experience of loss" (Davidson, 1984, p. 6). And Sanders, in her book *Grief, the Mourning After* (1989), distinguishes between the three concepts: bereavement is conceptualized as the overall experience one faces after a loss, grief is viewed as representing the physical and psychosocial reactions an individual experiences while in the state of bereavement, and mourning describes the culturally prescribed behaviors carried out after a death (p. 10).

Historically, the study of the bereavement experience, including the aspects of grief and mourning, began with the work of Eric Lindemann in 1944. His classic study of 101 bereaved survivors of Boston's "Coconut Grove" fire provided the benchmark for our contemporary understanding of the grieving process. Lindemann described the acute reaction to the death of a loved one as including such somatic responses as "a feeling of tightness in the throat; choking with shortness of breath; need for sighing; an empty feeling in the abdomen; lack of muscular power; and an intense subjective distress described as tension or mental pain" (p. 141).

Later scholars of bereavement such as Bowlby (1961) and Parkes (1972) viewed the grief reaction as being of longer duration and consisting of such phases as acute grief, chronic grief, conflicted grief or complicated grief, and prolonged or delayed grief. Writing in 1983, Colin Murray Parkes and Robert Weiss asserted that when grief was uncomplicated, recovery was generally accomplished within one year after the loss; this time period has been extended significantly in recent years, although the one-year anniversary may represent a milestone in the healing process for some mourners.

Extant research also supports the importance of a number of potentially mediating variables related to the bereavement experience: the meaning of the bereavement to the mourner; the relationship between the deceased and the bereaved; the physical, social, material, and psychological resources of the bereaved person; and the spiritual and religious beliefs of the family (Rando, 1988; Sanders, 1989). Sanders' (1989) model, labeled the "Integrative Theory of Bereavement," included the earlier-noted variables as well as the external mediator of religious practice. The work of identifying and meeting the spiritual or religious needs of bereaved persons is central to supporting positive coping with grief and loss.

Manifestations of an uncomplicated grief reaction are generally divided into four categories: physical, cognitive, emotional, and behavioral. Some of these as described by Worden (1982) include physical reactions such as stomach emptiness, shortness of breath, tightness in chest and throat, and fatigue; cognitive reactions of disbelief and mental confusion; emotional responses of sadness, guilt, anger, loneliness, numbness, and yearning for the deceased; and behavioral disruptions such as insomnia, loss of appetite, social isolation, crying, and restlessness (pp. 20–23). Worden described the four tasks of mourning during the bereavement experience as accepting "the reality of the loss," experiencing "the pain of the grief," adjusting "to an environment in which the deceased is missing," and reinvesting "emotional energy . . . in another relationship" (pp. 11–15). Rando (1988) suggested specifically that the bereaved person should not isolate himself or herself, accept the support of significant others, obtain information about what to expect in the grieving process, realize that grief may be expressed in a variety of ways, allow himself or herself to cry and to talk about the deceased, and trust that the pain will decrease after a time (pp. 242–248).

Bereaved persons need and will often accept spiritual support from the family's pastoral care provider, rabbi, minister, priest, or, in some cases, a nurse if he or she is skilled in bereavement counseling and support. Other significant persons who may provide spiritual support for the bereaved are church or faith group members who also understand the grieving person's or family's spiritual and theological perspective on the loss. Whether spiritual care is provided by the pastor, nurse, or church member, intervention should focus on supporting two major tasks of the bereaved individual: letting go of the deceased person and becoming reinvested in current life activities. The spiritual caregiver's challenge in grief and bereavement is to balance the activities of strengthening and disputing; the caregiver must "know when to comfort and support and when to challenge and confront" (Joesten, 1992,

p. 144). Joesten observed that an important dimension of spiritual intervention for bereaved persons is the presence of a caring other who is willing to be there and share in the grief and the pain (p. 145); he asserted that the spiritual caregiver assists the bereaved most by being someone who offers hope and honesty amid the darkness of the experience (p. 148).

Finally, it is important to remember, as noted by Young and Koopsen, that for those dealing with loss, "individuals in the early stages of spiritual development may need more external support and communication, while more spiritually developed individuals may use rituals, rites and symbols for comfort" (2005, p. 192).

DYSFUNCTIONAL AND DISENFRANCHISED GRIEF

Although normal grief encompasses many physical and psychosocial sequelae with which the bereaved must cope, complicated or dysfunctional grief may present even more suffering. Dysfunctional grief has many descriptions; it is generally believed to occur when the usual tasks of the grieving process are thwarted or blocked. Some factors that might be associated with a dysfunctional grief reaction are an unhealthy relationship between the deceased and the bereaved, poor coping skills on the part of the mourner, a lack of material and social support in the bereavement experience, and inadequate mental or physical health of the bereaved (Kemp, 1995, p. 77). Sudden or unexpected death may also result in complicated grieving (Rando, 1988; Smithe, 1990).

A more recently identified dysfunctional type of response to loss has been labeled "disenfranchised grief." Disenfranchised grief is defined as "the grief that persons experience when they incur a loss that is not, or cannot be openly acknowledged, publicly mourned, or socially supported" (Doka, 1989, p. 4). Doka posited that a survivor may be disenfranchised for three reasons: "the relationship is not recognized," for example, in the case of a child of an unwed mother who is unable to mourn a nonacknowledged father; "the loss is not recognized," such as the loss of a child to abortion or miscarriage; and "the griever is not recognized," as in the case of a mentally retarded or disabled survivor (pp. 5–7). In disenfranchised grief, as the tasks of grieving must be carried out privately without the support of family and friends, the bereaved person can be forced into a state of silent unresolved grief that may last for many years. Pastoral counselor Dale Kuhn (1989) pointed out that despite a negative or unsatisfactory experience with a church or faith group, a bereaved person experiencing disenfranchised grief may still continue to seek support from God; in this situation the individual spiritual caregiver may play an important role as a counseling and listening presence in the silent grieving process (p. 247).

Helen, the mother of a son who had died of AIDS, spoke about her experience of disenfranchised grief. "It was so hard with my church, to go to services. My minister suspects and some close friends, but with most of the church, I couldn't tell them. They would judge him; me too, I suppose. So I kept the pain inside me. What I wanted to do was cry and scream but I couldn't do that to him so I had to grieve his death alone." Helen concluded, "It shouldn't be like that; not for a mother, not for anybody!"

Elkin and Miller (1996) identified some nursing diagnoses reflecting spiritual problems occurring during a bereavement experience; the diagnoses include hopelessness, in which the bereaved feels that the grieving will never end, and spiritual distress, indicating that a mourner is unable to rely on his or her spiritual or religious beliefs to provide peace and hope for the future (p. 695). As noted earlier, a multiplicity of variables may mediate the pain and suffering of a bereavement experience; the quality and the nature of the relationship between the deceased and the bereaved is among them. Although any loss may be significant for those who survive, three especially significant bereavements are those that occur following the loss of a child, the loss of a spouse, and the loss of a parent.

Death of a Child

There is perhaps no loss so grievous for any person as the loss of a child. Most parents are devastated when one of their children dies, regardless of the age of the child. The common understanding of family, in virtually all societies, is that a child will survive his or her parents. Although family members attempt to find meaning and purpose in the life of the deceased offspring, the task is more difficult in the death of an infant or a very young child. The bereaved parents are often left with great frustration related to unfulfilled dreams and expectations. As Sanders (1989) observed, children represent a parent's legacy for the future; they are to be the bearers of the family tradition (p. 163). A parent may also experience guilt that he or she was somehow not able to protect the child from illness and death.

Sanders (1989) identified some parental responses to bereavement: despair, related to the ability to go on living following a child's death; confusion, related to the parent being unable to accept the reality of the death; guilt that the parent was not able to be responsible for the child's welfare; and anger, associated with the inability to prevent the child's death (pp. 165–169). Death of a child may also affect a marriage if the usual ways of interacting between the spouses are disrupted by the loss (Rando, 1988, p. 170). Many relationships end in separation or divorce as a result of the terminal illness and death of the couple's child.

Parents may find comfort in religious and spiritual beliefs, especially if they were able to integrate these into coping with the child's illness prior to the death experience. A nurse should not, however, attempt to impose such beliefs on a parent or parents with words such as "This must have been God's will," because the bereaved may still need to express feelings of anguish or anger over their loss (Amenta, 1995, p. 206). The nurse can, however, provide the spiritual care of presence by being available to the parents with a loving and listening heart.

Death of a Spouse

The death of one's life partner is a traumatic event, regardless of the number of years a couple has been together. The death of a spouse is recognized as emotionally overwhelming and is generally considered one of the most devastating human losses possible (Osterweis, Solomon, & Green, 1984, p. 71). Raphael (1983) posited that conjugal bereavement is one of the most disruptive and potentially stressful experiences that an adult can experience and may affect the essential meaning of the survivor's existence (p. 177). A particular difficulty for the surviving spouse is identity transition; that is, the change in self-image in beginning to view oneself as a single person rather than as one-half of a couple. In the case of a small number of bereaved partners, the inability to identify as a single person has generated feelings of helplessness so severe as to result in suicide (Raphael, 1983).

Some bereaved spouses experience physical symptoms of their grief. Parkes, Benjamin, and Fitzgerald (1969) coined the metaphor of the "broken heart" based on their findings that some widower deaths within six months of bereavement were due to heart disease related to the loss of one's spouse. An important mediator of such mortality and morbidity is the presence of spiritual and social support for the bereaved spouse. Shuchter's (1986) study of 70 bereaved spouses revealed that interaction with significant others helped the bereaved by providing emotional support and caring, and by giving the surviving spouse an opportunity to become involved in the concerns of others (p. 110).

Sanders (1989) found the practice of religion, particularly church attendance, to be a mainstay among bereaved spouses (p. 194). Nurses may have the occasion to provide spiritual care to bereaved spouses who stay in touch after the death of their partner in a hospital setting. If face-to-face interaction is not possible, a written note of condolence from a loved one's nurse can be very meaningful. During the dying process in a health care facility, staff nurses often become important significant others for the family of the ill person. Any expression of care and concern after the death, such as a letter or a phone call, will convey a deeply appreciated message of spiritual support.

Death of a Parent

The death of a parent frequently represents a loss of security on the part of the bereaved child or children. Although a surviving child may be chronologically an adult at the time of parental death, the loss of love and caring can be great. Even adult children who have undertaken complete support of a frail parent feel keenly the pain of a mother's or a father's death. The nature of the former parent–child relationship is, of course, a mediating variable in the bereavement experience of the offspring. Sanders (1989) believed, however, that even if a parent–child relationship has not been exemplary, a significant bond exists, which is traumatic when broken (p. 202).

The nurse assisting at the death of a parent, even an elderly parent, must be sensitive to the deep spiritual meaning of the parent–child bond. The grief associated with this death experience can be powerful and deep for surviving offspring of any age. Awareness of the significance of this loss will guide the nurse in his or her efforts to provide spiritual support for the grief experience of an adult child as well as that of a bereaved young child or teen.

SPIRITUAL CARE IN BEREAVEMENT: THE HEALING PROCESS

Clearly, the nurse seeking to provide spiritual care to a bereaved person will need to have some knowledge of the individual's spiritual and/or religious beliefs and practices related to loss and grieving. Respect for the religious attitudes and practices of the bereaved must be clearly communicated by one attempting to provide care and support (Doka, 1993a, p. 191). If a bereaved individual appears to have dysfunctional beliefs related to a particular religious tradition, referral to a clergyperson of the person's denomination or the use of religious books may be helpful (Doka, 1993a). Clinebell (1991) suggested that a caregiver attempting to facilitate the work of the grieving process may want to employ a ministry of caring and presence, responsive listening, counseling as the bereaved attempts to rebuild his or her life, facilitating of spiritual growth, and supporting the bereaved in reaching out to others with similar losses (p. 221). Although the funeral provides an important opportunity for the emotional expression of grief, Clinebell pointed out that it may take many months for the bereaved person to come to terms with a loss, and continued spiritual support is needed during that time. Some postfuneral questions that might encourage the expression of emotions are, "What have you been feeling since the funeral?", "What sort of memories keep coming back?", "How often have you let yourself cry?", "Have you had trouble keeping going?", and "Would you tell me more about the way he/she died?" (p. 224).

In order for healing to be completed, the bereaved person must be able to let go of the deceased. Although this may have appeared to occur at the time of death, when a family member verbally gives a dying person permission to give up, the emotional attachment may remain with the survivor. Many bereaved persons express significant distress at coming to a point at which they have difficulty remembering what the deceased looked like, or even at letting several hours pass without thinking about the deceased. Ruskay (1996) proposed an approach to bereavement care in which the griever is encouraged to incorporate the loss into daily activities and plans; the bereaved person is counseled to incorporate some of the deceased person's interests, for example, gardening, into their lives, thus adding a positive dimension to the grieving process (p. 5).

In discussing bereavement care, Bouton (1996) distinguished between the goals of grief counseling and bereavement care. Grief counseling is envisioned as facilitating the work of grieving to achieve a successful outcome by helping the bereaved person face the reality of the loss; cope with physical, psychological, and spiritual grief reactions; and reinvest himself or herself into life activities. Bereavement care is conceptualized as identifying and resolving the pain and conflict resulting from the loss that may block completion of the grieving process (p. 17).

Additionally, spiritual and religious beliefs are important considerations in the provision of bereavement care. Religious beliefs may be instrumental in defining right or acceptable attitudes and behavior in relation to the bereavement experience (Koenig, 1994, p. 405). Cullinan (1993) conceptualized spiritual care of the bereaved as a "sacred art." While acknowledging the existence of a multiplicity of theories related to the relationships among spirituality, religiosity, and bereavement, Cullinan (1993) viewed spirituality as undergirded and influenced by the individual's faith development, cultural background, and religious or denominational affiliation and practice (p. 197). Such an adaptive type of psychospiritual approach to care, Cullinan argued, will help the bereaved person to cope with the loss in a more positive and healthy way (p. 197).

Personal spirituality and religiosity or religious practice are important mediating variables in coping with death and bereavement. Dying persons' and their families' spiritual and religious beliefs about such concepts as the meaning of life and death, the existence of an afterlife, and the purpose of suffering can influence profoundly how the dying process is experienced. The nurse, sensitive to the spiritual and religious beliefs of a dying patient and his or her family, may be able to provide therapeutic spiritual support and intervention that will mediate the pain associated with the death and bereavement experiences.

REFERENCES

Amenta, M. O. (1995). Loss, death and dying. In D. D. Ignatavicus, M. L. Workman, & M. A. Mishler (Eds.), *Medical–surgical nursing: A nursing process approach* (pp. 195–212). Philadelphia: W. B. Saunders.

Angelucci, D., & Lawrence, M. (1995). Death and dying. In M. Stanley & P. G. Beare (Eds.), *Gerontological nursing* (pp. 400–414). Philadelphia: F. A. Davis.

Bouton, B. L. (1996). The interdisciplinary bereavement team: Defining and directing appropriate bereavement care. *The Hospice Journal, 11*(4), 15–24.

Bowlby, J. (1961). Processes of mourning. *The International Journal of Psychoanalysis, 42*(8), 317–340.

Burns, S. (1991). The spirituality of dying. *Health Progress, 72*(7), 48–52.

Charlton, R. G. (1992). Spiritual need of the dying and bereaved: Views from the United Kingdom and New Zealand. *Journal of Palliative Care, 8*(4), 38–40.

Clinebell, H. (1991). *Basic types of pastoral care and counseling.* Nashville, TN: Abingdon Press.

Cohen, K. P. (1979). *Hospice: Prescription for terminal care.* Germantown, MD: Aspen Systems.

Conrad, N. L. (1985). Spiritual support for the dying. *Nursing Clinics of North America, 20*(2), 415–426.

Cullinan, A. (1993). Bereavement and the sacred art of spiritual care. In K. J. Doka (Ed.), *Death and spirituality* (pp. 195–205). Amityville, NY: Baywood.

Davidson, G. W. (1984). *Understanding mourning: A guide for those who grieve.* Minneapolis, MN: Augsburg.

Derrickson, B. S. (1996). The spiritual work of the dying: A framework and case studies. *The Hospice Journal, 11*(2), 11–30.

Doka, K. J. (1989). *Disenfranchised grief: Recognizing hidden sorrow.* Lexington, MA: Lexington Books.

Doka, K. J. (1993a). The spiritual crisis of bereavement. In K. J. Doka (Ed.), *Death and spirituality* (pp. 185–194). Amityville, NY: Baywood.

Doka, K. J. (1993b). The spiritual needs of the dying. In K. J. Doka (Ed.), *Death and spirituality* (pp. 143–150). Amityville, NY: Baywood.

Doyle, D. (1984). *Palliative care: The management of far-advanced illness.* Philadelphia: The Charles Press.

Eisdon, R. (1995). Spiritual pain in dying people: The nurse's role. *Professional Nurse, 10*(10), 641–643.

Elkin, M. K., & Miller, R. M. (1996). Facilitating grief work. In M. K. Elkin, A. G. Perry, & P. A. Potter (Eds.), *Nursing interventions and clinical skills* (pp. 691–704). St. Louis, MO: C. V. Mosby.

Esposito, J. L. (1990). Islam. In J. A. Komonchak, M. Collins, & D. A. Lane (Eds.), *The new dictionary of theology* (pp. 527–529). Collegeville, MN: The Liturgical Press.

Featherstone, S. M. (1997). Coping with loss, death and grieving. In P. A. Potter & A. G. Perry (Eds.), *Foundations of nursing: Concepts, process and practice* (pp. 457–476). St. Louis, MO: C. V. Mosby.

Franco, V. W. (1985). The hospice: Humane care for the dying. *Journal of Religion and Health, 24*(1), 79–89.

Green, J. (1989a). Death with dignity: Hinduism. *Nursing Times, 85*(6), 50–51.

Green, J. (1989b). Death with dignity: Buddhism. *Nursing Times, 85*(9), 40–41.

Grey, R. (1996). The psycho-spiritual care matrix: A new paradigm for hospice caregiving. *The American Journal of Hospice and Palliative Care, 13*(4), 19–25.

Grollman, E. A. (1993). Death in Jewish thought. In K. J. Doka (Ed.), *Death and spirituality* (pp. 21–32). Amityville, NY: Baywood.

Hamel, R. P., & Lysaught, M. T. (1994). Choosing palliative care: Do religious beliefs make a difference? *Journal of Palliative Care, 10*(3), 61–66.

Hart, A., Kohlwes, R., Deyo, R., Rhodes, L., & Bowen, D. (2003). Hospice patients' attitudes regarding spiritual discussions with their doctors. *American Journal of Hospice and Palliative Care, 20*(2), 135–139; 160.

Harvey, T. (1996). Who is the chaplain anyway?: Philosophy and integration of hospice chaplaincy. *The American Journal of Hospice and Palliative Care, 13*(5), 41–43.

Hayes, Z. (1993). Death. In J. A. Komonchak, M. Collins, & D. A. Lane (Eds.), *The new dictionary of theology.* Collegeville, MN: The Liturgical Press.

Head, D. (1994). Religious approaches to dying. In I. B. Corless, B. B. Germino, & M. Pittman (Eds.), *Dying, death and bereavement: Theoretical perspectives and other ways of knowing.* Boston: Jones and Bartlett.

Hermann, C. P. (2001). Spiritual needs of dying patients: A qualitative study. *Oncology Nursing Forum, 28*(1), 67–72.

Highfield, M. F. (1992). Spiritual health of oncology patients: Nurse and patient perspectives. *Cancer Nursing, 15*(1), 1–8.

Highfield, M. E., Taylor, E. J., & Amenta, M. O. (2000). Preparation to care: The spiritual care education of oncology and hospice nurses. *Journal of Hospice and Palliative Nursing, 2*(2), 53–63.

Hittle, J. M. (1994). Death and spirituality: A nurse's perspective. *The American Journal of Hospice and Palliative Care, 11*(5), 23–24.

Hoy, T. (1983). Hospice chaplaincy in the caregiving team. In C. A. Corr & D. M. Corr (Eds.), *Hospice care: Principles and practice* (pp. 177–196). New York: Spring.

Irion, P. E. (1993). Spiritual issues in death and dying for those who do not have conventional religious belief. In K. J. Doka (Ed.), *Death and spirituality* (pp. 93–112). Amityville, NY: Baywood.

James, C. R., & MacLeod, R. D. (1993). The problematic nature of education in palliative care. *Journal of Palliative Care, 9*(4), 5–10.

Joesten, L. B. (1992). The voices of the dying and the bereaved: A bridge between loss and growth. In L. E. Holst (Ed.), *Hospital ministry: The role of the chaplain today* (pp. 139–150). New York: Crossroad.

Kalina, K. (1993). *Midwife for souls: Spiritual care for the dying.* Boston: St. Paul Books and Media.

Katz, J., & Sidell, M. (1994). *Easeful death: Caring for dying and bereaved people.* London: Hodder & Stoughton.

Kemp, C. (1995). *Terminal illness: A guide to nursing care.* Philadelphia: J. B. Lippincott.

Kinast, R. L. (1993). Death and dying. In M. Downey (Ed.), *The new dictionary of Catholic spirituality* (pp. 252–256). Collegeville, MN: The Liturgical Press.

Kirschling, J. M., & Pittman, J. F. (1989). Measurement of spiritual well-being: A hospice caregiver sample. *The Hospice Journal, 5*(2), 1–11.

Klass, D. (1993). Spirituality, Protestantism and death. In K. J. Doka (Ed.), *Death and spirituality* (pp. 51–74). Amityville, NY: Baywood.

Koenig, H. G. (1994). *Aging and God: Spiritual pathways to mental health in midlife and later years.* New York: The Haworth Press.

Kübler-Ross, E. (1969). *On death and dying.* New York: Macmillan.

Kuhn, D. (1989). A pastoral counselor looks at silence as a factor in disenfranchised grief. In K. J. Doka (Ed.), *Disenfranchised grief: Recognizing hidden sorrow* (pp. 241–256). Lexington, MA: Lexington Books.

Lindemann, E. (1944). Symptomatology and management of acute grief. *American Journal of Psychiatry, 101*(1), 141–148.

MacDonald, S. M., Sandmaier, R., & Fainsinger, R. L. (1993). Objective evaluation of spiritual care: A case report. *Journal of Palliative Care, 9*(2), 47–49.

Miller, E. J. (1993). A Roman Catholic view of death. In K. J. Doka (Ed.), *Death and spirituality* (pp. 33–50). Amityville, NY: Baywood.

Millison, M. B., & Dudley, J. R. (1992). Providing spiritual support: A job for all hospice professionals. *The Hospice Journal, 8*(4), 49–66.

Moller, D. W. (1990). *On death without dignity: The human impact of technical dying.* Amityville, NY: Baywood.

Murray, D., & Lyall, D. (1994). Pastoral care. In D. Doyle (Ed.), *Palliative care: The management of far-advanced illness* (pp. 414–427). Philadelphia: The Charles Press.

Murray, S., Kendall, M., Boyd, K., Worth, A., & Benton, T. F. (2004). Exploring the spiritual needs of people dying of lung cancer or heart failure: A prospective qualitative interview study of patients and their carers. *Palliative Medicine, 18,* 39–45.

The National Hospice Organization. (1996a). Hospice code of ethics. *The Hospice Journal, 11*(2), 75–81.

The National Hospice Organization. (1996b). Hospice services guidelines and definitions. *The Hospice Journal, 11*(2), 65–73.

Neuberger, J. (1994). *Caring for dying people of different faiths* (2nd ed.). St. Louis, MO: C. V. Mosby.

Olson, M. (1997). *Healing the dying.* New York: Delmar.

Osterweis, A., Solomon, F., & Green, M. (1984). *Bereavement reactions: Consequences and care.* Washington, DC: National Academy Press.

Parkes, C. (1972). Bereavement. *Studies of grief in adult life.* New York: International University Press.

Parkes, C. M., Benjamin, B., & Fitzgerald, R. (1969). Broken hearts: A statistical study of increased mortality among widowers. *British Medical Journal, 1*(1), 7400–7443.

Parkes, C. M., & Weiss, R. (1983). Recovery from bereavement. New York: Basic Books.

Praill, D. (1995). Approaches to spiritual care. *Nursing Times, 91*(34), 54–57.

President's Commission for the Study of Ethical Problems in Medicine and Biomedical and Behavioral Research. (1981). *Defining death* (Pub. No. 81-600150). Washington, DC: U.S. Government Printing Office.

Price, J. L., Stevens, H. O., & LaBarre, M. C. (1995). Spiritual caregiving in nursing practice. *Journal of Psychosocial Nursing, 33*(12), 5–9.

Raether, H. C. (1993). Rituals, beliefs and grief. In K. J. Doka (Ed.), *Death and spirituality* (pp. 207–215). Amityville, NY: Baywood.

Rando, T. A. (1988). *Grieving: How to go on living when someone you love dies.* Lexington, MA: Lexington Books.

Raphael, B. C. (1983). *The anatomy of bereavement.* New York: Basic Books.

Reese, D. J., & Brown, D. R. (1997). Psychosocial and spiritual care in hospice: Differences between nursing, social work, and clergy. *The Hospice Journal, 12*(1), 29–41.

Renard, J. (1993). Islamic spirituality. In M. Downey (Ed.), *The new dictionary of Catholic spirituality* (pp. 555–559). Collegeville, MN: The Liturgical Press.

Ruskay, S. (1996). Saying hello again: A new approach to bereavement counseling. *The Hospice Journal, 11*(4), 5–14.

Ryan, D. (1993). Death: Eastern perspectives. In K. J. Doka (Ed.), *Death and spirituality* (pp. 75–92). Amityville, NY: Baywood.

Sanders, C. M. (1989). *Grief: The mourning after, dealing with adult bereavement.* New York: John Wiley & Sons.

Saunders, C. (1981). The founding philosophy. In C. Saunders, D. H. Summers, & N. Teller (Eds.), *Hospice: The living idea* (p. 4). Philadelphia: W. B. Saunders.

Saunders, C. (1983). The last stages of life. In C. A. Corr & D. M. Corr (Eds.), *Hospice care: Principles and practice* (pp. 5–11). New York: Springer.

Sheldon, J. E. (2000). Spirituality as a part of nursing. *Journal of Hospice and Palliative Nursing, 2*(3), 101–108.

Shuchter, J. (1986). Dimensions of grief: Adjusting to the death of a spouse. San Francisco: Jossey-Bass.

Smithe, F. F. (1990). General health care ministry. In H. Hayes & C. J. van der Poel (Eds.), *Health care ministry: A handbook for chaplains* (pp. 114–130). New York: Paulist Press.

Stepnick, A., & Perry, T. (1992). Preventing spiritual distress in the dying client. *Journal of Psychosocial Nursing, 30*(1), 17–24.

Stoddard, S. (1978). *The hospice movement: A better way of caring for the dying.* Briarcliff Manor, NY: Stein and Day.

Taylor, E. J., & Amenta, M. (1994). Midwifery to the soul while the body dies: Spiritual care among hospice nurses. *The American Journal of Hospice and Palliative Care, 11*(6), 28–35.

Vassallo, B. M. (2001). The spiritual aspects of dying at home. *Holistic Nursing Practice, 15*(2), 17–29.

Worden, J. W. (1982). *Grief counseling and grief therapy: A handbook for the mental health practitioner.* New York: Springer.

World Health Organization. (1990). Cancer pain relief and palliative care: Technical report series 804. Geneva, Switzerland: World Health Organization.

Young, C., & Koopsen, C. (2005). *Spirituality and health and healing.* Thorofare, NJ: Slack Incorporated.

13 ◼ Parish Nursing: Caregiving within a Faith Community

"The role of parish nurses is basically a reaching out for more whole person ways of ministering to people who are hurting."

GRANGER WESTBERG, 1999

A parish nurse related the following anecdote: At a conference for religious pastors of urban churches, a presentation was given on the topic of parish nursing. Although the parish nurse presenter was described as well prepared and articulate, most of the clergy audience came away admitting that they still "did not know what parish nursing really was." This is a very telling story and reflects the lack of understanding of many contemporary nurses and pastors related to the place of the subfield of parish nursing within the larger profession. This chapter explores the philosophy of parish nursing, including the scope and standards of practice, and the historical background, models, educational preparation, spirituality, parish nursing research, and the present-day art and practice of parish nursing. In addition to literature review in the area, empirical examples of parish nursing are presented in data elicited through interviews with contemporary practitioners and recipients of parish nursing.

PARISH NURSING DEFINED

The Philosophy of Parish Nursing

Essentially, the philosophy of parish nursing is grounded in the relationship between spirituality or faith beliefs and the conduct of caring for the sick. This might be described best in the following paradigm of "Beatitudes for Parish Nurses," which combines the Scriptural beatitudes identified by Jesus in His Sermon on the Mount (Matthew 5:3–10) with the primary roles identified for contemporary parish nurses: health counselor, health educator (health promoter), health referral agent, health advocate, health visitor, integrator of faith and health, and coordinator of support and volunteer groups.

Beatitudes for Parish Nurses

Blessed are parish nurses who care for the poor, for theirs is
  The kingdom of heaven.
Blessed are parish nurses who mourn for parishioners lost, for they will
  Be comforted.
Blessed are parish nurses who visit the isolated and the elderly,
  For they will inherit the land.
Blessed are parish nurses who advocate for marginalized clients,
  For they will be satisfied.
Blessed are parish nurses who minister to those in pain and suffering,
  For they will be shown mercy.
Blessed are parish nurses who bring peace to patients who are anxious
  And afraid, for they will be called children of God.
Blessed are parish nurses who suffer misunderstanding for the sake of
  Their ministry, for they will see God.
Blessed are parish nurses who comfort and care in the Lord's Name, for
  Their reward will be great in heaven.

The former director of the International Parish Nurse Resource Center, Ann Solari-Twadell, suggests that the best way to answer the question "What is parish nursing?" is to study the philosophy of the discipline (1999, p. 3). Solari-Twadell notes that in calling the nurse to care for the "whole person," parish nursing includes and, in fact, highlights the individual's "spiritual dimension": "The pastoral dimensions of nursing care are emphasized, with particular attention to the spiritual maturity of the nurse. This begins to distinguish the practice from the traditional community health nurse and to set the parameters for the role" (1999, pp. 3–4). Two key points of Solari-Twadell's identified philosophy are that "parish nursing holds the spiritual dimension to be central to the practice," and "the focus of practice is the faith community and its ministry" (1999, p. 15). The philosophy of parish nursing has been described as the guiding principle to "promote the health of a faith community by working with the pastor and staff to integrate theological, sociological and physiological perspectives of health and healing into the word, sacrament and service of the congregation" (Lovinus, 1996, p. 7). The parish nurse serves as "a role model for the relationship between one's faith and health" (Solari-Twadell & Westberg, 1991, p. 24).

The parish nurse is considered by most parish nurse educators to be a registered nurse with well-developed clinical and interpersonal skills, a strong personal religious faith, and a desire or felt call to serve the needs of a parish or faith community. A parish nursing philosophy builds on the existing philosophy of caring and commitment already espoused by the nurse as a professional ethic. One parish nurse described her ministry as a vocation. "Nursing in a faith community is a calling, an absolute caring for people and a deep sense of personal faith" (Palmer, 2001, p. 17). Parish nurses are generally noted for their roles as educators and health promoters within a congregation. "They provide information on healthy life styles and ways to prevent illness" (Dunkle, 2000, p. 316); they also, however, tend to patients' "psychosocial and spiritual needs" (p. 316). It is pointed out that parish nurses practice within a specific "cultural community": "in a place of worship where the focus is on meeting spiritual needs; the nurses work with the community leaders as their professional partners" (Trofino, Hughes, O'Brien, Mack, Marrinan, & Hay, 2000, p. 60). As a final point in examining the philosophy of parish nursing, it is important to emphasize that the role or title of parish nurse does not limit one to working with any "particular faith community or religious denomination"; it has, therefore, been suggested by some that the label be changed from parish nursing to "health ministry" or "congregational nursing" (Pennsylvania Nurse, 2000, pp. 8–9).

Scope and Standards of Practice

Between 1996 and 1998, a document identifying the scope and standards of parish nursing practice was developed by the Practice and Education Committee of the Health Ministries Association (HMA). The HMA is a professional organization that represents parish nurses and other health ministers. The scope and standards document was acknowledged by the American Nurses Association, Congress of Nursing Practice, in Spring 1998. The introduction to the document states that "Parish nursing promotes health and healing within faith communities" (Scope and Standards of Parish Nursing Practice, 1998, p. 1). The purpose of the scope and standards document is to "describe the evolving specialty of parish nursing and to provide parish nurses, the nursing profession, and other health care providers, employers, insurers, and their clients with the unique scope and competent standards of care and professional performance expected of a parish nurse" (1998, p. 3). The parish nurse scope and standards are based on the ANA's 1991 Standards of Clinical Nursing Practice (p. 4). The definition of parish nurse, as articulated formally in the scope and standards of practice is, "The most common title given to a registered professional nurse who serves as a member of the ministry staff of a faith community to promote health as wholeness of the faith community, its family and individual members, and the community it serves through the independent practice of nursing as defined by the nurse practice act in the jurisdiction in which he or she practices and the standards of practice set forth in this document" (1998, p. 7).

Some of the parish nurse's roles, as identified in the scope and standards of practice include collecting client health data (health assessment); diagnosing, based on the data; identifying desired health outcomes; health care and promotion planning; implementing interventions; and evaluating client responses (1998, pp. 9–14). The nurse also participates in such activities as quality assessment, performance appraisal, education, collegial sharing, ethical decision making, collaboration with the community, research, and resource utilization (1998, pp. 15–22).

A HISTORY OF PARISH NURSING

The contemporary concept of parish nursing is usually attributed to Lutheran pastor Granger Westberg, as an outgrowth of his holistic health center project of the mid-1980s. This experimental program of care was supported by the Kellogg Foundation and the University of Illinois College of Medicine (Westberg, 1990). Although Pastor Westberg is appropriately acknowledged as the founder of the current parish nursing movement in the United States, one should also recognize the health care activities of the early Christian Church, as well as the European models of parish nursing, such as the 19th century German Christian Deaconesses, the *Gemeindeschwestern* (Zerson, 1994, p. 20). As described in chapter 2 of this book, the earliest deacons and deaconesses of the fledgling Christian community established immediately after the death of Christ considered care of the sick in their homes to be one of the primary ministries of the Church. Following those early centuries and throughout the Middle Ages, men and women felt their calling to minister to the ill and the infirm to be a vocation from God. St. Vincent de Paul, the great minister to the sick in 17th century France, established "societies of women of the Church who banded themselves together with some simple rules to tend the sick and the poor of the immediate neighborhood. They called themselves the 'servants of the poor' " (Woodgate, 1946, p. 43). These women could surely be considered forebears of contemporary parish nurses.

In the mid-20th century, an article was published in a religious nursing journal entitled *In the Parish* (Cummings, 1960). The nurse author begins the piece by relating the fact that in recent issues of the journal she had read about nurses "in hospitals, in clinics, in schools and in homes" but, she lamented, "Alas, I was not included, for in the parish, is my job" (Cummings, 1960, p. 26). Nurse Cummings describes her role as a parish health counselor in a parish of about thirty-five hundred families and asserts that, at this time, her Church believes that their multidisciplinary health program is "the only one of its kind in the United States" (p. 26). This innovative parish nursing program was focused on such things as care of the chronically ill elders in the parish, education for home care of the ill, referral to community agencies, volunteers service, and home visiting. Nurse Cummings' role as a parish health counselor reads very much like that of the parish nurse of today. Some other parish nursing activities described in the 20th century nursing literature included a Christian Church-affiliated "volunteer nursing program" to provide care for the ill and infirm in their homes (Martin & Lacoutre, 1953) and an "organized plan for visiting individuals who are ill and lonely" sponsored by a Church Diocesan Council of Nurses (*The Catholic Nurse,* 1956, p. 42).

In the era of the late 1970s and early 1980s, Pastor Granger Westberg's interest in and support of the concept of holistic health care, including the subfield of parish nursing, began to capture the attention of some members of the larger nursing community. With his support, a parish nursing program was sponsored by Lutheran General Hospital in Park Ridge, Illinois; parish nursing was also initiated at several parishes in the area. As the ministry developed, the International Parish Nurse Resource Center (IPNRC) was created in 1986 under the aegis of Advocate Lutheran General Hospital. Together with a committee of nurse consultants from across the country, the staff of the IPNRC developed a model curriculum for parish nursing education. The IPNRC also began to sponsor annual Westberg Symposiums to provide a forum for parish nurses from across the country to come together to discuss the emerging subfield and its practice. In an October 2001 letter addressed to the "Friends of the International Parish Nurse Resource Center," however, it was announced that the IPNRC would no longer be an agency of Advocate Health Care, the umbrella organization providing support for this parish nursing education effort. It was anticipated that the Westberg Symposiums and some other activities formerly conducted by the IPNRC would continue to be supported in other arenas.

Another parish nursing association, this one a volunteer membership group labeled the Health Ministries Association (HMA), was derived from the emerging parish nursing interest of the '70s and '80s. The HMA, author of the "Scope and Standards of Nursing Practice," is an association for those who serve in health ministry. The group "serves as the professional specialty organization for parish nurses and as such has been accepted by the American Nurses Association for membership in the Nursing Organization Liaison Forum (NOLF)" (FAQ about HMA & Parish Nursing, 2001, p. 1).

As the new millennium dawned, it was estimated that "200 institutions in the United States offered parish nurse education"; no curriculum has been endorsed by the American Nurses Association ("The ANA does not endorse curriculum"); "there is no process in place for parish nurses to become certified"; and "parish nursing" has been "designated a specialty practice by ANA," which means that "a parish nurse cannot practice without a license" in his or her state (Story, 2001, p. 3). It was also noted that it will probably take a number of years, and "a minimum of $80,000" before ANA certification exams can be offered (Story, 2001, p. 3).

CONTEMPORARY MODELS OF PARISH NURSING

Four models of parish nursing have been defined: congregation-based volunteer (CBV), congregation-based paid (CBP), institution-based volunteer (IBV), and institution-based paid (IBP) (Kuhn, 1997, p. 26). The terms congregational nurse practitioner (CNP) and congregational care nurse (CCN) have also begun to be used to describe the role of the nurse working primarily within a parish or faith community (Souther, 1997). A parish nurse may be employed by a church to work as a member of a ministerial team and provide some nursing services to parishioners; a hospital or other health care institution may also employ a parish nurse in partnership with a local parish, as a way of bringing health promotion into the community. Wilson (1997) described the parish nurse as "a community health nurse who also becomes God's representative of love, caring and healing on earth" (p. 13). The parish nurse does not compete with the public health nurse, but rather works in concert with other nurses in the community (Schank, Weis, & Matheus, 1996).

Lynda Whitney Miller (1997) developed a contemporary parish nursing model undergirded by the theological perspective of evangelical Christianity. The Miller Model of Parish Nursing contains four major components: "person/parishioner"; "health"; "nurse/parish nurse"; and "community/parish" (p. 18). Miller's goal is to provide Christian nurses with a theoretical base to support the practice of parish nursing (1997, p. 17). A separate parish nursing model called the "Circle of Christian Caring" was created by Dr. Margie Maddox (2001). In her model, Dr. Maddox incorporated a number of activities already in place when she began to serve as parish nurse at a large Presbyterian church. Dr. Maddox noted that as she "worked with the services in which the church was already engaged, the model began to emerge" (p. 11). The Circle of Christian Caring model focuses on the parish nurse roles of health educator, health counselor, referral resource/client advocate, and facilitator of groups and/or processes (pp. 12–13).

Parish Nursing Education

Related to the emerging models of parish nursing are a variety of educational programs that prepare one for the field of parish nursing. These educational offerings range from weekend or weeklong continuing education unit (CEU) programs, which may award from three to six CEUs, to academic courses in parish nursing, awarding from three to six credits for the overall program. There are also several post-baccalaureate and graduate programs that focus on the topic of nursing in a faith community. These programs are sponsored primarily by health care institutions, colleges and universities, seminaries, or other church-related associations. In some instances, community interfaith groups of churches have collaboratively put together parish nurse education programs to prepare nurses to serve in their various faith communities. The multiplicity of parish nurse preparation programs are, as noted earlier, conducted in a variety of ways; some of these include "one day to weeklong orientations, continuing education workshops, seminars, distance learning, and ongoing coursework over weeks and months, as well as credit-bearing coursework in BSN, MSN and M.Div. programs offered over the course of a semester or, for some, over several years" (McDermott, Solari-Twadell, & Matheus, 1999, p. 271).

Three examples of contemporary parish nurse programs are:

- A weeklong continuing education program, sponsored by a Christian nursing group, following which the participants are awarded three CEUs and are "commissioned" as parish nurses. Requirements for the course include having a state nursing license, some clinical nursing experience, and the desire to work with a faith community.
- A parish nurse preparation program, sponsored by a college and awarding the participants three CEUs, which holds classes on six alternating Saturdays. This program requires that the RNs have at least three years experience and be partnered with a faith community. The course ends with a "dedication ceremony."
- A university-affiliated program that covers nine days and awards the participants 5.4 CEUs. As well as including the usual topics described below, this longer program includes participation in several interfaith

services and provides student on-site observations and clinical experiences with parish nurses in the community.

Some basic components of most contemporary parish nursing programs include such topics as a theology of health and healing; the nurse's role in spiritual care; history, philosophy, and models of parish nursing; ethical issues in parish nursing; assessment of the individual, the family, and the congregation; documentation and accountability; the functions of the parish nurse, such as health counseling, health education, health referral, coordination of volunteers and support groups, patient advocacy, and integration of faith and health; working with a congregation; health promotion; dealing with grief and loss; and legal considerations in the conduct of parish nursing. Some programs also include classes focusing on such activities as prayer and worship leadership, research, grant writing, service among underprivileged people, and working with a ministerial team.

THE SPIRITUALITY OF PARISH NURSING

Although nurses from a variety of religious denominations are currently engaged in parish nursing, it is the nurse's personal spirituality and spiritual vocation to serve the ill that inspire and support the ministry. For Christian nurses, Jesus' blessing, related by the evangelist Matthew "I was ill and you cared for me" (25:36) provides both the catalyst and the reward for their caring for the sick within a faith community. Most parish nurses, many of whom serve on a volunteer basis, carry out their nursing within their own faith communities. This is usually desirable for both nurse and congregation, because the parish nurse is thus familiar with the spiritual and religious beliefs of the congregation and of the pastor. In the future, however, if parish nursing becomes "professionalized" to a greater degree, and if acceptable to a faith community, parish nurses may be hired to work with a church not of their own denomination. This kind of partnering does exist to some degree, in contemporary hospital-based parish nursing programs in which staff parish nurses provide consultation and support to developing church programs from a variety of religious traditions.

Perhaps one of the most critical elements in beginning a parish nursing program with a faith community is to *listen* to the needs and desires of the pastor and the parishioners. Lloyd and Ludwig-Beymer (1999) in discussing a concept they call VOC or "voice of the customer," note that "parishioners, whom we may think of as clients, patients, or in other terms, must be listened to. Clients are the ones who define quality and set the expectations of performance" (1999, pp. 108–109). A director of a large community-based health ministry program observed that when approached about the initiation of a parish ministry program in their churches, most pastors raise three immediate questions: "How much of my time will this involve?"; "How much money is it going to cost me?"; and "Can I be sued?" The goal is to be able to provide negative answers to all three questions to allay the pastors' anxieties about the burden of establishing a parish nursing program for their congregation.

In this era of continued change within the U.S. health care system, including such factors as short hospital stays, same day surgeries, and early discharges, parish nursing, or nursing provided to those in their homes by members of a local faith community, may be critical to a patient's recovery, and perhaps even to his or her survival. No longer are patients, especially older patients or those who live alone, allowed the luxury of remaining in the hospital until they are able to fully function on their own. Health insurance policies rarely cover such extended stays, even if a patient's recovery may be at risk. It is expected that many of the former hospital nursing care services will now be provided by relatives or friends in a home care setting. This makes the role of the contemporary parish nurse vitally important to recovering patients who have no extended family networks and who may depend on their churches for caring support in times of crisis or significant need. It is suggested that individuals of all ages can benefit from the "personal caring and attention offered by a parish nursing model" (Stewart, 2000, p. 116).

One of the first things a parish nurse may find helpful in beginning to work with a faith community, especially a church to which the concept of parish nursing is new, is to do a "needs assessment" of the parish. There are a variety of needs assessment schemas being developed; however, the assessment must take into account certain factors that vary in parishes, such as the mean age of the parishioners, the range of socioeconomic levels in the church, the parish size, and the availability of volunteers to assist with the development of a parish health ministry. Parish nurses report that a critical factor in beginning a new effort with a faith community is the support of the pastor; as noted above, he or she may have concerns about the time, financial, and/or legal burdens that the establishment of any new program may bring to the church. If however, the potential parish nurse or health ministry team can predict that the program will be a benefit, rather than a burden, to the church, most pastors are enthusiastic in their support of the effort.

An example of a professional parish needs assessment is that conducted by the University of Massachusetts, Amherst School of Nursing, at the
request of a large urban parish. The school was also asked to assess a newly
hired parish nurse. The assessment's aims were to "determine the health
status of parishioners; identify their perceived health needs and perceived
barriers in meeting those needs; and to assist the church and parish nurse
in developing a health program for their faith community" (Swinney, Anson-
Wonkka, Maki, & Corneau, 2001, p. 40). The assessment team concluded
that the health needs of this faith community were similar to those identified in the goals of "Healthy People 2000," that is, "increased life span in a
healthy state, reduced health disparities . . . and access to preventive care"
(p. 43). In another study of the health needs and preferences of an individual faith community, in which 67 church members, 6 parish nurses, and the
pastor participated, 80 percent of the services desired were educational, including education about such factors as health screening, disease, staying
well, spiritual health, and emotional health (Mayhugh & Martens, 2001,
p. 15). Some other parish nursing preferences of the faith community studied by Mayhugh and Martens were consultation about health problems, visiting (hospital, home, and nursing home), and coordination and training of
volunteers (p. 15).

Although existing church-based parish nursing programs are still new
to many faith communities, the number and scope of these ministries is expanding rapidly. In some churches, programs may be limited to such activities as monthly blood-pressure screenings, with occasional health
educational programs for the congregation and infrequent home or hospital visiting by members of an "on-call" volunteer team; there may or may
not be a parish nurse leading the effort. In other parishes, well-developed
parish health ministry programs exist, under the leadership of a paid part-
time or full-time parish or congregational nurse.

Depending on the interest and sophistication, in terms of health care
experience, on the part of a pastor and congregation, a church may require
that their parish nurse have specific training in parish nursing; be a nurse
practitioner; have a number of years of experience in nursing; or simply be
a registered nurse who has a commitment and desire to work with a faith
community. For example, one church in a moderately sized urban area ad-
vertised for a part-time parish nurse who would be a licensed RN in the state
with at least three years experience in nursing; the church also wanted the
candidate to have completed a parish nursing preparation course, although
the parameters of that course were not specified. It was noted that the nurse's
role would include health promotion, disease prevention, education, coun-

seling, advocacy, health screening, and referral. The parish nurse's hours could be "flexible."

Some congregations employing either paid or volunteer parish nurses try to schedule "office hours" at the parish, for example, Wednesdays and Fridays, 9 to 12 noon, so that parishioners can come for private consultation or education. In such a situation, the parish nurse will usually have "on call" hours also. Some of the activities associated with existing parish nursing or health ministry programs, in addition to parish nurse office hours and monthly blood-pressure screening, include exercise classes (especially for seniors), cardiopulmonary resuscitation (CPR) classes, foot care classes, nutritional education classes, diabetes education classes, prenatal classes, bike safety classes for children, self breast exam classes, substance abuse classes for parents and teens, healthy aging classes, family fitness classes, and classes preparing church volunteers for such ministries as hospital and nursing home visiting, homebound visiting, and respite family care.

The parish nurse may himself or herself also do some home and hospital visiting as time permits; the nurse's most important role, however, is to serve as the health ministry team leader and coordinator of non-medical health ministry volunteers. The parish nurse is an advocate for the ill parishioners of a faith community and a source of referral to needed and appropriate community health services.

PARISH NURSING RESEARCH

In an exploratory study of the parish nursing role, 48 practicing parish nurses identified ways in which they incorporated spiritual care into their activities, including prayer, if acceptable to the client; a caring and compassionate attitude; discussing illness-related spiritual concerns; and conducting or participating in rituals such as healing services and the distribution of Communion (Kuhn, 1997, p. 27). A nursing study of 40 parish nurses, who identified 1,800 client interactions, revealed that although approximately one-half of the nurses' activities dealt with physical problems, the other half related to spiritual–psychosocial issues (Rydholm, 1997). This latter finding is supported by the comments of parish nurse Linda Miles (1997), who asserted that in all of her nursing she included the spiritual dimension of care. "Spiritual nurturing contributes to improved life satisfaction and quality of life, improved health, reduced functional disability, and lower levels of depression" (p. 24).

A number of case study articles describing innovative experiences in parish nursing have been presented in the literature. For example, Dr. Margie

Maddox, in "Clinical Experience in Parish Nursing," described a newly created student clinical course in parish nursing (2003); and Gretchen Quenstedt-Moe, in "Parish Nursing and Home Care: A Blended Role?," explored parish nurses adopting a primary role of home visiting that she viewed as helping "fill the gaps left by the fragmented health care system" and that can "help parishioners to find meaningful connections that involve their needs, the parish nurse and God" (2003, p. 30).

In looking at parish nursing as meeting the spiritual needs of elders at or near the end of their lives, a qualitative study of 15 end-of-life older adults revealed the importance of the parish nurse's spiritual care interventions: "1) Sharing of prayer and scripture; 2) Spiritual presence (listening with the heart); and 3) Pastoral counseling (including facilitating participation in religious rituals)" (O'Brien, 2006, p. 30; details of the study method and nursing diagnoses related to spiritual need identified in the research are presented in chapter 11).

The Gift of Faith in Chronic Illness

The author conducted an exploratory pilot study of the impact of parish nursing on persons who were unable to practice their faith because of illness and disability. The aim of the study was to test the effectiveness of a model of parish nursing/health ministry on spiritual well-being, hope, and life satisfaction among persons marginalized from their churches, and to explore the relationship between spiritual well-being and quality of life (measured in terms of hope and life satisfaction) for chronically ill persons. For a study participant distanced from his or her church, or desirous of additional spiritual support, pastoral care intervention was carried out in the hope of increasing spiritual well-being and positive quality of life. Following an initial individual spiritual needs assessment, pastoral care interventions were tailored by the parish nurse for each study participant.

The sample group consisted of six chronically ill individuals: four men and two women whose ages ranged from 45 to 92, with a mean of 74 years. Three patients were married, two were widowed, and one was single. Five individuals were college graduates and one completed high school; one person lived alone, one resided in a nursing home, and four lived with spouses or adult children. Three of the study patients were Protestant (Protestant, Church of God, and United Church of Christ), two were Roman Catholic, and one patient was Jewish. In terms of church attendance, the group reported attending services from once a month (or even daily when possible) to two to three times a year. Church attendance was quite variable depending on illness symptoms and remission and exacerbation of disease conditions. Patients' diagnoses included glaucoma and lupus, cancer, renal failure (dialysis), myasthenia gravis, type II diabetes and hypertension, substance abuse, and stroke. The study group reported degrees of disability as being from minimal to complete; this again varied with exacerbation of illness symptoms.

The initial needs assessment was carried out using three quantitative tools and one qualitative tool: the *Spiritual Well-Being Scale* (O'Brien, 1999); the *Miller Hope Scale* (Miller & Powers, 1988; abbreviated with permission of the author); the *Life Satisfaction Index-Z* (Wood, Wylie, & Sheafor, 1969); and the *Spiritual Well-Being Interview Guide* (O'Brien, 1999). Following the collection of baseline data, three or more pastoral visits were planned by the parish nurse, with the nursing interventions geared to the health considerations of the study participant. As well as listening to, counseling, and praying with patients, small devotional items such as prayer books, Bibles, religious pictures, or other items requested by a patient were provided to assist in facilitating the practice of his or her faith. At a final pastoral care visit, study participants were again evaluated in terms of spiritual well-being and quality of life.

The sample population was identified through referrals from a local pastor and from a neighborhood parish, neither of whom had staff engaged in parish nursing, and through several informal referrals. All six individuals approached to participate in the study agreed with enthusiasm; appropriate informed consent procedures were carried out prior to initiation of the research.

The initial exploration of the impact of parish nursing on a group of chronically ill persons revealed that all benefited from the pastoral care interventions of the parish nurse. The quantitative measurement tools identified a number of spiritual needs and concerns amenable to pastoral counseling, such as "uncertainty that God might not take care of one's needs"; "getting angry" at God for "letting bad things happen" to oneself or to persons one cares about; frustration about not being able to attend church because of disability; fear of having done some things "for which God might not forgive"; and "uncertainty" about being at peace with God and with God's care. There were, however, a number of positive changes documented in response to these items following the parish nurse's intervention. One example is the case of a forty-five-year-old man, suffering from several chronic illnesses, who asserted that the parish nurse's visits had helped him a great deal. In his initial assessment, the patient agreed that there were "some things for which [he feared] God may not forgive [him]"; following the parish nursing intervention the study participant disagreed with the item, that is, he no longer was living with the fear that God would not forgive him for perceived transgressions.

The patient's spiritual well-being measures also changed positively on a number of other items following nursing intervention. For example, at baseline interview (Time 1 [T1]), he responded that he was "uncertain" about whether he was at peace with God but at follow up (Time 2 [T2]), he agreed that he was at peace. At T1 he admitted "uncertainty" about three other items: receiving strength and comfort from spiritual beliefs, believing God is interested in activities of his life, and spiritual beliefs supporting a positive image of himself and others as members of God's family, but at T2 the patient responded affirmatively to all three items. At T1, the study participant disagreed that he found "any satisfaction in religiously motivated activities" but at T2 he strongly agreed. At T1, he agreed to having "pain associated with spiritual beliefs," but at T2 he strongly disagreed. Finally, at T1 the study participant admitted to sometimes feeling "far away" from God, but at T2 he disagreed with having any such perception.

It is important to note that this patient also reflected a number of positive changes in terms of hope and life satisfaction following the parish nurse's intervention, including being positive about most aspects of life, being able to set goals, being positive about the future, being valued for who he was, looking forward to doing things he enjoyed, trying to do things important to him, things seeming better, being as happy as when younger, things being as interesting and being as satisfied with life as before his illness, and feeling that he had gotten most of the important things and what he had expected out of life.

In his responses to the qualitative study questions, this study participant also reported a very positive response to the interactions he had had with the parish nurse. The patient had asked for a devotional item that was unfamiliar to the parish nurse and to the study's principal investigator. It was called (he thought) a "prayer box" to help organize his prayers. The patient, who self-identified as Protestant, did not belong to any particular church but did have a strong belief in the existence of God. Through the use of a religious articles catalog, the research team located a small wooden box labeled a "God box"; the box came with a guide for use; it was suggested that the user write out thoughts, concerns, or prayers and place them in the box as one might make entries into a journal. The study participant reported at a follow-up interview that he was delighted with his prayer box. "I use that, I have something in it right now, in the box. The 'God box' I found extremely comforting. I put some real issues that I'm facing and the fact that I was trying to take my will back and get in [God's] way. I wrote it all down on a piece of paper, all my concerns and issues and fears, and then at the end I said 'God I'm putting this in Your hands.' Almost a ceremonial kind of thing. I put it in the box and I prayed over it and then put the box away and walked away."

The patient concluded, "It helped me to be able to put [my concerns and fears] someplace else; to, like, take it out of my head and put it there [in the 'God box']."

Comments of other study participants following the parish nurse's interactions reflected similar positive outcomes, such as "I am at peace with God"; "I don't know how people survive without a trust and faith in God"; "That [practice of faith] is what keeps me going"; "Without your religion, you would be nowhere"; and "God will not let us have more than we can bear without His help; what a peace that gives you."

A participant in a separate study exploring the functions of parish nursing, Angela, a parish nurse for the past five years, described her understanding of the parish nursing role:

> I think being a parish nurse is being a "be-er," rather than a "do-er." We are there to listen, to be a facilitator, to assess and refer. We're not getting into the doctor's or the community health nurse's turf. Here's an example: You see somebody who's had a headache for weeks and they can't sleep and they have been to the doctor. I look at the spiritual dimension. Maybe there's some spiritual problem that is causing the headaches and the not sleeping; something else may be going on. Maybe they need to talk with the pastor. The parish nurse goes into a house and sees that maybe the dishes are not done, or the steps are starting to crack. Maybe there is someone in the church who can help with that. Or you can see that your client is getting confused and leaving the stove on; maybe you need to do a referral to the VNA. A lot of us work with volunteers also; you can teach them to take blood pressures and vital signs. I do that, as a representative of my church; and arranging for transportation for people who maybe need to go to a doctor or dentist.

Finally, Angela explained how spirituality was incorporated into her parish nursing interventions:

> Spirituality is all encompassing. Sometimes, these people, it's all they need. They need somebody to listen and to say "let's talk about this." Then you can assess their needs and minister to them if they need

that; counseling or referral or whatever comes up. Sometimes it is just that something is wrecking their spiritual equilibrium; something is attacking their spiritual base. It might be guilt or anxiety about something they feel they did wrong. Sometimes it's easier for a person to talk to a nurse before they go to the pastor. . . . I think parish nursing is caring; it is a caring ministry. It's spiritual care, and it's health promotion and it's illness prevention. If we could get people to a healthier lifestyle, a more spiritual lifestyle, then they wouldn't get into trouble and need secondary and tertiary care.

This chapter has explored briefly the basic dimensions of parish nursing, including the philosophy, scope, and standards of practice; the history of parish nursing; contemporary models and parish nursing education; working with a faith community; and parish nursing research. Parish nursing is presently a developing subfield within the larger nursing community, but interest in the area is growing rapidly. New parish nursing education programs continue to be developed by colleges and universities and by church-related organizations. It is hoped that eventually there will be ANA certification for parish nurses. Until this comes about, however, professional nurses who feel called by God to serve within a faith community continue to support and enhance the parish nursing role through their vision and their dedication. The concept of parish nursing is very new and it is also very old; contemporary parish nurses have embraced their ministry with the caring and commitment of the first century deacons and deaconesses and with the wisdom and understanding of present-day nursing knowledge. Parish nursing, however it develops in the coming decades, is definitely here to stay.

REFERENCES

Council projects: Plan for friendly visiting. (1956). *The Catholic Nurse, 5*(1), 42–44.

Cummings, A. L. (1960). In the parish. *The Catholic Nurse, 8*(3), 26–29.

Dunkle, R. E. (2000). Parish nurses help patients, body and soul. In R. Hunt (Ed.), *Readings in community based nursing* (pp. 316–320). Philadelphia: Lippincott.

FAQ about HMA & parish nursing. (2001). *Connections, The Health Ministries Association Information & Contacts, 1*(2), 1.

Kuhn, J. (1997). A profile of parish nurses. (2001). *Journal of Christian Nursing, 14*(1), 26–28.

Lloyd, R., & Ludwig-Beymer, P. (1999). Listening to faith communities. In P. Solari-Twadell & M. McDermott (Eds.), *Parish nursing: Promoting whole person health within faith communities* (pp. 107–121). Thousand Oaks, CA: Sage Publications.

Lovinus, B. (1996). A healer in the midst of the congregation. *The Journal of Christian Healing, 18*(4), 3–18.

Maddox, M. (2001). Circle of Christian caring: A model for parish nursing practice. *Journal of Christian Nursing, 18*(3), 11–13.

Maddox, M. (2003). Clinical experience in parish nursing. *Journal of Christian Nursing, 20*(2), 18–20.

Martin, G., & Lacoutre, C. (1953). Volunteer nursing. *The Catholic Nurse, 2*(2), 13–14.

Mayhugh, L. J., & Martens, K. H. (2001). What's a parish nurse to do: Congregational expectations. *Journal of Christian Nursing, 18*(3), 14–16.

McDermott, M., Solari-Twadell, P., & Matheus, R. (1999). Educational preparation. In P. Solari-Twadell and M. McDermott (Eds.), *Parish nursing: Promoting whole person health within faith communities* (pp. 269–276). Thousand Oaks, CA: Sage Publications.

Miles, L. (1997). Getting started: Parish nursing in a rural community. *Journal of Christian Nursing, 14*(1), 22–24.

Miller, J., & Powers, M. (1988). Development of an instrument to measure hope. *Nursing Research, 37*(1), 6–10.

Miller, L. W. (1997). Nursing through the lens of faith: A conceptual model. *Journal of Christian Nursing, 14*(1), 17–20.

O'Brien, M. E. (1999). *Spirituality in nursing: Standing on holy ground,* 1st ed. Sudbury, MA: Jones and Bartlett Publishers.

O'Brien, M. E. (2001). *The nurse's calling: A Christian spirituality of caring for the sick.* Mahwah, NJ: Paulist Press.

O'Brien, M. E. (2006). Parish nursing: Meeting spiritual needs of elders near the end of life. *Journal of Christian Nursing, 23*(1), 28–33.

Palmer, J. (2001). Parish nursing: Connecting faith and health. *Reflections on Nursing Leadership, 27*(1), 17–19; 45–46.

Parish nursing: Building on the spiritual dimensions of nursing. (2001). *Pennsylvania Nurse, 55*(6), 8–9.

Quenstedt-Moe, G. (2003). Parish nursing & home care: A blended role? *Journal of Christian Nursing, 20*(3), 26–30.

Rydholm, L. (1997) "Patient focused care in parish nursing," *Holistic Nursing Practice, 11*(3), 47–60.

Schank, M. J., Weis, D., & Matheus, R. (1996). Parish nursing: Ministry of healing. *Geriatric Nursing, 17*(1), 11–13.

Scope and standards of parish nursing practice. (1998).Washington, DC: American Nurses Publishing.

Solari-Twadell, P. (1999). The emerging practice of parish nursing. In P. Solari-Twadell & M. McDermott (Eds.), *Parish nursing: Promoting whole person health within faith communities* (pp. 3–24). Thousand Oaks, CA: Sage Publications.

Solari-Twadell, P., & Westberg, G. (1991). Body, mind and soul: The parish nurse offers physical, emotional and spiritual care. *Health Progress, 72*(7), 24–28.

Souther, B. (1997). Congregational nurse practitioner: An idea whose time has come. *Journal of Christian Nursing, 14*(1), 32–34.

Stewart, L. E. (2000). Parish nursing: Reviewing a long tradition of caring. *Gastroenterology Nursing, 23*(3), 16–20.

Story, C. (2001, April). Carol's corner. *Puget Sound Parish Nurse Ministries, 3*.

Swinney, J., Anson-Wonkka, C., Maki, E., & Corneau, J. (2001). Community assessment: A church community and the parish nurse. *Public Health Nursing, 18*(1), 40–44.

Trofino, J., Hughes, C., O'Brien, B., Mack, J., Marrinan, M., & Hay, K. (2000). Primary care parish nursing: Academic, service and parish partnership. *Nursing Administration Quarterly, 25*(1), 59–74.

Westberg, G. (1990). *The parish nurse: Providing a minister of health for your congregation.* Minneapolis, MN: Augsburg.

Westberg, G. (1999). A personal historical perspective on whole person health and the congregation. In P. Solari-Twadell & M. McDermott (Eds.), *Parish nursing: Promoting whole person health within faith communities* (pp. 35–41). Thousand Oaks, CA: Sage Publications.

Wilson, R. P. (1997). What does a parish nurse do? *Journal of Christian Nursing, 14*(1), 13–16.

Wood, V., Wylie, M., & Sheafor, B. (1969). An analysis of a short self-report measure of life satisfaction. *Journal of Gerontology, 24*(2), 465–469.

Woodgate, M. V. (1946). *St. Louise de Marillac.* London: B. Herdor Book Company.

Zerson, D. (1994). Parish nursing: 20th century fad? *Journal of Christian Nursing, 11*(2), 19–22.

14 ✵ Spiritual Needs in Mass Casualty Disasters

"I have not a moment. The whole army is coming into the hospitals. The task will be gigantic. Alas, how will it all end? We are in the hands of God. Pray for us. We have at the moment five thousand sick and wounded. My only comfort is, God sees it, God knows it, God loves us."

FLORENCE NIGHTINGALE, December 1854

This final chapter is dedicated to the New York City firefighters and police officers who gave their lives on September 11, 2001; they made the ultimate sacrifice in the hope of helping thousands of their brothers and sisters trapped in a towering inferno. As nurses, they too are anonymous ministers. The firefighters and police officers indeed "stood on holy ground" before God, deeply present in the "burning bush" of the mortally wounded World Trade Center. While the world witnessed, in horror, the absolute evil of the September 11th attack, it also witnessed, in awe, the absolute goodness embodied in the courage and heroism of these ministers of commitment and compassion. They have truly taught us the meaning of spiritual caring in mass casualty disasters. Their fallen comrades now rest in the loving arms of our Father in heaven. They answered His call to serve with the precious gift of their lives; they are, among all persons, most blessed!

This chapter was written several months after the September 11, 2001, terrorist attack on America; the attack that resulted in three simultaneous mass casualty disasters situated at the World Trade Center in New York City; the Pentagon, located in a Virginia suburb near Washington, DC; and a rural area southeast of Pittsburgh, Pennsylvania. The chapter begins with a brief overview of disaster nursing, including the types and phases of disasters, and selected key disaster service agencies: the Federal Emergency Management Agency (FEMA), the American Red Cross, and the Salvation Army. Following are discussions of the psychosocial impact of mass casualty trauma, spiritual needs in the aftermath of a disaster, and the nurse's role in the spiritual care of disaster victims. The heart of the chapter, however, which includes many examples of spiritual need and spiritual care in a mass casualty disaster, is based on the case example of the terrorist attack on America, particularly at the sites of the World Trade Center (WTC) and the Pentagon. Data were obtained through news reports, writings published after the attack, and the author's personal interviews and experiences with chaplains, firefighters, police officers, and other witnesses of the attack.

DISASTER NURSING

Most books on the topic of disaster nursing were published in the era of the mid-20th century, the 1950s and 1960s. They included concerns about disasters such as hurricanes, tornados, fires, floods, accidents, and nuclear radiation incidents, such as those caused by an atomic bomb explosion. Although there was some discussion of biological and chemical warfare, suicidal terrorist attacks, as occurred in the United States on September 11, 2001, were not considered. Some of the early works devoted specifically to disaster nursing include *Disaster Nursing* (Francis Nabbe, RN, 1960); *Disaster Nursing Preparation* (Mary V. Neal, RN, 1963); *Disaster Handbook for Physicians and Nurses* (American Red Cross, 1966); *Disaster Handbook* (Solomon Garb, M.D. & Evelyn Eng, RN, 1969); and *Emergency and Disaster Nursing* (Robert Mahoney, RN, 1969). In 1985, Loretta M. Garcia, RN, MSN, edited a book entitled *Disaster Nursing: Planning, Assessment and Intervention.* Although these earlier disaster nursing books do include discussions of the psychosocial impact of a disaster, spiritual or religious needs in mass casualty trauma are not included as key topics of discussion. In that era, the assessment of a patient or family member's spiritual or religious need was still considered by many nurses to fall within the role of the pastoral caregiver only; that thinking has changed, and a number of nurses have developed spiritual assessment scales to be used as nursing tools.

Disaster nursing poses multiple challenges in terms of assessment and intervention. As Susan Gardner notes, "The nurse does not have the luxury of a leisurely assessment; every second counts" (1985, p. 18). Most disaster scenes also include elements of danger and confusion; thus, the "physical and emotional stress factors may be extreme" (Brown, 1985, p. 45). Although disaster nursing is a unique area of nursing, only a modest number of journal articles on the topic are found in the literature; this is probably related to the fact that the majority of nurses have never had disaster nursing experience and never expect to become engaged in such nursing. Publications extant in the nursing literature primarily involve reports of care given in individual disaster situations; these experiences are reflected in such titles as "When the Tornado Hit Worcester: Heroic Nurses Play a Vital Role" (*The Catholic Nurse*, 1953); "Nurses Respond to Hurricane Hugo: Victims' Disaster Stress" (Weinrich, Hardin, & Johnson, 1990); "In the Wake of Hurricane Andrew: The Development of a Community-Based Primary Care Center" (Horner, Pfeifer, & Clunn, 1994); "Community Health Nursing: Shelter from the Storm" (Christopher & McConnell, 1994); "Disaster Nursing in the Oklahoma City Bombing" (Atkinson, Keylon, Odor, Walker, & Hunt, 1995); "Disaster Relief Efforts After Hurricane Marilyn: A Pediatric Team's Experience in St. Thomas" (Damian, Atkinson, Bouchard, Harrington, & Powers, 1997); "Multiple Accident Victims, All Elderly: Would Our Disaster Plan Be Up to the Challenge?" (Walhout, Tubergen, & Cook, 1998); and "The City of New Orleans Amtrak Train Disaster: One Emergency Department's Experience" (Mickelson, Bruno, & Schario, 1999).

A disaster has been described as "any man-made or natural event that causes destruction and devastation and that cannot be alleviated without assistance" (Hassmiller, 2000, p. 401), and as testing "the adaptive responses of communities or individuals beyond their capabilities and lead[ing] to at least a temporary disruption of function" (Clark, 1999, p. 704). Disasters are generally categorized as falling within two broad categories: natural disasters, such as tornadoes, hurricanes, floods, avalanches, earthquakes, volcanic eruptions, and communicable diseases; and human-generated disasters, including warfare, riots, mass demonstrations, and accidents (Lundy & Butts, 2001, p. 551). A disaster is classified as a "multiple patient incident" if less than 10 casualties have occurred; as a "multiple casualty incident" if there are less than 100 casualties but stress is placed on local health care facilities; and as a "mass casualty incident or disaster" if the occurrence involves more than 100 casualties and "significantly overtaxes existing health care facilities" (Demi & Miles, 1984, p. 64).

Disaster phases have been identified in various ways, including such stages as predisaster preparation, warning, impact, emergency, and recovery (Taggart, 1985, p. 7); and prevention, preparedness, response, and recovery (Tait and Spradley, 2001, p. 394). Regardless of terminology, the disaster phases are generally considered to include some period of disaster planning or preparation, a time of immediate impact and emergency response, and a recovery period. It is important to remember that nurses involved in responding to a disaster impact may themselves be victims of the disaster, especially if the incident involves an entire community, as in the case of a tornado or flood. Often the nurse will have to put personal or fam-

ily concerns on a "back burner," to carry out his or her professional responsibilities.

The nurse's role in a disaster response may depend on where the nurse
happens to be at the time of impact, such as at home, a hospital, a clinic, or
somewhere in the community. If a nurse is in the immediate location of the
disaster, he or she may be able to make a direct nursing response through
such activities as "assisting in evacuation, rescue, and first aid efforts until
the immediate needs of the situation are met" (Taggert, 1985, p. 11). An example is given later in this chapter in the report of a non-native New York
nurse who was visiting the city at the time of the terrorist attack on the World
Trade Center. She was able to provide emergency care to rescue workers in
need of a variety of kinds of first aid in the initial hours following the collapse
of the twin towers.

As noted, there may be a multiplicity of first aid and other emergency
care needs at a disaster site that will fall within the purview of the nurse.
Some related activities that professional nurses might assist with include
providing leadership; maintaining a communication network; organizing
the provision of food, warmth, shelter, and social support; and counseling
victims who appear to display "panic or hysterical behavior" (Reichsmeier
& Miller, 1985, p. 191). Another important role of the nurse responding to a
disaster situation is awareness and assessment of the needs of the rescue
workers. If the disaster is particularly devastating in terms of multiple injuries or loss of life, "psychological reactions can easily overwhelm relief
teams of caregivers unless careful attention is given to meeting basic biological needs, especially the need for rest and sleep" (Reichsmeier & Miller,
1985, p. 199).

Disaster Services

Three agencies are charged with the provision of relief services in mass casualty disasters in the United States: the Federal Emergency Management
Agency (FEMA), the American Red Cross, and the Salvation Army. Each
group has specific responsibilities in times of disaster and mass trauma.

Federal Emergency Management Agency (FEMA)

The Federal Emergency Management Agency (FEMA) is an agency of the
federal government that is charged with planning for and responding to disasters, both natural and man-made. Since March 2003, it has been a part of
the U.S. Department of Homeland Security. The organization "has also been

active in the development of nationwide contingency systems for disaster re-lief" (Switzer, 1985, p. 318). FEMA staff provide leadership in recovery efforts and support to the victims of disasters through both direct and indirect fund-ing of services to provide the necessities of daily life and functioning. FEMA, founded in 1979, has a staff of several thousand full-time workers, supported by reservists who can be activated if needed. FEMA is called in whenever a situation is declared a disaster or in need of emergency services.

The American Red Cross

The American Red Cross, initiated under the direction of nurse Clara Barton in 1881, received its charge from the 58th Congress of the United States to "continue and carry on a system of national and international relief in time of . . . suffering caused by pestilence, famine, fire, floods and other great na-tional calamities" (Nabbe, 1961, p. 10). Thus, the American Red Cross, al-though not a government agency, has a national mandate to provide relief services in times of great calamity and disaster in our country; the group is also mandated to provide services for the armed forces of the country as needed. The Red Cross is primarily a volunteer organization supported by private contributions and the volunteer work of a number of individuals. A significant role of the American Red Cross is the provision of blood supplies to hospitals in need of supplemental stocks for disaster victims. Other ac-tivities carried out by Red Cross nursing staff and volunteers include pro-viding first aid at disaster sites, feeding rescue and recovery workers, providing food and shelter for disaster victims, communicating with fami-lies of disaster victims, providing mental health services, and assisting sur-vivors with accessing available resources. The Red Cross suggests that "community health skills and psychological support skills are important as-sets for a nurse to possess when helping victims after a disaster" (Hanson, Jesz, & Baldwin, 1991, p. 391).

The Salvation Army

The Salvation Army is an international religious organization founded in London in 1865 by William Booth. The "Army" adopted, early on, a military style of organization and dress; this reflects the group's war against evil as well as its witness of the Christian gospel, to which all Army members adhere. Many people think of Salvation Army members primarily as the "bell-ringers," seen on city street corners with their classic red collection buckets. In fact, this activity of collecting money for the poor is only a small part of the Army's ministry. As well as carrying out a number of services for those in need, the Salvation Army embraces the commitment of assisting any community following a disaster incident. Army members can usually be seen at disaster sites involved in such works as feeding survivors and rescue workers, counseling those in need of psychological and social support, providing grief and bereavement counseling, praying with persons desiring spiritual support, and generally assisting victims and their families with whatever needs they present, in attempting to cope with the disaster experience and its aftermath.

PSYCHOSOCIAL IMPACT OF MASS CASUALTY TRAUMA

Support provided by the above-identified organizations is critical in managing a mass casualty trauma, because in such situations, the problems, especially the psychosocial problems experienced by both victims and responders, frequently "exceed the medical community's resources to deal with them" (Baker, 1980, p. 149). Two broad categories of disaster victims are identified: primary victims, who "directly experience physical, material and personal losses from the disaster event"; and secondary victims, who "witness the destructiveness of the disaster but do not experience the actual impact" (Bolin, 1985, p. 6). Secondary victims may include both family members and rescue workers involved in a disaster incident. The American Psychiatric Association's DSM-IV Classification now identifies "bearing witness to a trauma or being confronted by the traumatic experience of a family member or close friend" as a stressor that may have "psychiatric consequences" (Fullerton & Ursano, 1997, p. 59).

It is suggested that "the impact of victimization" may threaten or even "shatter" certain basic assumptions of the survivor: "the belief in personal invulnerability; the perception of the world as meaningful and the perception of oneself as positive [or as being a worthy person]" (Janoff-Bulman, 1985, p. 15). This psychological impact of a disaster has important implications for spiritual need and spiritual care, which are discussed later in this chapter. Obviously some victims of a disaster will be affected by the victimization to a greater degree than others. Some factors that may negatively influence a survivor's ability to cope both physically and psychologically include a history of "previous traumatic life events"; "recent ill health"; the "experience of severe stress and loss"; loss of "social and psychological supports"; and "lack of coping skills" (Cohen & Ahearn, 1980, p. 9). Especially vulnerable, of course, are the elderly, the young, and those with cognitive or mental disabilities (Cohen & Ahearn, 1980, pp. 9–10).

Another group particularly at risk of both physical and psychosocial stress following a mass casualty disaster are the "responders": police officers, firefighters, EMTs and other medical personnel (physicians and nurses), rescue personnel such as iron or steel workers, and any other individuals who witness the human carnage brought about by a major disaster. In many major disasters, the responding personnel face such traumatic sights as burned, dismembered, or mutilated bodies; these experiences put disaster workers at great risk "for the development of posttraumatic stress" (McCarroll, Ursano, & Fullerton, 1997, p. 37). Thus, it is important for disaster nurses to remember to assess the needs of disaster workers and to provide care for the caregivers as well as the "primary victims" in the days following a major disaster (Newburn, 1993, p. 127).

In one study, a group of firefighters who had been involved in mass casualty disasters were asked what incidents bothered them most in order of significance. They identified as most stressful: (1) "dead or injured children"; (2) "high rise fires with threat to life involved"; (3) "multi-casualty incidents"; (4) "death"; (5) "threat of personal mutilation or death" (Hodgkinson & Stewart, 1998, p. 197). Heroically, the firefighters placed their own potential injury or death at the lowest end of the scale in terms of significance. This fact, in itself, has important implications for the kinds of stressors that surviving firefighters or other rescue personnel might experience in terms of the concept of "survivor guilt." Some rescue workers may question their own survival in the face of massive losses of life at a disaster and even fear a "mission failure" (Hartsough, 1985, p. 27). Emergency workers may also have trouble sleeping or "winding down" after a disaster in which they were exposed to "almost daily horrors of death, destruction and coping with the needs of hurting human beings" (Mitchell, 1986, p. 109). A discussion of the "psychological aftermath" of a disaster for EMT personnel suggests that some negative feelings identified by responders to a mass casualty incident may include "feelings of frustration and powerlessness," "fear," "guilt" ("over real or imagined misjudgements" or "over casual handling of the dead"), and "insecurity" (Butman, 1982, pp. 149–150). Again, the disaster workers' stressors provide important implications for spiritual care in the aftermath of the incident.

For both victims and responders, as well as the planning of long-term care and counseling, "psychological first aid" may be needed at or near the disaster site. This consists of such activities as "instilling confidence," "showing warmth and caring," "providing guidance in stress reduction," and "attempting to assess [the individual's] need for counseling" (Mahoney, 1969, p. 208).

A final group that needs to be considered as having unique and special needs in the wake of a disaster incident is children. Obviously the child's degree of involvement in the disaster, as well as such factors as age, developmental stage, past life experience, and family support, will significantly influence his or her response to a traumatic event. In one nursing study of children who had experienced Hurricane Andrew in 1992, it was reported that children ages 5 to 12 described life as "weird" after the storm; the children's families and schools, however, served as primary resources in helping them cope with the life changes necessitated by the disaster (Coffman, 1994, p. 363). There are a number of books that might help parents or disaster nurses working with children who survive a mass casualty incident in which loved ones were lost; one example is *Your Grieving Child* (Dodds, 2001).

A great deal has been written about posttraumatic stress disorder (PTSD) following a disaster; the physical and psychological signs and symptoms vary widely among victims and responders. Dr. Michele Davidson, RN, pointed out that because Americans were exposed to incredible "images of death and destruction at the hands of the terrorists" in the September 11th attack, some may continue to experience some degree of PTSD "for months or even years to come" (2001, p. 10). Some common symptoms of PTSD include fatigue, irritability, restlessness, fear, anxiety and depression, nightmares, difficulty sleeping, lack of appetite, difficulty concentrating, headaches, GI upsets, and a multiplicity of other physical complaints. After the WTC disaster, some New Yorkers reported anxiety at hearing loud noises, especially if they involved an aircraft passing overhead. A variety of therapeutic interventions may be employed to ameliorate these symptoms and help the sufferer on the road to recovery; some basic steps in therapy include "initial exploration of the stress event," "establishing the therapeutic alliance," and "working through thoughts and feelings" about the event (Marmar & Horowitz, 1988, pp. 93–97).

The "critical incident stress syndrome (CISS)" is a fairly recent concept identifying a stress reaction of disaster workers appropriate for psychological intervention. This may occur in EMTs, physicians, nurses, police, firefighters, and other rescue workers after a traumatic incident causes interference with their ability to function, or later results in a strong emotional reaction (Kennedy & Charles, 2001, p. 391). The CISS is defined as "responding to a scene and becoming overwhelmed by what one sees, hears, touches, or smells; and experiencing normal reactions of an abnormal event" (Kennedy & Charles, 2001, p. 391) such as can occur at the site of a mass casualty trauma. A therapy recommended to counter the stress of emergency workers in a disaster is the psychological debriefing process labeled the

"Critical Incident Stress Debriefing (CISD)" (Mitchell, 1986, p. 109). In this process, the emergency workers are allowed to vent their emotions after a disaster through a peer support group led by a mental health professional. CISD is reported to assist "emergency personnel in understanding their re-actions" and reassuring them "that what they are experiencing is normal and common to most of those who were involved in the incident" (Mitchell, 1986, p. 109).

SPIRITUAL NEEDS IN THE AFTERMATH OF A DISASTER

The topic of spiritual needs immediately after, and in the long term follow-ing, a mass casualty disaster is vast. A disaster victim's or a responder's spir-itual needs may involve a desire for personal prayer or prayer with a clergy person; a loving hug or words of support from a relative, friend, or caregiver; formal religious rituals in cases of death or critical wounding of loved ones; and myriad other kinds of spiritual or religious support. Much will have to do with the nature of the disaster, the role of the individual in the disaster, and the personal spiritual or religious orientation of the victim or responder. Examples of need and kind of spiritual/religious care provided are best pre-sented in context of a specific disaster incident. Thus, much of the pastoral care literature addressing disaster response is described in such a context. The same is true of this chapter, which, as noted earlier, focuses on the spir-itual need and spiritual care involved in the September 11th attack on America. Prior to discussion of the spiritual needs of Pentagon and World Trade Center victims and responders, however, an overview of the extant literature on spiritual care in earlier mass casualty disasters is presented.

In 1966, a tornado devastated a large area near Topeka, Kansas, taking 17 lives and destroying over 800 homes; thousands were left homeless. A chaplain from the Menninger Foundation summarized the reports of the spiritual care provided by local pastors as primarily involving counseling survivors in terms of their everyday needs. The pastors' interventions rep-resented loving, caring church support, and it was noted that "no one re-ported . . . a discussion on God's will or providence" (Klink, 1966, p. 200). Another widely explored early disaster was that of the 1972 Buffalo Creek experience, in which a local coal mine waste heap collapsed, killing 125 peo-ple and leaving hundreds homeless. Shortly after the disaster, local chaplains responded to the scene to provide whatever emergency pastoral care the victims desired; a plan for long-term care was also initiated to focus on "in-tense unresolved grief; disaster syndrome; and loss of community" (Jordan, 1976, p. 160). A 1974 tornado in Louisville, Kentucky, killed 40 people and left over 900 homeless. Some of the pastoral care strategies reported after this disaster included assisting victims to verbalize the "trauma" (i.e., getting the person to talk), helping victims deal with the stress of "uprootedness" and "loss of possessions," and dealing with problems of "isolation and disillusionment" (Reed, 1977, pp. 98–106). Also in 1974, another Kentucky tornado left 77 people dead and more than 1,000 injured. Some of the key spiritual ministries provided by local pastors included visiting victims in hospitals, attending a mass funeral service, helping rebuild homes, giving last rites and conducting individual funeral services, and collecting money for victims (Chinnici, 1985, p. 248).

Following a 1980 tornado in Grand Island, Nebraska, in which more than 1,000 homes were destroyed, a pastor found that his congregation particularly needed to deal with the meaning of the event. His sermons thus dealt with such topics as the stages of loss, empathy for the victims, and the challenge to help those in need (Allen, 1982, p. 464). Hurricane Hugo devastated areas of Florida in August of 1992, leaving many injured and homeless; there were a number of stress-related deaths following the storm. Florida pastors reported that stress was reduced with the help of two spiritual orientations: humility, or the ability to admit that one was not "in charge" in a disaster, and the sharing of disaster experiences with a "community that understood and empathized" (Dudley & Schoonover, 1993, pp. 588–589). Sometimes, the pastors note, these communities were made up of "Christian congregations, but just as often . . . of old friends, neighbors or strangers" (1993, p. 589). Two other disasters described in the pastoral care literature are those of the 1992 impact of Hurricane Iniki, west of Honolulu, and the 1997 Red River flood that devastated Grand Forks, North Dakota. Spiritual care following these disasters included pastors' encouraging victims to take care of each other "reinforcing a living community that became a living reminder of God's love and care" (Moody & Carr, 1996, p. 27), and encouraging citizens to become a community of Christ "by planned and random acts of kindness" (Hulden, 1997, p. 31).

The descriptions of spiritual care and spiritual need included in the reports described above focus primarily on the actual ministries of pastors and congregations in meeting the early needs of disaster victims and their families. Several pastors, however, admit that the question of "why" begins to be articulated as initial stressors fade and long-term coping begins. A victim's or survivor's request for an answer to the "why" of evil or suffering is perhaps the most difficult issue for a spiritual caregiver to address, quite simply because there is no clear answer. The question of why becomes even more sensitive when a disaster or trauma affects the very young. Following a 1989 school disaster in Hudson Valley, New York, in which 10 children died and many others were injured, questions were reported such as "They were so innocent: how could God allow this?" (Cullinan, 1993, p. 227). It is generally believed that "religion can play a role in assigning meaning" to disasters (Kroll-Smith & Couch, 1987, p. 26); yet, an individual, even a religious person, may be left questioning his or her "trust in God's benevolence" following a devastating disaster (Pedraja, 1997, p. 7).

In discussing the theology and "theodicy or Divine Justice" (Kropf, 1988, p. 57) of disasters, theologians note the difficulty of reconciling three propositions generally held by most religious people: "God is loving and perfectly good"; "God is omnipotent"; and "There is evil and suffering in the world" (Chester, 1998, p. 488). This is the problem presented in the Old Testament book of Job, which, in fact, concludes without giving the reader a satisfying answer as to why Job, ostensibly a good man, had to suffer; the focus of the book is on Job's faith in the midst of suffering. It is suggested, however, that although Job's God may be "inscrutable . . . he speaks and he cares" (Cohn, 1986, p. 276). As movingly put by author David Toole in an essay on the theology of natural disasters, "But what must we ask of the suffering of the innocents . . . we mourn the deaths and cheer only the possibility that somewhere amidst disaster God is at work judging and saving the world" (1999, p. 561).

In his best-selling book *When Bad Things Happen to Good People*, Rabbi Harold Kushner took a similar position. "God does not cause our misfortunes," he notes. "Some are caused by bad luck, some are caused by bad people, and some are simply an inevitable consequence of our being human and being mortal, living in a world of inflexible natural laws" (1981, p. 134). Rabbi Kushner adds that because a tragedy that befalls us is "not God's will. . . . We can turn to Him for help in overcoming it, precisely because we can tell ourselves that God is as outraged by it as we are" (p. 134). Rabbi Kushner's position is strikingly reminiscent of a mother's comment at the time of her son's dying. "Even when I was screaming at God, because, you know, why and why and why? Even when I was angry with him, I knew that God was crying with me" (O'Brien, 1992, p. 67).

THE DISASTER NURSE'S ROLE IN SPIRITUAL CARE

Perhaps the most important thing that a nurse caring for a disaster victim can do, in terms of spiritual care, is to reinforce the fact that the trauma a patient has experienced was not caused by God, or brought about by any behavior on the victim's part. This can free a victim from possible feelings of guilt, help restore his or her faith in God, and allow the individual to, as Rabbi Kushner suggests, "turn to God for help" in overcoming the suffering caused by the disaster. Before attempting to provide more specific spiritual care such as praying with a patient or clergy referral, a nurse can do an on-the-spot spiritual assessment by asking a few simple questions related to a disaster victim's spiritual or religious tradition, such as finding out what kind of pastoral care or prayer life they have been used to and what might support them both immediately and in future coping with the disaster. Family members, if available, can provide much of this information. Also, a variety of volunteer clergy members are usually present at disaster sites; their intervention may be very helpful in assisting the nurse with both assessment and planning for a patient's future, especially if the victim is to be hospitalized.

As suggested in chapter 3, not all nurses will or need to feel comfortable in providing such spiritual care as praying with a patient; they may, however, feel at ease giving a supportive hug. Nurses in disaster situations should, however, be prepared to assess a patient's spiritual needs, especially if the victim is seriously or mortally wounded. For example, a critically injured Roman Catholic victim would be greatly comforted to receive an anointing or "the Sacrament of the Sick"; this could be done on the spot, if a priest is available. It is doubtful that any priest would come to a disaster site without bringing the holy oil needed for the sacrament. If the patient should die either at the disaster site or in transport to a hospital, the fact that the "last rites" of the Church had been administered prior to his or her death would be very meaningful to a Catholic family.

It can also be helpful for a disaster nurse to provide clergy referral to less seriously injured victims for future spiritual care and counseling. It is very important to refer patients to pastors who are willing and able to listen to the sometimes graphic and gruesome reports of a disaster scene "in a nonjudgmental and practical way but with a sensitivity to the theological implications for the victim" (Williams, 1998, p. 330). Because of the "trust many people have in ministers" they often become natural crisis counselors (Clinebell, 1991, p. 183). Nurses also are "natural crisis counselors" and natural providers of spiritual care, because they are often the people most closely involved with a victim immediately after a disaster. Guidelines suggested for pastoral caregivers working with trauma victims can also be useful for disaster nurses regarding the provision of spiritual support and spiritual care; some of these include "non-judgmental acceptance of the survivor," a posture of "support and advocacy," an understanding of "post-traumatic distress," "willingness to be exposed to the survivor's recounting of the traumatic experience," and recognition that grieving may be a life-long process (Foy, Drescher, Fitz, & Kennedy, 1993, p. 631). The authors also note that the spiritual caregiver should provide for "pastoral self-care" (p. 631). Pastoral or spiritual self-care is a given for any nurse attempting to provide spiritual care for victims of a mass casualty disaster.

SEPTEMBER 11, 2001: THE TERRORIST ATTACK ON AMERICA: SPIRITUAL NEEDS AND SPIRITUAL CARE

The Attack

Although explorations of spiritual needs and spiritual care at the Pentagon and the World Trade Center (WTC) disaster sites are addressed separately, an overview of the terrorist attack on America, including that of the Pennsylvania plane crash, is initially presented; this is to set the tone for that day of tragedy for the citizens of the United States.

In the early hours of September 11, 2001, four large passenger jet aircraft were hijacked by terrorists intent on causing death and destruction in key areas of the United States. At approximately 8:45 A.M., a hijacked American Airlines jetliner, Flight 11 out of Boston, bound for Los Angeles and carrying 20,000 gallons of fuel, crashed into the 110-story north tower (Tower 1) of New York City's WTC at a level between floors 90 and 100. The building immediately burst into flames. At 9:03 A.M., a hijacked United Airlines jet, Flight 175 from Boston, bound for Los Angeles and also fully loaded with fuel, crashed into the south tower (Tower 2) of the WTC between floors 78 and 87 and exploded. Both buildings were now on fire. At 9:45 A.M., American Airlines Flight 77 from Washington, DC, bound for Los Angeles and fully fueled, crashed into the western side of the Pentagon, exploding into flames; a huge section of the building soon collapsed. At 10:10 A.M., United Airlines Flight 93 from Newark, New Jersey, and bound for San Francisco crashed into a field in rural Somerset County, Pennsylvania. It is hypothesized that this fourth hijacked plane may have been headed for the United States Capitol or the White House. It is believed that only the actions of some courageous passengers—who, according to reported cell phone conversations, overpowered the hijackers and took control of Flight 93—prevented a fourth major mass casualty disaster from happening on September 11th. At 10:05 A.M., the 110-story south tower of the WTC collapsed in on itself from the heat of the fire melting its steel structure; at 10:28 A.M., the north tower of the WTC also collapsed from the top down. Hundreds of people raced through the streets of Manhattan, fleeing the deluge of debris raining down on the city from the collapsing towers. Some trapped WTC employees leapt to their deaths, perhaps in hope of a miraculous escape from the flames engulfing their offices. Later that afternoon, WTC Building 7, a 47-story structure, also collapsed from the fire.

The country's initial reaction to the first jet crash into the north tower of the WTC was one of shock over a terrible accident. Eighteen minutes later, after the second tower was hit, it was clear that this disaster was not accidental, and all nonmilitary planes in U.S. airspace were immediately grounded. The Port Authority of New York closed all tunnels and bridges into the city and many buildings near the WTC were evacuated. There was a recall of all New York City firefighters to respond to the WTC disaster site. Forty minutes after the second WTC tower was hit, and the Pentagon had been attacked, the country knew that an "act of war" had occurred. President Bush was temporarily evacuated aboard Air Force One; many government office buildings in Washington, DC, were also evacuated. Fighter jets were deployed from military air bases across the country, and all inbound transatlantic flights were diverted to Canada. The Pentagon announced that five warships and two aircraft carriers had been deployed from a Virginia naval station to protect the east coast from further attack. The president informed the country that a national emergency had been declared, and U.S. military worldwide were placed on high alert. The number of casualties was unknown in the immediate aftermath of the attacks, but the estimates were staggering; the entire country was in shock. The president begged for prayers for the thousands of victims and their families.

Some months after the attack on America, the numbers of missing, dead, and wounded were still changing, but it had generally been determined that 266 people, including the hijackers, lost their lives in the four plane crashes; 189 people were killed in the Pentagon attack; and close to 3,000 became victims of the World Trade Center disaster. Of the WTC lives lost, 343 represented fallen members of the New York City Fire Department, 75 were New York Port Authority officers and staff members, and 23 were New York City police officers. The City of New York was overwhelmed with funerals and memorial services and with bereaved and grieving families. All of America, and indeed the world, grieved for so many innocent lives lost in this unbelievably painful mass casualty disaster that struck the country with such force and such surprise. Everyone had a story to tell: where they were when the attack occurred; who they knew in New York or Washington that they had worried about; how they expressed their pain, their grief, and their sympathy for the suffering victims. Some of these anecdotes, as well as the author's own experiences and insights in gathering data for this chapter, are woven throughout the following pages describing spiritual needs and spiritual care following the attack on America.

The Pentagon

On September 11th, the famous Pentagon, an east coast hub of U.S. military operations, located only a few miles from the nation's capital, was grievously damaged by the terrorist attack. The disaster resulted in the loss of 189 lives and numerous injuries. American Airlines Flight 77 slammed into the western side of the Pentagon between corridors 4 and 5: "The plane blasted through rings E, D, and C, and parts of it were found between rings C and B" (Cannon, 2001, p. 31). Newscasters across the country noted, with awe, that only the fact that the plane happened to hit a portion of the Pentagon that had recently been renovated, saved hundreds, if not thousands, of lives. The newly reinforced side wall kept the floors from collapsing for about half an hour, thus allowing many Pentagon staffers to escape before that portion of the building came down.

I live and work at The Catholic University of America in Washington, DC, about four miles from the Pentagon. And I, like everyone else in the area, worried and grieved and prayed with and for the victims of September 11th. The Pentagon attack seemed like a lesser disaster, compared to the carnage at the World Trade Center, but the impact was in no way minor to the victims, their families, and the brave responders to the disaster site. My university held a moving candlelight memorial service the week of September 11th for those who died at the Pentagon and also those who died in Pennsylvania and New York; we desperately needed to do something, and turning to God in prayer seemed the most important step in coping with what had befallen our country.

Washington, DC, as New York, never got the huge number of mass casualties initially expected; nursing students and faculty at Catholic University were ready to help but the call never came; sadly, there were not enough survivors at either site to overwhelm the existing health care systems. To view the Pentagon disaster site in the early days was shocking; to see the gaping hole left in this so familiar building, the distinguished center of military operations. To view the grieving families, waiting at the perimeter of the Pentagon disaster site in the hope that a missing loved one might be found alive, was heartbreaking. The wife of one missing soldier asserted, "I'm not going home without him."

The Chaplains

"It's not the collar, it's the color."

Washington, DC, Fire Department Chaplain

One of the first people I spoke with about the spiritual needs of Pentagon disaster victims was Reverend "Smith" (all names used in reporting interview data are pseudonyms), a Washington, DC, police and fire chaplain. He had been paged with the DC Fire Department immediately after the attack and had been at the site, ministering to the wounded, to their families, and to the rescue workers each day for weeks. Chaplain Smith reported that there had been a spiritual presence at the Pentagon disaster site 24/7 since the attack. When I asked whether the religious denomination of a person providing spiritual care to disaster survivors mattered to the victims and rescue workers, he replied, "No, it's not the collar; it's the color!" Rev. Smith explained that what was important, especially to rescue workers, was the "color" of his badges, representing the police and fire departments of Washington, DC; he was "their chaplain" and, thus, the chaplain for the survivors and families following a disaster. Rev. Smith explained that "working with people of diverse religious backgrounds is one of the challenges of disaster response chaplaincy. My role is to coordinate with chaplains of other faiths, ministering to victims and rescue workers; being there and dispensing hugs and thank you's." Rev. Smith also added that a primary ministry, in his role as fire and police chaplain, is for the emergency responders. "You are there for them."

Rev. Smith described his "church" at the Pentagon disaster site as a "tent" that had been set up for the chaplains to provide spiritual care; this was also a place where a stressed-out rescue worker could come for a massage or just to "talk." The chaplains' tent was a "safe place where people could come for refuge." The chaplain explained that "Spiritual care is critical in such a setting; a situation that was that traumatic." He noted, "It was three days before a secure perimeter was established. The fire burned from 9 A.M. on Tuesday to 6 P.M. on Wednesday; lots of people were there waiting for survivors, praying for them." An additional witness of the importance of spiritual need and spiritual care at a disaster site was reflected in FEMA's designating a room for "Meditation and Prayer" (a "Quiet Room") for any staff members seeking a place apart.

Chaplain Smith reported that the spiritual care staff were assisted by staff members from the Red Cross and the Salvation Army who also prayed with and counseled victims and disaster workers at the site. He observed that spiritual counseling after a disaster may also bring out a victim's other life problems, such as with their marriage or relationship with God. Rev. Smith reported that volunteer chiropractors were also a "real asset for those lifting and carrying," especially steel workers and plumbers. This kind of human caring seemed relevant to the topic of spiritual care in the post-disaster situation; the roles of steel workers and plumbers were critical in attempting to rescue survivors who might be trapped in the rubble.

Chaplain Smith admitted that some people he spoke with did "ask why?" "There's nothing wrong with that," he asserted. "I don't have the answers. Some people may be angry with God but that's where faith and prayer come in. My job is to be," he added, "being present." A great deal of his ministry involved "listening, praying and saying 'thank you' to the rescue workers."

When I asked Chaplain Smith how he coped with his own stress in the face of ministering at the Pentagon disaster site, he commented, "My anxiety was that I could not rush to New York to assist my brother chaplains there, but here they said to me 'Who will care for us if you go to New York?' " Rev. Smith added that his faith, his family, and his friendships with other chaplains who were close friends provided his personal spiritual support. Finally, Rev. Smith suggested three pamphlets helpful in responding to spiritual need and providing spiritual care in mass casualty disasters: *Bringing God's Peace to Disaster* (Church World Service, 2001); *Bringing God's Presence to Survivors* (Church World Service, 1997); and *Cooperative Faith-Based Disaster Recovery in Your Community* (Church World Service, 2001).

The Firefighters

> "It's more like eagerness, not really fear; you can't wait to get in there. Like we were itching to get in there. It's like: 'Let's go; let's go; let's go! Let's get in there! We gotta get in there. C'mon; c'mon!' "

> Washington, DC, firefighter on arrival
> at the Pentagon site on September 11th

I was truly hesitant to ask to speak with any firefighters because of the incredible trauma they had recently experienced in witnessing the human carnage at the September 11th disaster sites, as well as because of the great losses they had suffered within their ranks in the City of New York. Nevertheless, my desire to try and understand, even a little, the heroism and spiritual caring of these men and women who rush to enter those places others rush to leave overcame my shyness. Through informal networking, I met a DC firefighter who graciously agreed to speak with me. Michael was a young firefighter, but seasoned through a number of years of volunteer experience and also through a number of years of "only wanting to be a firefighter," before actually beginning his firefighting career.

Michael belongs to one of the DC engine companies that was off-duty on September 11th when they were called in to respond to the Pentagon alarm. I'll let Michael take up the story from here:

> I drove to the firehouse as fast as I could. We keep our gear at the firehouse; I changed into my uniform, got my stuff. They had called in everybody off-duty and put us into groups; what we were supposed to do. They had additional engines and ladder trucks to operate throughout the city; about 130 firefighters were sent to the Pentagon. We served as relief to the companies that were at the initial alarm. There was still a good amount of fire throughout the building. The companies that were there were saying it was "pretty bad" inside; just bodies and people charred pretty bad. So, I was expecting it to be pretty bad. One of the guys I came with, we were talking about it and pretty much expecting the worst so we tried to be prepared for it.

Mike paused, "Something like this; you pretty much couldn't believe what had happened. It's like the whole world's changed after this. It's still hard to take in, even now." He continued:

> By the time we went in we really weren't expecting to find people alive but we had hope that we'd find somebody; I had hope. Not right around the exact impact of the plane because it was pretty much uninhabitable; it looked like a big fireball had gone through that entire ring of the building and you knew that pretty much everybody in that area, it looked like they had died. But areas around there where the plane didn't exactly hit, it looked like they might have been habitable by people so we started doing searches, and hoping. Mostly around the impact area we found bodies, badly charred; sometimes it was really difficult to tell where the bodies were or if we were really seeing bodies.
>
> But if you know that somebody's in there; if you have the slightest inclination that somebody might be alive in there, you go above and beyond. You're pushing it as far as you can go to try and save whoever might be in there. I had some hope that somebody might be in there; alive still! I was talking with one of the guys and

we said: "somebody's got to be in there; we're going to find somebody. We gotta keep going!" And I remember being so exhausted;
just so exhausted. The heat; the concrete in that building was just
containing the heat. I mean I've been in worse fire conditions but we
were looking for fire in the walls, hot spots, you don't have a lot of vis-
ibility and we wear about 40 pounds of gear; we also have an air
bottle and carry some kind of tool like an axe to have the ability to
cut through something if you need to. And the guy I was with, we
kept encouraging each other. We were just like: "Let's go; let's go."

At this point in our meeting, I asked Michael if he had been afraid on
arriving at the Pentagon disaster site and preparing to enter the burning
building. His response, as cited above, bears repeating, because it reflects so
beautifully the spiritual caring of the firefighter:

It's more like eagerness; not really fear. You want to get in there. Like
we were really itching to get in there. It's like: "Let's go, Let's go, Let's
go! Let's get in there! We gotta get in there! C'mon, c'mon!"

At the point of arrival at a fire, or to use Mike's expression, "when we
roll up on a fire," the firefighter employs all of his training to put aside fear
and direct his energies to the task of rescue at hand; the lives of the victims
always come before the firefighter's own safety.

A final question that I had for Michael was about his personal faith;
how it supported his ministry as a firefighter and whether experiences such
as that of the Pentagon disaster response were something that firefighters in
general wanted or needed to talk to a spiritual counselor about. Mike replied,
"Well, most guys don't really talk about the stuff that bothers them too much.
What I've noticed is guys kind of joke after something like this just kind of
to get your mind off it; try to not think about the bodies or whatever. I talked
a little bit to a guy I was with; he's pretty spiritual so I felt kind of comfortable talking with him; he's kind of on the spiritual level." Mike continued:

And I pray a lot. There was one thing that was kind of burned into my
head at the Pentagon. There was this one man; you could tell that
when the place was hit he wasn't killed right away, like the other people. It looked like he had been trying to make it to a doorway and he
had his ID out and I thought 'Oh, man. I think he was trying to keep
his ID out so somebody could identify him.' And I said that to my
friend; it was like I wanted to say that to somebody. I wanted to say

something about it. And then, that was it. I didn't tell anybody else or say anything more. But, seeing that guy trying to get out of the Pentagon, that'll probably stay with me forever. And he was going the right way, too. Oh, man, this guy was heading the right way!

Michael completed his response to my question about his own faith life, "I do pray. I pray every morning before I go to work. I pray every night. I always pray the night before I go to work. When I pray I just ask God to be with me, for Jesus to be with me, to just guide me and help me; that's all. And I know a couple of other guys who pray a lot; I think a lot of others do too but they might not want anybody to know that."

Mike summarized his experience, "Like I tell [family] all the time, I'm glad I was able to be part of it [the Pentagon response]; to do something because it would have crushed me if I couldn't do anything. And every time I see the World Trade Center, I think, 'Oh, I wish I could have been there; to do something.' " He concluded, "I mean I wanted to be part of the Pentagon [response] but at the same time I wish I could have been part of the World Trade Center too. It's just frustrating! I mean I wish I could have done something!"

As a postscript to my meeting with Michael, he told me after our interview that he had recently been to New York to attend the funeral of one of his FDNY friends whose life was lost in the World Trade Center response.

A Prayer for Firefighters

Dear Father in Heaven, guide and protect your beloved firefighters
  who daily risk their lives in ministry to brothers and sisters in
  need.
Grant them courage in the face of danger, strength in times of
  challenge, and compassion in the midst of suffering.
Guard all firefighters with the power of your loving care, Dear Lord,
  for they are truly Your own. Bless these heroic men and women
  who bravely rush to enter the places others rush to leave.
Amen.

There were many post-September 11th stories, in both the local and national news, describing the heroic efforts of firefighters, police, military personnel, and civilians who assisted others to escape during the early minutes of the attack on the Pentagon. As well as the chaplains, these heroic rescuers provided spiritual care in responding to both the physical and psychological needs of disaster victims at the site. Most survivors interviewed by the media attributed their escape from the disaster to God and to his "ministers" who had led them out of the fiery building.

The World Trade Center

It is difficult to know how to begin to describe the myriad kinds of spiritual needs and spiritual care manifested at the site of the overwhelming mass casualty disaster that occurred at the WTC on September 11th. As soon as the impact of the first plane on the WTC's north tower was witnessed in New York, chaplains began to head to the scene. One of the first to arrive was the now-famous Franciscan New York Fire Department chaplain, Father Mychal Judge. According to accounts, Father Mike, as he was known by the fire-fighting community, immediately rushed into the burning north tower to begin ministering to the injured. As he knelt to give the last rites, the anointing of the sick, to a fallen firefighter, he removed his helmet in reverent prayer; he was struck in the head by falling debris and killed instantly while engaged in the ministry he loved. A group of firefighters picked up Father Mike's body, carried it to a nearby church, and laid him down before the altar; a fitting place for Father Mychal to begin his eternal rest.

I was told by a New Yorker friend that another New York priest quickly made his way to the disaster site and began blessing and giving absolution to firefighters, en masse, as they rushed into the burning building to search for survivors. This is a very consoling thought, spiritually, for the families of those who lost their lives in the effort to save others. A young firefighter, being transported to the World Trade Center with 50 other firefighters, is quoted as saying, "There was this chaplain on the bus and he was giving absolution to everyone" (Sullivan, 2001, p. 5). Father Benedict Groeschel, also a New York Franciscan, wrote, "I am sure that the first priests on hand, like Father Mychal Judge, the fire chaplain who lost his life ministering to the dying, gave general absolution as soon as they arrived on the scene. It may have been the biggest general absolution in history" (2001a, p. 242).

The Recoveries

Medical personnel poured into New York City with plans to set up triaging facilities near the disaster site, and also to help staff local hospitals. The volunteers were initially welcomed but, after a few hours, it became clear that, as in the Pentagon attack in Washington, DC, there would not be an overwhelming number of live casualties; the mortality would be much higher than the morbidity following the disaster. Those who did not get out of the towers quickly would not be getting out at all. The most critically important spiritual care, at that point, aside from that needed by rescue workers and family members, was the need for religious rituals to accompany the recovery of victims' bodies. To that end, a temporary morgue site, staffed by an interdenominational group of chaplains, was set up at the nearby Chelsea Piers.

Heart-wrenchingly tender scenes began to be replayed over and over on TV screens across the country, as news cameras at "Ground Zero" recorded the finding of bodies in the days following the September 11th attack. When the body of a uniformed police officer or a firefighter was identified, the deceased was draped in an American flag, and rescue workers stopped their digging to form two long lines of honor guards before which the heroic victim's remains were carried. One journalist reported that some of the men prayed as a fallen brother's remains passed by; others sang hymns. "Some of the men have beautiful voices," she wrote, "and sing the ancient chants; I heard one softly singing the *Dies Irae"* (Vitullo-Martin, 2001, p. 8). Many staid police officers', firefighters', steel and construction workers', and EMTs' eyes were moist with tears during these impromptu memorials carried out at the WTC disaster site.

The disaster victims' remains were immediately taken from the site to the makeshift morgue set up at Chelsea Piers. There, volunteer chaplains waited to receive the recovered bodies with a prayerful ritual of remembrance. One chaplain reported, "We were about a block away from 'Ground Zero.' All around us were huge piles of rubble, and a tremendous amount of work was going on with diggers and power shovels" (Groeschel, 2001b, p. 23). He continued, "Our task was to conduct a short service each time the remains of a victim's body were brought into the morgue. In the course of . . . six hours we held a service eight times" (pp. 23–24). Another clergyman who had ministered at the Chelsea Piers morgue, Father Philip Murnion, described the ritual. "Most of the time is spent in waiting . . . Then when a rescue worker arrives with remains, we all jump to our feet and a chapel-silence fills the air . . . . all wait as one or two of the clergy step forward and call all to prayer; all the other workers want to make sure this is done. We pray briefly, using our own words and the words of our ritual for the deceased, committing the person to God's love, and perhaps praying for the family . . . all remain quiet for a few seconds" (2001a, p. 1). Father added, "The respect, actually reverence, shown to each remain, however small, is extraordinary. It is as if the very fact that full bodies are only rarely retrieved has made the least part of a body all that much more important. The sacred character of each life is so fully honored" (2001a, p. 2). Father Murnion concluded his reflections from the WTC morgue site by poignantly expressing a spiritual response to the disaster. "The magnitude of the tragedy and the complexity of forces involved in the attack make almost any response seem inadequate. The hymn lines that occurred to me are from the *Stabat Mater:* 'Is there one who would not weep, whelmed in misery so deep?' Yet the powerful exertion of compassion-seeking-understanding evident at the site looks to faith and church for grounding, bonding, and action worthy of us as a people" (2001a, p. 2).

Manhattan churches of all denominations opened their doors to those in need: to exhausted rescue workers and to family members searching desperately for a loved one missing in the disaster. Quickly, victims' families began to establish personal prayer sites "mounting photos of their loved ones in nearby parks, at the receiving hospitals, at the medical examiner's office . . . and at the armory that served as a clearing house for the names of those missing" (Murnion, 2001b, p. 2). When some asked, "Where was God on September 11th?", clergymen answered with such responses as, "God was there in the seat with every person who went down in the fiery inferno . . . He was in the fireman's suit and behind the police badge. God was there in the elevators and the stairwells of the World Trade Center" (Stover, 2001, p. 79).

For many survivors and families, the Internet became a spiritual "lifeline" to access information, search for survivors, and share personal stories of pain, suffering, hope, and survival in the aftermath of the attack (Terrell & Perry, 2001, p. 67). Spiritual and religiously affiliated organizations and churches providing services to victims and families of the WTC disaster were listed on the Internet; they included such groups as The Salvation Army, Catholic Charities, Healing Works, the Southern Baptist Convention, Church of God Ministries, Christian Reformed Church, United Jewish Appeal Federation, United Methodist Committee on Relief, Evangelical Lutheran Church of America, National Presbyterian Church, Episcopal Church Center of N.Y., YMCA, World Vision, Association of Gospel Missions, World Relief, the Society of St. Vincent de Paul, and many others. Services offered on Web sites by these organizations included prayer and counseling (crisis and grief counseling), financial support, pastoral counseling (spiritual ministry), emergency services for survivors (food, clothing, shelter), school outreach to children, help with burial costs, emergency day care, legal counseling, job counseling, mental and physical health care, and general assistance for rescue and recovery workers. Approximately three months after the disaster, there were 7,450 Web sites listed under the heading WTC disaster and spiritual need. Especially in the aftermath of mass casualty disasters, churches and other religiously affiliated groups include provision for physical and mental health needs, as well as materials needed to sustain daily life, as part of their spiritual ministry to victims and survivors.

As noted, another source of spiritual support provided by the Internet was the opportunity for survivors, especially those who had escaped from the World Trade Center, or nearby areas, to tell their stories. Many disaster victims posted lengthy accounts of their experiences, their fears, their horror at the devastation, and their narrow, for some, escapes. Sharing experiences on Web sites, sometimes anonymously, gave the survivors a chance to vent painful emotions, to say thank you to sometimes unknown rescuers, and to express gratitude, often to God, for simply being alive. Some of the Internet writers ended their narratives with an expression of gratitude for the Web site and the opportunity it provided to share their experiences. It was interesting to discover that although the majority of stories, especially the most emotional anecdotes, were authored by New Yorkers who were intimately involved with the disaster, a number of people from as far away as California and Washington State felt the need to express their thoughts and feelings. One writer from Kirkland, Washington, ended a narrative with the words, "Thank you for this Web site!"

Many people from both New York and elsewhere visited the disaster site, "Ground Zero," in the days after the attack. There were mixed feelings about this both on the part of victims' families and rescue workers. No one wanted this sacred place, where so many suffered and died, to become a "tourist attraction"; most visitors, however, came out of a desire to grieve, to pray, and to pay homage to the victims, especially to those who gave their lives so heroically in a mission of rescue. It was admitted shortly after the attack, by psychologist and spiritual writer Eugene Kennedy, that "We cannot deal with this event. We can only respond to it and that requires that we enter into the mystery of loss" (2001, p. 17). Kennedy points out the importance of people expressing their grief over such a massive loss of life. "Nothing is more human," he asserts, "than our need to do that work of mourning that nobody can do for us" (p. 17).

The Chaplains

Aside from the stories of absolution given to rescue workers, and rituals provided at the morgue site, there are a number of accounts of other ministries provided by chaplains at the disaster site on the day(s) of and weeks after September 11th. Father James Martin, a New York Jesuit, described his arrival at the disaster site when he came to provide spiritual support two days after the attack. He reported that he was attempting to minister to a soldier at the site but could hardly tear his eyes away from the overwhelming scene before him. "I make an effort to ask after the soldier's welfare. But instead he ministers to me. 'That's OK, Father,' he says, 'Everybody stares when they see it. It's hard to see, isn't it?' He hands me a face mask" (2001a, p. 8). As he went about the disaster site listening and supporting and caring for the rescue and recovery workers, some of whom had lost friends and co-workers in the attack, Father Martin reported, "Suddenly I realize that I am standing beside grace. Here are men and women, some of whom tell me 'I lost a buddy in there,' who are going about their business; the business that includes the possibility of dying. 'Greater love has no person,' said Jesus, 'than the one who lays down his life for another.' And that is what this looks like. Here it is" (Martin, 2001a, p. 9).

Five days after the attack, Father Martin and several fellow priests went back to the disaster site to say Mass for the rescue workers in a make-shift chapel at the World Trade Center "Ground Zero" ruins. "In a dusty plaza, we discover a cast off table, which we cover with a sheet. Borrowed chalices and patens from a nearby Jesuit church sit next to a Poland Springs water bottle, a hardhat and a gas mask . . . we assemble . . . with our gas masks. In a few minutes a small group of people gathers around the table—all visibly tired, all covered with sweat, all blanketed in ash" (2001b, p. 29). Father Martin noted that the gospel reading for the day was "heartbreakingly appropriate": "the shepherd who rescues his lost sheep . . . we speak of searching, rescuing, hoping and loving . . . many come to receive communion" (2001b, p. 29). After Mass, one of Father Martin's companions came to him and said, "Have you seen the sign?" Large poster boards had been placed around the disaster site with spray-painted messages to indicate services or activities: " 'Morgue', says one sign. 'Eye Wash Station,' says another" (p. 29). And, a sign written by someone unknown to us, Father Martin reported, had been placed "a few feet from our little altar. It reads: *'Body of Christ' "* (p. 29).

There was so much written and replayed on national news reports about the hundreds of funerals in New York that attempting to describe even a few would take up a chapter in itself: the haunting bagpipe melody of "Amazing Grace," which accompanied the fire engine–borne caskets of so many of New York's bravest; the tears of the widows, the children, the parents, the co-workers, the ministers; the moving sermons on pain and suffering and hope in eternal life. An excerpt from a homily offered by Edward Cardinal Egan at a Memorial Mass for rescue workers at St. Patrick's Cathedral reflects the spirituality of those who gave their lives in attempting to save others:

All of us have our fears. These heroes of ours had theirs too. But they conquered them. Millions of tons of stone and steel were falling all around them. Hurricanes of dirt, dust and debris were engulfing them. There was no light with which to see. There was no air with which to breathe. All the same, they did what they always do. The guided, they protected, they defended, they shielded, they rescued. And in so doing they handed over their lives for the safety and well being of others. If this is not triumph, I do not know what triumph might be. Triumph over fear. Triumph over caring only for oneself. Triumph over all that makes us less than the Lord would have us be. Triumph that defines heroes; wondrous, glorious heroes. (Groeschel, 2001b, p. 133; cited with permission of Edward Cardinal Egan)

The account of one Catholic parish in Staten Island gave some idea of the enormity of the loss for individual communities and of the need for spiritual rituals in the aftermath of the attack on America. St. Clare's parish lost 30 parishioners in the disaster; 11 were firefighters. It was reported that "Some of the most heart-rending funerals and memorial Masses have been in St. Clare's red-brick church, like the one for Louis J. Modaferi, the Captain of Staten Island's Rescue Company 5. . . . Rescue Company 5 was wiped out on September 11" (Golway, 2001, p. 6).

Several weeks after the disaster, I had the opportunity to interview a New York City chaplain who had been working with FDNY, the city fire department, since the attack. One of the first things Chaplain Kelly commented on was the fact that so many victims of the WTC disaster were young; that was especially true among the ranks of the police and firefighters, of whom a great number were in their forties, thirties, and even twenties. Another particularly heart-wrenching aspect of the losses among the 343 firefighters was the fact that some were from the same families, for example, a father and son. It was incredibly difficult for families that so many WTC victims' bodies were never recovered.

At the initial alarm, Father Kelly commented, "No one thought the buildings would collapse. One small engine company, with only seven men, was assigned to the 40th floor of Tower 2. The elevator, with all seven firefighters, went up and the building came down. They have never been heard from since. Another trauma was the terrorist nature of the disaster: the homicide, the mutilated bodies, and the loss of public safety personnel; people think 'if policemen and firemen are killed, who will protect us?' "

Father Kelly related the difficulty of ministry at the morgue. Although he had not done the work himself, several clergy he knew were involved and he noted that when they came back from a six-hour tour at the morgue, they said it "felt like six months": "It was very hard; they had to wear masks and gowns, they saw the mutilated bodies . . . we saw the indignity of death."

Father Kelly, whose role was to provide information, in conjunction with the fire department, on CISD and available counseling services, commented on the firefighters' culture. "You know, firemen don't have a choice. You don't stand by and watch the World Trade Center burn down; you go in and fight the fire. Also, if a firefighter is down [if he is dead or injured] he is never left alone. If a firefighter is injured in the line of duty, there will be an intense search for that person and the firefighters reserve the right and honor and privilege of retrieving and removing the body. They do it with a sense of ritual and dignity. They never canceled their presence at the site even for the Thanskgiving and Christmas holidays."

Father Kelly described the experience of "numbing" after the WTC disaster:

> People saw terrible trauma; people jumping out windows, that will be replaying over and over but you selectively process; you can't take it all in. Some people at the site saw the WTC come down but said they didn't hear anything. The site of the WTC disaster looks like one of those movies where you see the world after an atomic bomb had dropped and you say "this cannot be real." You say to yourself "this cannot be the World Trade Center; where I'm standing, right now!" You just can't take it in. Everyone is in shock about the situation. I met a widow outside a firehouse and she just said: "I'm not going home until my husband comes home."

People needed to tell their personal stories over and over again, Father Kelly noted. And the question of "Where was God?" came up. He added:

> Some people can fall back on their faith, for others that doesn't work. There were so many memorial services with similar messages being preached. Some may say: "It's not enough." It was especially hard on the firefighters' widows because they all go to each other's husband's services to be supportive and then have to live their own pain all over again. Some people are angry with God and questioning God. They know we don't have the answers but what they want is for us to be with them in the questioning: to give them the freedom, the permission to question.

Another very difficult dimension of this tragedy, in terms of the grieving process, Father Kelly pointed out, was the absence of remains for so
many victim's families.

> Physical remains give us a sense of how someone died. In the initial
> weeks there were a number of people living in hope; they were sus-
> tained by a belief that "my loved one is trapped in a void. There are
> a lot of cafeterias, so he's in a cafeteria and has food and water; he's
> safe." But at the end of two weeks, the operation seemed to move
> from rescue to recovery and there was little hope of survivors. There
> was some controversy over it but finally the city decided to issue
> death certificates for those who were missing; some families didn't
> want to come and pick them up because it was the end of hope.

Finally, Father Kelly observed that to be a compassionate minister in
a disaster such as that of the WTC attack, "you have to walk a fine line; to be
able to grieve with those you serve yet not break down completely. You must
exercise some boundaries or compassion fatigue can creep up. Some of the
survivors will tell you that they just don't know if they can cope. I tell them
if you can just borrow some of my strength, I know you can make it. I have
faith in you. I have no doubt you will survive with time."

Father Kelly concluded his sharing with an assessment of the firefighters' spiritual mission. "Firefighters are physically very strong, very fit
but their gift is compassion. They have selected a profession where the primary and most important skill is to save people, and they fight fires too. But
the most important concern of any fireman fighting a fire is are there any
people trapped inside. They are there to save lives; there is great sensitivity.
They have a compassion orientation."

The Firefighters

On that fateful day, life changed for everyone in America; but for none more
than for the citizens of New York City; and surely for none more than the
renowned FDNY, the Fire Department of New York City. The entire country
cried and grieved and prayed with the victims and their families. As a col-
league from the Midwest said in a phone call on the afternoon of September
11th, "Today we are all New Yorkers!" On September 11th, the world witnessed, in horror, the absolute, unmitigated evil of the terrorist destruction
of the World Trade Center; on September 11th, the world also witnessed, in
awe, the absolute, unmitigated goodness of the hundreds of New York City

firefighters and police officers who rushed into the towering inferno in the hope of saving at least some of the thousands of men and women trapped in the burning building. A *Newsweek* report described the scene immediately after the attack. "Scores of firemen were pouring in [to the Trade Center] . . . the men were climbing the stairs under staggering loads of state of the art gear . . . helmets . . . turnout coats . . . boots . . . compressed air cylinders for breathing . . . radios . . . and assorted axes and hand tools [that] weighed between 80 and 100 pounds per man" (Thomas, 2001/2002, p. 54).

Initially, those at the site hoped that the buildings would remain standing. When the towers collapsed, they took with them not only thousands of WTC workers but also hundreds of firefighters who were so bravely climbing the stairs in search of survivors. Many deaths, especially those of the uniformed officers of the New York City Police Department and the New York City Port Authority, occurred in the midst of great courage and caring. The details of a multitude of brave rescues and rescue attempts, carried out by both police officers and civilians, have been documented; many others remain known only to God, who has now welcomed these courageous men and women into His loving arms. By far, however, the greatest loss of life among uniformed rescuers occurred within the heroic ranks of the Fire Department of the City of New York. In that one rescue effort, 343 firefighters were lost, including 21 fire station captains; 19 battalion chiefs; 46 lieutenants; 251 firefighters; the fire department chaplain, Father Judge; a fire marshall; a deputy commissoner; two assistant chiefs; and the chief of FDNY, Chief Peter J. Ganci. New York Mayor Rudolph Giuliani described the spiritual commitment of his firefighters. "When firefighters run into a burning building, they don't stop to wonder whether the people inside are rich or poor, what race they are, or what religion they practice. Their thoughts are focused solely on the individuals inside that need to be saved." The mayor concluded poignantly, "Their actions represent the purest example of love for humanity" (2001a, p. 8).

Many bodies of these caring and compassionate men were entombed in the smoldering ruins of the disaster site. In the days and weeks following the disaster incident, New York City firefighters worked tirelessly, alongside police officers, EMTs, iron workers, construction engineers, and a variety of other rescue workers, to attempt to retrieve the bodies of their fallen brothers. This was risky and dangerous work because the remaining WTC skeletal structure was unstable and the air was toxic with dust and fumes from the fallen concrete and the fires that smoldered for more than 100 days after the attack. The task was critically important to the New York City firefighters, however, because the firefighter's code is to never leave a fallen brother. The

WTC site was never without the presence of New York City firefighters during the weeks and months in which the rescue and recovery efforts were carried out. Twenty-four hours a day, seven days a week, FDNY members kept vigil over the place, the "sacred ground," where the bodies of so many of their brother firefighters, "New York's bravest," rested beneath the enormous pile of rock and rubble. The need to find a spiritual dimension to the horror of the disaster, especially for those involved in the recovery efforts, was evident from the beginning of the work. One powerful spiritual symbol embodied in the ruins was a twenty-foot cross, which had evolved naturally out of the intersection of two fallen beams, part of the wounded WTC steel structure. "This cross," it was noted, became "a startling witness to faith for hundreds of thousands of people who were deeply grieved by the terrorist attack" (Groeschel, 2001b, p. 13). A chaplain offered a blessing of the cross and prayed with the workers at its foot.

It was reported that FDNY's engine 54 "sent fifteen men to the first call for help; none returned. The forty-five firefighters left behind worked 24-hour shifts and returned to the attack site on their own time to search for their comrades" (McBride, 2001, p. 15). In reflecting on the behavior of his firefighters after September 11th, Mayor Rudolph Giuliani explained the firefighters' spiritual philosophy and mission. "It is human instinct to run away from a fire. Firefighters train themselves to run toward fire, determined to save . . . lives" (2001b, p. xvi); and Fire Commissioner Thomas Von Essen described the FDNY as a family: ". . . a family of men and women linked by a unique bond and a noble calling: to save lives at whatever cost" (2001, p. xix). It is important to remember that, as well as the professional and human commitment to save lives and fight fires, the "legal responsibility for the command of a disaster scene usually rests with the Fire Chief and his officers" (Brown, 1985, p. 51). At the WTC disaster, one of the first firefighters lost was the courageous and respected FDNY Chief, Peter J. Ganci, who was reportedly in the center of the disaster scene providing leadership and support for his men when the first building collapsed.

So many brave firefighters were lost . . . so many stories warrant telling. One exquisitely beautiful and yet heartbreaking account of the disaster's impact on the FDNY is reflected in the book *Brotherhood* (Hendra, 2001). Included in *Brotherhood* are pictures of all of the New York City firehouses that lost members at the WTC site. The fronts of many fire stations were turned into religious shrines by neighbors who left flowers, candles, prayer cards, pictures, and statues to honor the dead and the missing. The firefighters' personal spirituality is reflected over and over in the messages they, themselves, posted over fire station doors. Some examples include Rescue

4, Engine 292: "Pray for Our Brothers" (nine names of missing firefighters are listed); Squad 18 FDNY: "We Pray and Hope for Our Brothers" (the names of seven firefighters follow); Engine 290, Ladder 103: "God Bless Our Heroes; Gone But Not Forgotten" (nine firefighters' names are identified); Engine 165, Ladder 85: "To All Our Lost Brothers; Forever Rest in Peace. God Bless You"; FDNY Engine 23: "We Are Missing the Following Members (six fire-fighters' names listed—Please Keep Them in Your Prayers"; Engine 230: "Please Say a Prayer for Our 6 Missing Brothers"; and Engine 37, Ladder 4: "God Bless Our FDNY Brothers." Many of the signs thanked the neighbors for their care, their support, and their prayers. The firefighters at Engine 37, Ladder 4, added a touching comment; after thanking the community for their support, the sign concluded with the words: "We Are Still Here for You!" (Hendra, 2001).

The Police Officers

NYPD, the New York City Police Department, proudly referred to as "New York's Finest," lost 23 of its members in the WTC disaster. While overshad-owed in numbers by the FDNY mortality, the loss of that many officers in one incident was a grievous assault to the NYPD; and, of course, to the loved ones they left behind. One New York police officer interviewed several months after the attack commented, "I pray more now but I don't ask for anything; I just say 'thank you' for being alive!"

I was able to speak with an NYPD officer who, although not at the WTC site on September 11th, had worked with victims and families in Manhattan immediately after the attack and later at the Staten Island recovery landfill. Officer Kevin O'Connor, who also has a brother in the NYPD, was off duty at the time of the attack; as with the firefighters, he immediately reported to duty. Officer O'Connor's role in the first days following the disaster was to as-sist several local hospitals to help with family notification as patients were coming in, and to work with family members in taking missing person re-ports. Officer O'Connor admitted that, although he knew the work he was doing was important for the victims' families, it was difficult not to be down at the site. "You want to be down there helping out. I mean, there could be people trapped that you want to help but with the police department, you don't know what else is going to happen so you have to do other things too." Officer O'Connor noted that an NYPD buddy also shared a similar desire. "We both were going through the same thing; like you want to be down there helping out; we should be down there digging. You want to be in the heart of it."

A site had been set up for family members to come and report missing loved ones, and Officer O'Connor commented that having a social worker there to work with the families was helpful; he added, "I've been doing this for 18 years and you just try to be as consoling as you can."

A part of Officer O'Connor's investigation did take him to the WTC site in the early days and he described his initial reaction. "I remember the first time I went down there, it was nighttime with the lights all lit up; it looked like a movie set. I mean, it was so huge, and to see all those guys working, it was like 'Holy Smokes,' this is unbelievable!" I suggested to Officer O'Connor that he must see a lot as an officer with the NYPD; his response was simply, "This tops anything I've seen before!" He also commented on the gratitude of New Yorkers for the police, firefighters, and other rescue workers. "You see people cheering along the road for all the workers. It was a travesty but I tell you, you saw New York coming together. We got donations at the police stations, the firehouses; there was stuff coming in to go down to the site, because the cops were doing 12 hour tours, 7 days a week. You really didn't have time to go home, so people were sending in all kinds of stuff: food, toothbrushes, toothpaste, change of clothes, shampoo. Soup to nuts, you name it. What we needed, we got it. There were just tables full of stuff."

After Officer O'Connor acknowledged the support of the New York citizens, I commented that the entire country had, in effect, laid a mantle of heroism on the NYPD and FDNY for their response to the WTC attacks; I suggested that they probably did not, however, walk around feeling like "heroes." Officer O'Connor just gently replied, "Nah!"

In the later weeks after the terrorist attack, Officer O'Connor's role was to work with sometimes as many as 500 other NYPD officers at the Staten Island landfill where the debris from the WTC site was taken for processing and investigation. The officers were still looking for body parts and/or crime scene objects such as the black box from the hijacked aircraft. Officer O'Connor did not complain about the mission but when I asked if the work was difficult, he did admit that "As dreary as the site is, the landfill is just as dreary a place. It's a dreary place to be. You do 12 hour shifts; you go and leave in the dark." He added, "The first couple of weeks it was set up with army tents; you would have thought it was Desert Storm." Officer O'Connor observed that the presence of the Salvation Army was helpful because they cooked for the recovery teams; he also said he had met several chaplains who were providing a spiritual presence at the landfill.

I asked Officer O'Connor if personal spirituality was helpful to him and his family coping with the WTC disaster; he replied:

Oh, sure. We're Roman Catholic and we go to church every Sunday. My [eight-year-old] daughter goes to Catholic school and I know some kids in her school lost parents. The religion helps when we talk to her and the school helped. She's very smart and the day it happened she knew about it and she knows that her daddy is a police officer but she said: 'Oh my daddy is [on vacation].' She knew I wasn't there. But it is a concern of hers; she's brought it up a couple times, and not that we don't want her to know about it [the attack] but we try to make it that it is not something she has to be worried about; that's for us as parents to worry about and we wouldn't let anything happen to her.

A last question I had for Officer O'Connor was whether counseling or debriefing groups, such as CISD, would be helpful to him. He replied that "talking to people that are going through the same emotions that you are is helpful; it helps to hear that somebody else has the same things going through their mind that you do. The buddy that I traveled with that day [September 11], we were going through the same things; we wanted to be down there to help."

In summary, I believe that Officer Kevin O'Connor's response to the WTC disaster modeled that of many other officers and firefighters in primarily wanting to "be there" to help others; yet, also, of being willing to "carry on" with whatever tasks were assigned, as part of the overall commitment of service reflected in the commonly used descriptor of the NYPD as "New York's Finest."

A Prayer for Police Officers

Dear Father in heaven, guide and protect Your beloved police officers who daily risk their lives in the service of those in need. Grant them strength in conflict, courage in danger, and compassion for those who suffer. Hold all police officers in Your loving arms, Dear Lord, for they are truly Your own. Bless these brave men and women whose call to serve preserves the peace and justice of our world. Amen.

The Nurses

Because the number of living casualties was, sadly, not great, much of the nursing of survivors was carried out by regular hospital staff nurses, especially those working in burn and surgical ICUs, both in New York and

Washington, DC. One trauma nurse from St. Vincent's Hospital in New York commented that the unit was much less busy than she expected, "the victims just didn't have a chance to get out" (Ostrowski, 2001, p. 36). Overall, "St. Vincent's treated 264 patients in the first hours after the attack; 51 were in critical condition" (Ostrowski, 2001, p. 36). Some volunteer nurses and EMTs were involved in caregiving at both disaster sites. Pamela Charles, a pediatric oncology nurse visiting New York on September 11th, provided basic first aid at the WTC site, especially the washing of rescue workers' eyes and treating cuts and burns in the hours immediately after the attack. One young firefighter broke into tears and told her that he had just lost his whole unit; she reported, "All I could do was hug him" (2001, p. 44). Charles admitted that at first she wondered why a FEMA director had requested three nurses as well as three doctors to come to the site, when he could have had all surgeons. At the end of her tour, she concluded that the FEMA official "understood what traumatized, weary rescue workers needed was caring. And that," she noted, "is what nursing is all about" (2001, p. 44).

Nurses at St. Vincent's opened a Family Support Center the day following the disaster, to provide a place where victims' loved ones could come to try to locate survivors. The center also gathered a group of volunteer mental health professionals to help "people cope with a range of experiences related to the tragedy, from losing a family member to being displaced" ("The Road Back," 2001, p. 94).

Much of the spiritual care provided by nurses immediately after the attack on America will remain known only to those individuals involved in the nurse–patient interactions and to God. Spiritual caring on the part of nurses will continue for these disaster victims and their families for years, however, as the long-term stress reactions influence the lives and functioning of many of their patients.

Now, having passed the five-year anniversary of the devastating 9-11 attack on America, the case study articles by nurses involved in caring for survivors has dwindled. More contemporary disaster nursing literature has begun to focus on the tremendous medical and nursing caregiving needs engendered by Hurricane Katrina, which devastated the city of New Orleans and several other gulf coast regions in the fall of 2005. Joyce Martin, a family nurse practitioner working in a 120-bed hospital in "the oldest part of New Orleans," documented her experience in an article entitled "Riding out Hurricane Katrina." Martin admitted at one point, "I cried, feeling hopeless and abandoned. 'Where is God?' I asked" (2006, p. 37). In the end, however, her personal spirituality and biblical faith in Psalm 107 supported her. "Then they cried unto the Lord in their trouble and he delivered them out of their distresses. And he led them forth by the right way, that they might go to a city of habitation." Listening to those words, Martin observed, she knew that "God had not abandoned us" (p. 37).

This chapter was challenging to write, because the topic of spiritual need in mass casualty disasters is vast and variable. Spiritual needs in the immediate and long-term periods following a disaster are very much related to the particular disaster incident and to the overall needs of the victims and their families. Little has been written recently on disaster nursing in general; I found virtually nothing in the nursing literature specifically exploring the spiritual needs of the survivors. The heart of the chapter is, as noted earlier, focused on the spiritual needs of those involved in the September 11th attack on America. That topic is also vast and we are only beginning to explore the impact of the disaster on those more directly involved as victims, family members, and rescue workers. It is believed, however, that this beginning examination of spiritual need and spiritual care following the terrorist attack on America will help nurses caring for all victims of trauma, especially those involved in mass casualty incidents.

REFERENCES

Allen, R. J. (1982). How we respond to natural disaster. *Theology Today, 38*(1), 458–464.

American National Red Cross. (1966). *Disaster handbook for physicians and nurses.* Washington, DC: Author.

Anderson, M. B., & Woodrow, P. J. (1998). *Rising from the ashes: Developmental strategies in time of disaster.* Boulder, CO: Lynne Rienner Publishers.

Atkinson, P., Keylon, K., Odor, P. S., Walker, G., & Hunt, L. (1995). Disaster nursing in the Oklahoma City bombing. *Insight, 20*(3), 30–31.

Baker, F. J. (1980). The management of mass casualty disasters. In H. W. Meislin (Ed.), *Priorities in multiple trauma* (pp. 149–157). Germantown, MD: Aspen Systems.

Bolin, R. (1985). Disaster characteristics and psychosocial impacts. In B. J. Sowder (Ed.), *Disasters and mental health: Selected contemporary perspectives* (pp. 3–28). Rockville, MD: National Institutes of Mental Health.

Brown, R. L. (1985). Management and triage at the disaster site. In L. M. Garcia (Ed.), *Disaster nursing: Planning, assessment and intervention* (pp. 45–70). Rockville, MD: Aspen Systems.

Butman, A. M. (1982). *Responding to the mass casualty incident: A guide for EMS personnel.* Akron, OH: Emergency Training.

Cannon, A. (2001). The other tragedy: The attack on the Pentagon left heroes, victims, survivors. *U.S. News & World Report, 131*(24), 20–32.

Charles, P. (2001). What I learned at ground zero. *RN, 64*(12), 42–44.

Chester, D. K. (1998). The theodicy of natural disasters. *Scottish Journal of Theology, 51*(4), 485–505.

Chinnici, R. (1985). Pastoral care following a natural disaster. *Pastoral Psychology, 33*(2), 245–254.

Christopher, M. A., & McConnell, K. (1994). Community health nursing: Shelter from the storm. *Caring, 13*(1), 37–39.

Church World Service. (2001). *Bringing God's peace to disaster.* New York, NY: Author.

Church World Service. (2001). *Bringing God's presence to survivors.* New York, NY: Author.

Church World Service. (2001). *Co-operative faith based disaster recovery in New York.* New York: Author.

Clark, M. J. (1999). *Nursing in the community.* Stamford, CT: Appleton & Lange.

Clinebell, H. (1991). *Basic types of pastoral care and counseling.* Nashville, TN: Abingdon Press.

Coffman, S. (1994). Children describe life after Hurricane Andrew. *Pediatric Nursing, 20*(4), 363–368; 375.

Cohen, R. E., & Ahearn, F. L. (1980). *Handbook for mental health care of disaster victims.* Baltimore, MD: The Johns Hopkins University Press.

Cohn, R. L. (1986). Biblical response to catastrophe. *Judaism, 35*(3), 263–276.

Cullinan, A. (1993). Spiritual care of the traumatized: A necessary component. In K. J. Doka and J. D. Morgan (Eds.), *Death and spirituality* (pp. 227–242). Amityville, NY: Baywood Publishing Company.

Damian, F., Atkinson, C., Bouchard, A., Harrington, S., & Powers, T. (1997). Disaster relief efforts after Hurricane Marilyn: A pediatric team's experience in St. Thomas. *Journal of Emergency Nursing, 23*(6), 545–549.

Davidson, M. (2001). Not-so-frightening facts about posttraumatic stress disorder. *Nursing Spectrum, 11*(24), 10–11.

Demi, A., & Miles, M. S. (1984). An examination of nursing leadership following a disaster. *Topics in Clinical Nursing, 6*(1), 63–78.

Dodds, B. (2001). *Your grieving child.* Huntington, IN: Our Sunday Visitor Publications.

Dudley, C. S., & Schoonover, M. E. (1993). After the hurricane: Pastoral lessons from Andrew. *Christian Century, 110*(6), 588–590.

Egan, Edward Cardinal. (2001). Homily at the Mass for deceased police officers, fire-fighters, healthcare and emergency service workers. In B. J. Groeschel (Ed.), *The cross at ground zero* (pp. 129–135). Huntington, IN: Our Sunday Visitor.

Foy, D. A., Drescher, K. D., Fitz, A. G., & Kennedy, K. R. (1993). Posttraumatic stress disorder. In R. J. Wicks and R. D. Parsons (Eds.), *Clinical handbook of pastoral counseling, volume 2* (pp. 621–637). Mahwah, NJ: Paulist Press.

Frederick, C. J. (1987). Psychic trauma in victims of crime and terrorism. In G. R. Vandenbos & B. K. Bryant (Eds.), *Cataclysms, crises and catastrophes: Psychology in action* (pp. 55–108). Washington, DC: American Psychological Association.

Fullerton, C. S., & Ursano, R. J. (1997). Posttraumatic responses in spouse/ significant others of disaster workers. In C. S. Fullerton & R. J. Ursano (Eds.), *Posttraumatic stress disorder: Acute and long-term responses to trauma and disaster* (pp. 59–75). Washington, DC: American Psychiatric Press.

Garb, S., & Eng, E. (1969). *Disaster handbook* (2nd ed.). New York: Springer Publishing Company.

Garcia, L. M. (Ed.). (1985). *Disaster nursing: Planning, assessment and intervention.* Rockville, MD: Aspen Systems.

Gardner, S. S. (1985). Skills in rapid field assessment. In L. M. Garcia (Ed.), *Disaster nursing: Planning, assessment and intervention* (pp. 17–43). Rockville, MD: Aspen Systems.

Giuliani, R. W. (2001a). Introduction. In R. Sullivan (Ed.), *In the land of the free: September 11 and after* (pp. 6–10). New York: Life.

Giuliani, R. W. (2001b). Prologue. In T. Hedra (Ed.), *Brotherhood,* (pp. xv–xvi). New York: American Express Publishing Corporation.

Golway, T. (2001). An advent of mourning. *America, 185*(18), 6.

Groeschel, B. J. (2001a). Divine mercy at ground zero. In J. Farina (Ed.), *Beauty for ashes: Spiritual reflections on the attack on America* (pp. 242–250). New York: Crossroad.

Groeschel, B. J. (2001b). *The cross at ground zero.* Huntington, IN: Our Sunday Visitor.

Hanson, C., Jesz, B. L., & Baldwin, S. S. (1991). The American Red Cross: A nursing oriented overview of services. *Journal of Emergency Nursing, 17*(6), 390, 394.

Hartsough, D. M. (1985). Effects of stress on disaster workers. In D. M. Hartsough & D. G. Myers (Eds.), *Disaster work and mental health: Prevention and control of stress among workers* (pp. 27–34). Rockville, MD: National Institutes of Mental Health.

Hassmiller, S. B. (2000). Disaster management. In M. Stanhope and J. Lancaster (Eds.), *Community and public health nursing* (pp. 400–415). St. Louis, MO: Mosby.

Hendra, T. (2001). *Brotherhood.* New York: American Express Publishing Corporation.

Hodgkinson, P. E., & Stewart, M. (1998). *Coping with catastrophe, a handbook of post-disaster psychological aftercare* (2nd ed.). London: Routledge.

Horner, D., Pfeifer, D., & Clunn, P. (1994). In the wake of Hurricane Andrew: The development of a community-based primary care center. *Nursing and Health Care, 15*(2), 61–63.

Hulden, J. (1997). The Red River rises. *Sojourners, 26*(4), 31.

Janoff-Bulman, R. (1985). The aftermath of victimization: Rebuilding shattered assumptions. In C. R. Figley (Ed.), *Trauma and its wake* (pp. 15–35). New York: Brunner/Mazel Publishers.

Jordan, C. (1976). Pastoral care and chronic disaster victims: The Buffalo Creek experience. *The Journal of Pastoral Care, 30*(3), 159–171.

Kennedy, E. (2001). Ancient rituals of grief must not be hurried. *National Catholic Reporter, 38*(5), 17.

Kennedy, E., & Charles, S. C. (2001). *On becoming a counselor.* New York: Crossroad.

Klink, T. W. (1966) Pastoral work in a disaster: Debriefing with comments. *The Journal of Pastoral Care, 20*(2), 194–199.

Kroll-Smith, J. S., & Couch, S. R. (1987). A chronic technical disaster and the irrelevance of religious meaning: The case of Centralia, Pennyslvania. *Journal for the Scientific Study of Religion, 26*(1), 25–37.

Kropf, R. W. (1988). National disaster or "act of God"? The search for the missing link in theodicy. *Dialogue & Alliance, 2*(1), 57–65.

Kushner, H. S. (1981). *When bad things happen to good people.* New York: Avon Books.

Lindemann, E. (1944). Symptomatology and management in acute grief. *American Journal of Psychiatry, 101*(1), 141–148.

Lundy, K. S., & Butts, J. B. (2001). The role of the community health nurse in disasters. In K. S. Lundy and S. Janes (Eds.), *Community health nursing: Caring for the public's health* (pp. 546–573). Sudbury, MA: Jones and Bartlett Publishers.

Mahoney, R. F. (1969). *Emergency and disaster nursing* (2nd ed.). Ontario, Canada: The Macmillan Company.

Marmar, C. R., & Horowitz, M. J. (1988). Diagnosis and phase-oriented treatment of post-traumatic stress disorder. In J. P. Wilson, Z. Harel, & B. Kahana (Eds.), *Human adaptation to extreme stress* (pp. 81–103). New York: Plenum Press.

Martin, J. (2001a). The laying down of life (at the World Trade Center). *America, 185*(9), 7–9.

Martin, J. (2001b). World Trade Center Journal. *America, 185*(10), 28–29.

Martin, J. (2006). Riding out Hurricane Katrina. *Journal of Christian Nursing, 23*(2), 34–37.

McBride, J. (2001). Kindness at ground zero. In J. Waldman (Ed.), *America September 11th: The courage to give* (pp. 9–15). Berkeley, CA: Conari Press.

McCarroll, J. E., Ursano, R. J., & Fullerton, C. S. (1997). Exposure to traumatic death in disaster and war. In C. S. Fullerton & J. R. Ursano (Eds.), *Posttraumatic stress disorder: Acute and long-term responses to trauma and disaster* (pp. 37–58). Washington, DC: American Psychiatric Press.

Meichenbaum, D. (1955). Disasters, stress and cognition. Cited in M. J. Clark (1999). *Nursing in the community.* Stamford, CT: Appleton & Lange.

Mickelson, A. S., Bruno, L., & Schario, M. E. (1999). The City of New Orleans Amtrak disaster: One emergency department's experience. *Journal of Emergency Nursing, 25*(5), 367–372.

Mitchell, J. T. (1986). Healing the helper. In Center for Mental Health Studies of Emergencies (Ed.), *Role stressors and supports for emergency workers* (pp. 105–118). Rockville, MD: National Institutes of Mental Health.

Moody, J., & Carr, C. (1996). After the hurricane. *The Christian Ministry, 27*(1), 25–27.

Murnion, P. J. (2001a). Bleecker & Elizabeth. *Church, 17*(4), 2.

Murnion, P. J. (2001b). Reflections from WTC morgue site, 15 October, 2001. Unpublished report cited with permission of the author.

Nabbe, F. C. (1961). *Disaster nursing.* Paterson, NJ: Littlefield, Adams & Company.

Neal, M. V. (1963). *Disaster nursing preparation.* N.Y.: National League for Nursing.

Nightingale, F. (1854). To Caroline Fleidner, December 1854. Cited in B. M. Dossey (2000). *Florence Nightingale: Mystic, visionary, healer.* Springhouse, PA: Springhouse Corporation.

Newburn, T. (1993). *Disaster and after.* London: Jessica Kingsley Publishers.

Ostrowski, M. (2001). Terrorism at home: A nurse's view from ground zero. *RN, 64*(11), 35–37.

Pedraja, L. G. (1997). In harm's way: Theological reflections on disasters. *Quarterly Review, 17*(1), 5–24.

Reed, J. P. (1977). The pastoral care of victims of major disaster. *The Journal of Pastoral Care, 31*(2), 97–108.

Reichsmeier, J. L., & Miller, J. K. (1985). Psychological aspects of disaster situations. In L. M. Garcia (Ed.), *Disaster nursing: Planning, assessment and intervention* (pp. 185–202). Rockville, MD: Aspen Systems.

Sanderson, L. M. (1997). Fires. In E. K. Noji (Ed.), *The public health consequences of disasters* (pp. 373–396). New York: Oxford University Press.

Stover, S. (2001). God was there. In *In the line of duty, a tribute to New York's finest and bravest* (p. 79). New York: Regan Books.

Sullivan, R. (Ed.). (2001). In the land of the free: September 11 and after. *Life: A commemorative, 1*(8), 1–128.

Switzer, K. H. (1985). Disaster planning: Assessing and using community resources. In L. M. Garcia (Ed.), *Disaster nursing: Planning, assessment and intervention* (pp. 307–344). Rockville, MD: Aspen Systems.

Taggert, S. B. (1985). Background and historical perspective. In L. M. Garcia (Ed.), *Disaster nursing: Planning, assessment and intervention* (pp. 1–16). Rockville, MD: Aspen Systems.

Tait, C., & Spradley, B. (2001). Communities in crisis: Disasters, group violence and terrorism. In J. A. Allender & B. W. Spradley (Eds.), *Community health nursing: Concepts and practice* (pp. 391–407). Philadelphia: Lippincott.

Terrell, K., & Perry, J. (2001). The day the web was a lifeline. *U.S. News & World Report, 131*(15), 67.

The road back: A new center in New York's Greenwich Village helps people to cope with the World Trade Center attack. (2001). *American Journal of Nursing, 101*(11), 94.

Thomas, E. (2001/2002). The day that changed America. *Newsweek* (Special Issue; December 31, 2001–January 7, 2002), 40–71.

Toole, D. C. (1999). Divine ecology and the apocalypse: A theological description of natural disasters and the environmental crisis. *Theology Today, 55*(1), 547–561.

Tumelty, D. (1990). *Social work in the wake of disaster.* London: Jessica Kingsley Publications.

Vitullo-Martin, J. (2001). Firefighters and cops: What provoked the shuffle? *Commonweal, 128*(20), 8.

Von Essen, T. (2001). Foreword. In T. Hedra (Ed.), *Brotherhood* (p. xix). New York: American Express Publishing Corporation.

Walhout, M. F., Tubergen, C. R., & Cook, K. J. (1998). Multiple accident victims, all elderly: Would our disaster plan be up to the challenge? *Nursing 98, 28*(11), 56–60.

Weinrich, S., Hardin, S. B., & Johnson, M. (1990). Nurses respond to Hurricane Hugo: Victims' disaster stress. *Archives of Psychiatric Nursing, 4*(3), 195–205.

When evil strikes: The Catholic response to terrorism. (2001). Huntington, IN: Our Sunday Visitor.

When the tornado hit Worcester: Heroic nurses play vital role. (1953). *The Catholic Nurse, 2*(1), 43–45.

Williams, T. (1998). Diagnosis and treatment of survivor guilt. In J. P. Wilson, Z. Harel, & B. Kahana (Eds.), *Human adaptation to extreme stress* (pp. 319–336). New York: Plenum Press.

☀ Epilogue

SPIRITUALITY IN NURSING: STANDING ON HOLY GROUND

The title of this book, *Spirituality in Nursing: Standing on Holy Ground*, reflects the theme that emerged from an analysis of the author's nursing research carried out over the past two decades. A variety of studies explored the spiritual needs of acutely and chronically ill children and adults, as well as those of their families. In their own poignant words, patients and family members documented the importance of spiritual beliefs and practices in coping with a multitude of illness conditions. Spiritual needs related to the dying process for patients, and grief and bereavement for families, were also identified. The significance of the relationship between faith beliefs and illness adaptation is beautifully exemplified in the faith of Peter, a long-term survivor of HIV infection, who said, "God is the one reliable constant in my life," and in the trust of Nora, mother of a dying child, who related, "Even when I was screaming at God . . . why, and why, and why? I knew that God was crying with me."

The personal spiritual beliefs and spiritual care experiences of professional nurses emerged from research with a cadre of contemporary practitioners of nursing. The many profound and touching examples of spiritual caring among the reported nursing therapeutics resulted in the author labeling the nurses "anonymous ministers."

Ultimately, the data on patient and family spiritual need and those describing nurses' attitudes and experiences revealed that whenever a nurse stands before an ill child, an ill adult, or a patient's family member, he or she is indeed, like Moses before the burning bush, standing on holy ground. For as Florence Nightingale asserted so many years ago, "God's precious gift of life is often placed literally" in the nurse's hands. This is spirituality in nursing; this is standing on holy ground.

❄ Index

key concepts of, 136

Hippocrates, 23

history. *See* Spiritual history of nursing

HIV. *See* Human immunodeficiency virus

HIV/AIDS nurses, 113, 116

HIV/AIDS patients, 103, 164, 165, 189

  ritual needs of, 199–201

  spiritual care for, 175–176

HIV Infection Interview Guide, 78–79

Hoeman, S. P., 209

holidays, and ill child, 229

holism, 4, 9

holistic care

  for dying persons, 309

  spiritual care in, 182

holistic health movement, spiritual care in, 129

holistic nursing

  body, mind, spirit connection in, 8–9

  model for, 4

  prayer in, 147

  spirituality and, 5–7

holistic practice, spiritual care in, 130, 131

Holland, B. E., 254

Holst, L. E., 120, 121

Holy Cross Monastery, 28

Holy Spirit, in Christian theology, 112

Homberg, Maria, 10

homebound elderly, spiritual needs of, 268–270

home health care

  defined, 211

  primary component of, 211

spiritual needs, 56

home health care client, spiritual needs of, 211–213

home health nurses, 212

homeless client, spiritual needs of, 213–215

homeless families

  health problems of, 244–245

  spiritual needs of, 245–246

Homeless Families Program, 245

homelessness, defined, 213

hope, 192–193

  as healing force, 167

  for old adults, 262–263

  sources of, 242, 263

  in spiritual well-being, 61

hopelessness

  bereavement, 323

  in chronic illness, 191

hospice

  during medieval period, 312

  modern concept of, 313

  spiritual care, 313–314

hospice care

  philosophy of, 312–314

  in United States, 313

Hospice Code of Ethics, 313

hospice nurses, 102, 106–107, 123–124, 243, 311, 314

hospitals

  children in, 232

  Muslim, 135

  parish nursing, 340

  precursors to, 26

  religiously affiliated, 3

Hotel-Dieu of Lyon, 29

Hotel-Dieu of Paris, 29–30, 38

Howe, Dr. Samuel, 44

Hoy, Chaplain Trevor, 313